Using Rational-Emotive Therapy Effectively
Therapy Effectively
A Practitioner's Guide

APPLIED CLINICAL PSYCHOLOGY

Series Editors:
Alan S. Bellack, *Medical College of Pennsylvania at EPPI, Philadelphia, Pennsylvania,* and Michel Hersen, *University of Pittsburgh, Pittsburgh, Pennsylvania*

Current Volumes in this Series

ACTIVITY MEASUREMENT IN PSYCHOLOGY AND MEDICINE
Warren W. Tryon

BEHAVIORAL CONSULTATION AND THERAPY
John R. Bergan and Thomas R. Kratochwill

BEHAVIORAL CONSULTATION IN APPLIED SETTINGS
An Individual Guide
Thomas R. Kratochwill and John R. Bergan

THE CHALLENGE OF COGNITIVE THERAPY
Applications to Nontraditional Populations
Edited by T. Michael Vallis, Janice L. Howes, and Philip C. Miller

CLINICAL PSYCHOLOGY
Historical and Research Foundations
Edited by C. Eugene Walker

ETHNIC VALIDITY, ECOLOGY, AND PSYCHOTHERAPY
A Psychosocial Competence Model
Forrest B. Tyler, Deborah Ridley Brome, and Janice E. Williams

HANDBOOK OF BEHAVIOR MODIFICATION WITH THE MENTALLY RETARDED
Second Edition
Edited by Johnny L. Matson

HANDBOOK OF CLINICAL BEHAVIOR THERAPY WITH THE ELDERLY CLIENT
Edited by Patricia A. Wisocki

PSYCHOLOGY
A Behavioral Overview
Alan Poling, Henry Schlinger, Stephen Starin, and Elbert Blakely

USING RATIONAL–EMOTIVE THERAPY EFFECTIVELY
A Practitioner's Guide
Michael E. Bernard

A Continuation Order Plan is available for this series. A continuation order will bring delivery of each new volume immediately upon publication. Volumes are billed only upon actual shipment. For further information please contact the publisher.

Using Rational-Emotive Therapy Effectively

A Practitioner's Guide

EDITED BY

MICHAEL E. BERNARD

The University of Melbourne
Parkville, Victoria, Australia

Plenum Press • New York and London

Library of Congress Cataloging-in-Publication Data

Using rational-emotive therapy effectively : a practitioner's guide /
   edited by Michael E. Bernard.
        p.   cm. -- (Applied clinical psychology)
   Includes bibliographical references and index.
   ISBN 0-306-43754-6 (hardbound). -- ISBN 0-306-43755-4 (paperbound)
   1. Rational-emotive psychotherapy.   I. Bernard, Michael Edwin,
1950-   . II. Series.
   [DNLM: 1. Psychotherapy, Rational-Emotive--methods.   WM 420 U85]
RC489.R3U85   1991
616.89'14--dc20
DNLM/DLC
for Library of Congress   91-3749
                                                                   CIP

ISBN 0-306-43754-6 (Hardbound)
ISBN 0-306-43755-4 (Paperbound)

© 1991 Plenum Press, New York
A Division of Plenum Publishing Corporation
233 Spring Street, New York, N.Y. 10013

Printed in the United States of America

Contributors

MICHAEL E. BERNARD, School of Education, University of Melbourne, Parkville, Victoria, Australia 3052, and Australian Institute for Rational-Emotive Therapy, P.O. Box 1160, Carlton, Victoria, Australia 3053

ROBERT W. DAWSON, Australian Institute for Rational-Emotive Therapy, P.O. Box 1160, Carlton, Victoria, Australia 3053, and Community Training Systems, 459 Swanston Street, Melbourne, Australia 3000

RAYMOND DiGIUSEPPE, Department of Psychology, St. John's University, Jamaica, New York 11432, and Institute for Rational-Emotive Therapy, 45 East 65th Street, New York, New York 10021

DOMINIC J. DiMATTIA, Department of Counseling and Human Resources, University of Bridgeport, Bridgeport, Connecticut 06602, and Institute for Rational-Emotive Therapy, 45 East 65th Street, New York, New York 10021

WINDY DRYDEN, Department of Psychology, Goldsmiths' College, University of London, New Cross, London, England SE14 6NW

ALBERT ELLIS, Institute for Rational-Emotive Therapy, 45 East 65th Street, New York, New York 10021

RUSSELL M. GRIEGER, 818 East High Street, Charlottesville, Virginia 22901

PAUL A. HAUCK, 1800 Third Avenue, Suite 302, Rock Island, Illinois 61201

MARIE R. JOYCE, Centre for Family Studies, Australian Catholic University, Oakleigh, Victoria, Australia 3168

Hedwin Naimark, Institute for Rational-Emotive Therapy, 45 East 65th Street, New York, New York 10021

Mary W. Rader, The Kennedy Family Center, 1235 East Monument Street, Baltimore, Maryland 21202

Susan R. Walen, Department of Psychology, Towson State University, and Baltimore Center for Cognitive Therapy, 6303 Greenspring Avenue, Baltimore, Maryland 21209

Janet L. Wolfe, Institute for Rational-Emotive Therapy, 45 East 65th Street, New York, New York 10021

Paul J. Woods, Department of Psychology, Hollins College, Roanoke, Virginia 24020

Preface

The initial conceptualization of this book was much more narrow than the final product that has emerged. I started out believing that it would be enlightening to have a group of acknowledged rational-emotive therapy (RET) expert practitioners with well-established literary credentials write about how they approach the problem of modifying client irrationality. Many RET practitioners of all levels of experience are, on the one hand, enamored of the economy, the precision, and the accuracy of psychological insight that RET theory offers, but they are, on the other hand, equally frustrated by their own inability to "persuade" or otherwise change some of the clients they work with more quickly or even at all. Indeed, clients themselves frequently express the view that RET is illuminating, yet they find themselves at the same time puzzled and perplexed by their inability to make the substantial changes that RET invites.

It became clearer as I discussed the project with many of the contributors that to practice RET effectively requires more than just innovative and persistent assessment and intervention techniques. For example, Russell Grieger expressed the view that more prerequisite work needs to be done on the value and philosophical systems of clients—including personal responsibility and the philosophy of happiness—before many clients can show significant shifts in their thinking. Susan Walen raised the general issues of how effective RET can be in the treatment of biologically driven affective disorders. Windy Dryden spoke of the importance of the therapeutic relationship and taking into account client expectations in determining how to bring out the best in RET and in the client. It became obvious to me before I even read the chapters that RET practitioners were doing as much "outside" traditional RET as "inside" RET to help clients to use RET to make changes in their lives.

The organization of the chapters flows from general considerations in improving RET's effectiveness to using RET with specific populations and problems. In Chapter 1, Albert Ellis summarizes why RET is an effective and efficient form of therapy and includes many do's and don'ts in using RET effectively. The second half of the chapter contains the transcript of an interview I conducted with Ellis covering the client, therapist, and therapy characteristics that he takes into account when he practices RET.

In Chapter 2, Russell Grieger, well-known RET author and practitioner (*Rational-Emotive Therapy: A Skills-Based Approach*, with John Boyd; *Handbook of Rational-Emotive Therapy*, with Ellis) presents a guide he uses with his clients to ensure that they will understand and follow the basic RET steps to change, beginning with Step 1, "Committing Oneself to Change," and ending with Step 6, "Going Forward." He argues that educating clients in a structured way about the theory and practice of RET tremendously enhances most clients' ability to use RET effectively. He also views as an important therapeutic task the education of clients about the concept of *personal responsibility.*

In my opinion, Paul Woods, coeditor (with Russell Grieger) of the *Journal of Rational-Emotive and Cognitive Behavior Therapy,* has made tremendous advances in the teaching methods that he uses with his clients to bring about RET-induced change. In Chapter 3, Woods presents the impressive array of RET visual-graphic aids that he uses with his clients and the introductory RET explanations that he uses with his clients.

Robert Dawson is one of Australia's foremost RET practitioners and trainers. In Chapter 4, Dawson presents a model he calls "REGIME," which he designed to improve RET's effectiveness. Rejecting what he terms the "mad-dog disputing" model, Dawson illustrates the importance of using basic microcounseling skills (e.g., empathy) in the relationship-building phase of RET. He goes on to discuss the importance of therapist–client goal setting as a prerequisite to disputation and of using Arnold Lazarus's multimodal theory to ensure that the clinician will not overlook important assessment information.

Windy Dryden continues to be a prolific generator not only of books on RET and allied cognitive-behavioral approaches, but also of creative and innovative ideas. In Chapter 5, using clinical case material, Dryden offers advice on the importance of the therapeutic alliance and of being prepared to make compromises with clients in order to bring about change.

One of RET's most prodigious thinkers is Raymond DiGiuseppe, author of countless thought-provoking pieces on aspects of the philosophy, theory, and practice of RET. In Chapter 6, he presents for the first time his view of RET's unique hypothesis-driven form of assessment as well as different methods for assessing client irrationality. In Chapter 7, DiGiuseppe discusses the nature of cognitive disputation and, again, offers the practitioner new techniques for identifying, challenging, and changing clients' irrational thinking.

Paul Hauck has been writing books on RET for three decades (e.g., *The Rational Management of Children*, 1967; *Overcoming Worry and Fear*, 1975; *Brief Counseling with RET*, 1980; *The Three Faces of Love*, 1984). Always thinking of and offering the RET practitioner new perspectives, in Chapter 8 he addresses the issue of how RET can be used by a client to solve interpersonal as distinct from intrapersonal problems and, specifically, how RET can help clients get what they want from others.

Susan Walen is regarded by her contemporaries as a leading RET practitioner-theoretician who is stimulated by model building, likes to write on sex and women's issues, and is most well known as the senior author of the popular RET training text *The Practitioner's Guide to Rational-Emotive Therapy* (coauthored by Richard Wessler and Raymond DiGiuseppe). Chapter 9, cowritten with Mary Rader, is the most moving and powerful of all the chapters in this collection. It is affectively moving and at the same time therapeutically challenging. Walen and Rader write poignantly of their own experiences of severe depression and offer illuminating insights into the phenomenology of the "disease" and the care with which RET needs to be offered to severely depressed clients.

Janet Wolfe has for many years been responsible for tailoring RET to the particular characteristics of women. As early as 1975, when she presented RET as an effective feminist therapy, she has been a driving force behind the development of RET for women. In Chapter 10, coauthored with Hedwin Naimark, the latest advances in the application of RET to the understanding and amelioration of "women's problems" are presented.

The person most responsible for the current increase in interest in the use of RET in organizational settings is Dominic DiMattia. In Chapter 11, he outlines ways in which rational effectiveness training can be used to boost the performance of individuals working in organizations and in sales training. He points out ways in which RET can be made more "user friendly" to big business.

Finally, in Chapter 12, Marie Joyce and I update our insights into how to use RET with younger populations, which we presented in our 1984 book *Rational-Emotive Therapy with Children and Adolescents: Theory, Treatment, Preventative Methods.*

Let me now try to summarize briefly some of the major conclusions about how to improve the way in which RET is practiced.

The generalizations that follow are based on a simple observation: *Certain clients require prerequisite work before they can profit from cognitive disputation and the allied RET change techniques.* There are many reasons for this phenomenon, most of which have to do largely with client characteristics. Perhaps the most relevant of these to the practice of RET has to do with clients' entering level of preparedness to change. Prochaska and DiClemente (1986) pointed out that, whereas some clients are "ready for action," others are in a "precontemplation" stage. RET may well be best suited to clients in the contemplation and action stages:

1. RET is best practiced when the practitioner has an in-depth understanding of the current RET theory of mental health problems, for it is this theory that drives RET assessment and intervention procedures (see Ber-

nard, 1991; Bernard & DiGiuseppe, 1989; Ellis, 1988; Ellis & Dryden, 1987, 1990).

2. RET practitioners need to pay more attention to the nature of the therapeutic relationship and how to go about forging a relationship with clients that will minimize client anxieties about the practitioner and RET. In particular, it is important to discard the "patient uniformity" myth and to recognize that different client characteristics, including gender, sex role, culture, personality, problems, and previous experience in therapy, require and lead to different types of practitioner–client relationships.

3. In building a therapeutic relationship, it is vital that the RET practitioner be able to successfully use basic microcounseling skills such as empathy and listening (e.g., Egan, 1990), as well as be supportive and caring when required. That is, simply showing clients how RET conceptualizes problems, "telling" them what they are thinking (advanced accurate empathy), and providing them with a minilecture on the ABCs of RET are not enough for many clients, who either require trust and understanding and/or may not be ready for RET action.

4. Multimodal assessment techniques (e.g., Lazarus, 1981, 1986) can be extremely useful adjuncts to the basic RET assessment regime. Conceptualizing client problems by using the BASIC ID framework can help to isolate the noncognitive aspects of problems surrounding dysfunctional thought–feeling links that may prevent RET from being used effectively. For example, the treatment of painful sensations through relaxation methods can clear the way for cognitive disputation. Further, a careful and thorough assessment of sensation may lead more quickly to the discovery of biologically driven emotional disorders, which, when discovered, will have a direct bearing on the way RET is introduced in therapy.

5. RET assessment effectiveness is enhanced by the practitioner's knowledge of RET and of the hypotheses that RET offers concerning the nature of the irrational beliefs that underlie different client problems. RET assessment techniques can also be augmented by a directive and active style of hypothesis testing. Using this approach, the RET practitioner not only permits the full force of RET theoretical schemata to direct the assessment process but also frequently offers hypotheses to the client concerning relationships among events, irrational beliefs, and feelings. The client's reaction (acceptance or rejection) to RET hypotheses helps to guide the practitioner's assessment interview.

6. RET attempts to empower clients by providing them with disputational skills that will enable them to modify their own emotional states and behaviors. RET also provides clients with a set of rational values (e.g., self-acceptance, other-acceptance, and involvement in creative pursuits; see Ellis & Bernard, 1985) that RET hypothesizes will lead to increased happiness. The use of disputational methods by clients as well as the adoption of new values would appear to demand from clients a sense of personal

responsibility, that is, a belief that it is possible, through their own efforts, to do something about their problems. A fair proportion of clients arrive in therapy with low personal responsibility, feeling helpless to change themselves or their circumstances. It is therefore vital for RET practitioners to provide their clients with an awareness of the importance of the attitude of personal responsibility and to provide their clients with experiences that will start to combat clients' attitudes of helplessness.

7. For some, but not all, clients, spending time explaining the theory of RET as well as the role and nature of disputation can be extremely helpful. For those who are experiencing extreme emotional pain, however, the exposition of the RET model, especially during initial treatment sessions, can do more harm than good by both alienating the client from the practitioner and increasing the emotional pain for clients who find themselves unable to be rational. This is especially the case for clients experiencing biologically driven affective disorders. However, for those clients who arrive in therapy ready for action, a clear discussion of RET will be helpful.

8. In attempting to modify irrational thinking through disputation, the RET practitioner needs to be aware that what leads clients to generate irrational thoughts in particular situations are frequently nonspoken, implicit irrational beliefs, which are collectively referred to as an *assumptive framework* or a *personal paradigm*. To produce changes in client thinking beyond specific environmental circumstances, it is necessary for the client to dispute and modify these more implicit irrational beliefs.

9. RET practitioners should not be exclusive in their use of traditional RET cognitive restructuring methods. RET also regularly employs many cognitive, emotive, and behavioral methods that are sometimes used in non-RET therapies. It particularly emphasizes forceful, emotive methods such as forceful coping statements, rational-emotive imagery, and shame-attacking exercises; and it gives its practitioners full leeway to use, especially with difficult and resistant clients, some nonrational and "irrational" methods, such as Pollyannaism, religious conversion, extreme active listening, and unusual and tricky paradoxical interventions. It also regularly uses practical problem solving, family therapy interventions, relaxation methods, and other useful techniques but adds to them the revealing and active disputing of clients' basic musturbatory philosophies. Arnold Lazarus (1989) illustrated how "time tripping" and certain imagery techniques can emotionally "unblock" clients concerning past events, freeing them to consider here-and-now issues by using RET.

I have tried to ensure that the material contained in this book will be useful to practitioners. As a rough guess, the practitioners who are contributors to this book have over 225 years of collective experience in using RET with clients. I am very pleased with the quality of the contributions and hope that readers will find many ideas that will help either reinforce some of the ways they have been working with their clients or introduce some new approaches that will have a significant impact on their professional functioning. There is little doubt that RET continues to be a dynamic and extremely effective therapy that offers challenges to the practitioner and the client alike.

MICHAEL E. BERNARD

Melbourne, Australia

REFERENCES

Bernard, M. E. (1991). *Staying rational in an irrational world: Albert Ellis and rational-emotive therapy.* New York: Carol Publishing.
Bernard, M. E., & DiGiuseppe, R. (Eds.). (1989). *Inside rational-emotive therapy: A critical analysis of the theory and practice of Albert Ellis.* New York: Academic Press.
Egan, G. (1990). *The skilled helper* (4th ed.). Pacific Grove, CA: Brooks/Cole.
Ellis, A. (1988). *How to stubbornly refuse to make yourself miserable about anything—Yes anything!* New York: Lyle Stuart.
Ellis, A., & Bernard, M. E. (Eds.). (1985). *Clinical applications of rational-emotive therapy.* New York: Plenum Press.
Ellis, A., & Dryden, W. (1987). *The practice of rational-emotive therapy.* New York: Springer.
Ellis, A., & Dryden, W. (1990). *The essential Albert Ellis.* New York: Springer.
Lazarus, A. (1981). *The practice of multi-modal therapy.* New York: McGraw-Hill.
Lazarus, A. (1986). Multimodal therapy. In J. C. Norcross (Ed.), *Handbook of eclectic psychotherapy* (pp. 65–93). New York: Brunner/Mazel.
Lazarus, A. (1989). The practice of rational-emotive therapy. In M. E. Bernard & R. DiGiuseppe (Eds.), *Inside rational-emotive therapy: A critical analysis of the theory and practice of Albert Ellis* (pp. 66–94). New York: Academic Press.
Prochaska, J. O., & DiClemente, C. C. (1986). The transtheoretical approach. In J. C. Norcross (Ed.), *Handbook of eclectic psychotherapy* (pp. 163–200). New York: Brunner/Mazel.

Contents

Chapter 1. Using RET Effectively: Reflections and Interview 1

ALBERT ELLIS

How RET Can Be Effectively Brief 2
How RET Can Be Effectively Elegant and Long-Lasting 8
Interview 11
References 32

Chapter 2. Keys to Effective RET 35

RUSSELL M. GRIEGER

Organizing and Guiding the Client 36
Helping Clients Take Responsibility 53
Therapist Checklist for RET Effectiveness 62
Summary 66
References 66

Chapter 3. Orthodox RET Taught Effectively with Graphics,
    Feedback on Irrational Beliefs, a Structured Homework Series,
    and Models of Disputation 69

PAUL J. WOODS

Introductory Minilectures 70
Report Booklet on the Client's Irrational Beliefs: Homework 83
Analyzing an Emotional Episode: Homework 85
Examples of Irrational Beliefs (iBs) with Disputational Responses
    and Rational Alternatives: Homework 95
Building Positive Self-Regard: An Inelegant Step along the Way to
    Unconditional Self-Acceptance 103
Evidence of the Effectiveness of the Above Strategies 104
References 108

Chapter 4. REGIME: A Counseling and Educational Model for
Using RET Effectively 111

ROBERT W. DAWSON

REGIME: Objectives, Therapist Strategies, and Client Behaviors .. 112
REGIME: Stages of Therapeutic Process 113
REGIME Intervention Matrix 127
Transcript 127
Conclusion 131
References 132

Chapter 5. Flexibility in RET: Forming Alliances and Making
Compromises 133

WINDY DRYDEN

The Therapeutic Alliance 133
Compromises in RET 140
Conclusion 148
References 148

Chapter 6. A Rational-Emotive Model of Assessment 151

RAYMOND DIGIUSEPPE

Overview of Rational-Emotive Assessment Procedures 152
RET versus Traditional Models of Assessment 153
Medical Model of Assessment 154
Static versus Dynamic Assessment 157
Therapeutic Relationships and Self-Disclosure 157
Epistemology 160
Hypothesis-Driven Assessment 162
Assessing Irrational Beliefs 165
References 169

Chapter 7. Comprehensive Cognitive Disputing in RET 173

RAYMOND DIGIUSEPPE

An Expanded Model 174
The Target of the Dispute 176
The Nature of the Dispute 177
Rhetorical Disputing Styles of Therapists 182
Level of Abstraction 186

Multiple Irrational Belief Processes 188
Comprehensive Cognitive Disputing in RET 191
References 194

Chapter 8. RET and the Assertive Process 197

PAUL A. HAUCK

Two Types of Problems 197
The Two Principles of Human Interaction 199
To Be or Not to Be Assertive: The JRC Principle 201
The Three Rules of Assertion 203
The Four Objections 206
When RET Is Especially Called For 208
The Four Options 209
Making a Choice 212
Wider Applications 213
A Case Study 217
References 218

Chapter 9. Depression and RET: Perspectives from Wounded
    Healers 219

SUSAN R. WALEN AND MARY W. RADER

Overview 219
The Self-Disclosure Part 220
Depressive Illness: The Uniformity Myth 232
Clinical and Treatment Implications 240
Conclusion 260
Some Recommended Books on Depression for Patients 261
References 261

Chapter 10. Psychological Messages and Social Context: Strategies
    for Increasing RET's Effectiveness with Women 265

JANET L. WOLFE AND HEDWIN NAIMARK

The Vicious Cycle of Sex-Role Stereotypes 267
The Vicious Cycle and the RET Process 275
Building Awareness of and Challenging Sex-Role Stereotypes 277
Case Study 279
Strategies and Exercises That Challenge Sex-Role Stereotypes 283
Conclusion 298
References 299

Chapter 11. Using RET Effectively in the Workplace 303

DOMINIC J. DIMATTIA

Problems in the Workplace 303
Applications of RET in the Workplace 305
General Issues When Using RET in the Workplace 314
Case Study 314
Summary 316
References 317

Chapter 12. RET with Children and Adolescents 319

MICHAEL E. BERNARD AND MARIE R. JOYCE

Theoretical Perspectives 319
RET Treatment Levels 321
The RATE Model 322
Keys to Successful RET Child Treatment 336
Working with Parents 337
Recommendations for Treating Specific Childhood Disorders 341
Conclusion 344
References 345

Index 349

Using RET Effectively
Reflections and Interview

ALBERT ELLIS

I would never have created rational-emotive therapy (RET) had I not been very interested in efficiency. From 1943 to 1953, I was mainly psycho-analytic, but after training in classical psychoanalysis and using it for six years, I fully realized how ineffective it was (even though my clients liked it and thought they had significantly improved). So in 1953, I began to call myself a psychotherapist rather than an analyst and became eclectic in my approach (Ellis, 1955a,b). But I still found most theories and techniques much less effective than I thought therapy could be and, at the beginning of 1955, combined philosophical with behavior therapy to start RET and become the grandfather of the cognitive-behavioral therapy (CBT) movement (Ellis, 1957a,b, 1958, 1962, 1972c).

Since I founded RET, its practitioners have adopted a wide variety of styles, some of which I am not enthusiastic about, such as doing it in a mamby-pamby manner, worrying too much about clients' approval, and diluting it considerably with other kinds of therapy (such as psycho-analysis and Gestalt therapy) that often are opposed to it. RET, of course, doesn't *have* to be done in the active-directive way that I usually do it. Like many therapies, it is tailor-made to each individual client and can be done quite differently with a cooperative, eager-to-learn than with a stubbornly resistant individual. Even when, in my estimation, it is done badly, I think that it often considerably helps people. But having had more experience in using it than any other therapist, I naturally think that it usually (not always) can be done in a manner that is effective for more of the people more of the time. This chapter presents my personal view of effectively

ALBERT ELLIS • Institute for Rational-Emotive Therapy, 45 East 65th Street, New York, New York 10021.

using RET, but being an empiricist as well as a theoretician, I hope that all the "effective" systems I make will be experimentally checked.

How RET Can Be Effectively Brief

As an analyst, I objected to the length of conventional psychoanalysis, as well as to its poor history of real cure (Ellis, 1950; Phillips, 1956). Also, disturbed people are in pain and sometimes suicidal. So I designed RET to be a relatively brief form of treatment, which in some cases takes only from 5 to 15 sessions and can still result in significant and profound change. To effect brief change with RET, I use the following techniques.

Quickly Teach the ABCDEs of RET

From the first session onward, I show most clients that unfortunate Activating Events (As) contribute to but do not really upset them or make them disturbed (self-defeating) at point C (emotional and behavioral Consequence). Instead, they mainly upset themselves by their Beliefs (Bs) *about* their As. I quite quickly also try to show them the vast difference between rational Beliefs (rBs), such as their wishes and preferences that Activating Events (As) be better, and irrational Beliefs (iBs), such as their absolutist demands and insistences that these As *should* and *must* be improved. And even in the first few sessions, I usually show them how to actively Dispute (at point D) their irrational Beliefs (iBs) and thereby arrive at E, an Effective New Philosophy and the Effective New (self-helping) Feelings and Behaviors that normally accompany strongly believed preferential, undogmatic philosophy.

Active-Directive RET

The more active-directive and persuasive I am about teaching the ABCDEs of RET, the more quickly many of my clients learn to use them to help themselves. Some, of course, are slow learners or resisters. Discovering this, I then slow down, use simpler language, repeat myself, give little tests of comprehension, and use other teaching techniques to speed the therapy process.

Encouragement

I show confidence that RET works and *can* work quickly. I don't give the impression that it *always*, but only that it *sometimes*, produces quick results. I try not to oversell it, lest clients think that there is something radically wrong with them if they do not improve rapidly.

Homework

I push clients, as soon as feasible, to do cognitive, emotive, and behavioral homework. I show them that if they want to change quickly and profoundly, they had better regularly, persistently follow what I often call RET Insight No. 3: There is no way but work and practice—yes, work and practice—to change themselves (Ellis, 1962, 1973, 1977a,b, 1988). I agree with them that they will do suitable homework, monitor their actually doing this homework, and check and Dispute (D) what irrational Beliefs (iBs) they have when they fail to carry out this agreement. I help them to challenge these iBs and then to get back to keeping the agreement.

Implosive Homework

Most therapies, and especially cognitive-behavioral therapy, use gradual homework assignments, such as encouraging clients to do imaginal or *in vivo* desensitization once or a few times a week (Wolpe, 1983). RET often does this, too. But I often encourage suitable (and sometimes even difficult) clients to do the homework implosively, if feasible, 10 or 20 times a day. Thus, I may induce cigarette addicts to make a list of the disadvantages of smoking and to forcefully go over this list 10 or 20 times every day. Or I persuade elevator phobics to take elevator rides 25 times every day while they are also telling themselves, "I don't *need* a guarantee that this elevator won't fall, but there is very little probability that it will. I *can* stand the discomfort of riding in elevators, and if I do so, I will soon feel comfortable!" I find that, when this kind of implosive homework is done, therapy frequently is briefer and more effective.

Forceful Disputing and Action

I show my clients how to *forcefully* and *vigorously* Dispute their iBs and how to *strongly* act against them. I try to convince them that mild Disputing and weak action will often lead to "intellectual" but not "emotional" insight and hence to little or temporary change. I show them how to Dispute and act in a forceful, determined, persistent manner.

Discriminating between Appropriate and Inappropriate Feelings

Right from the start, I show clients how to discriminate between appropriate negative feelings when Activating Events are seen as unfortunate (e.g., sorrow, regret, and frustration) and inappropriate feelings (e.g., panic, depression, and self-hatred) when these "unpleasant" Activating Events occur. I show that their rational, preferential Beliefs lead to the former and that their irrational, commanding Beliefs lead to the latter feelings. I teach them to acknowledge and have strong appropriate feelings and to replace their inappropriate ones. I indicate that it is often appropriate to have strong emotions but not necessarily to express these emotions to powerful people (such as bosses or teachers) who may penalize clients for having such feelings.

Helping Clients Be Realistic, Logical, and Antimusturbatory

Practically all clients hold unrealistic Beliefs (i.e., "Because you refused to have dinner with me, you think I did something wrong and hate me") and illogical Beliefs (e.g., "Because I treat you nicely, you absolutely *have to* treat me equally well"). But behind these unrealistic and illogical inferences, they almost always seem to have Jehovian demands (e.g., "I must, under all conditions, and at all times, win your approval and have you treat me well"). To help clients quickly and elegantly improve, I don't only show them how to be realistic and logical but also show them their underlying, tacit grandiose must's and how to discover and surrender these for themselves. I teach them how to be fairly consistent, scientific, and flexible and to be alternative-seeking thinkers, so that they rarely upset themselves in the future and quickly can stop upsetting themselves when they are disturbed.

Pushing Psychoeducational Methods

We have found, at our psychological clinic at the Institute for Rational-Emotive Therapy in New York, that therapy is hastened and deepened when clients read RET pamphlets and books; listen to cassettes; attend talks, workshops, and intensive seminars, and use other psychoeducational methods. Some of my clients, for example, significantly improve in a few sessions largely because they have read, often several times, *A New Guide to Rational Living* (Ellis & Harper, 1975) and *How to Stubbornly Refuse to Make Yourself Miserable about Anything—Yes, Anything!* (Ellis, 1988). So I encourage most of my clients to supplement their therapy with audiovisual materials and presentations. Having them listen several times to cassette recordings of their own therapy sessions often proves particularly useful in this regard.

Forceful RET

Shortly after I started using RET, I discovered that many clients *intellectually* or *lightly* agreed with rational, self-helping Beliefs but simultaneously *strongly* held on to their disturbance-creating irrationalities. Thus, they might lightly agree, "Yes, there's no reason why I *must* be loved by my mate," but much more solidly believe, "But I still *need* his or her love to be a worthwhile person!" So I incorporated the concept of vigor or force into RET (Ellis, 1962, 1971, 1972c, 1973, 1977a,b, 1979, 1988; Ellis & Abrahms, 1978; Ellis & Becker, 1982; Ellis & Dryden, 1987; Ellis & Whiteley, 1979). I find that, by using some of the forceful and dramatic RET techniques— such as rational-emotive imagery (Maultsby, 1971; Maultsby & Ellis, 1974), shame-attacking exercises (Ellis, 1969), and powerful coping statements (Ellis, 1988; Ellis & Abrahms, 1978)—with my clients, I often help them start thinking, feeling, and acting better after relatively few sessions.

RET Group Therapy

RET group therapy, by itself or in addition to individual therapy, frequently helps clients improve more quickly (and more thoroughly) because when they participate in a group, people tend to see that others have emotional problems; see how others solve these problems; learn to talk group members out of their irrational beliefs; gain support from others; are often encouraged to do the homework that they agree with the group to do; often talk to each other during the week to remind each other to use RET; learn to take risks in speaking up in the group; participate in RET exercises—such as shame-attacking exercises—right in the group; benefit from the Disputing of their irrational Beliefs by both the group leader and the other members; learn socialization skills; and benefit from other aspects of therapy that the group particularly provides (Ellis, 1974, 1990; Ellis & Dryden, 1987).

Avoidance of Inefficient and Inelegant Procedures

RET may be used in conjunction with many other procedures that are commonly used in psychoanalysis, Gestalt therapy, family systems therapy, transactional analysis, existential therapy, and other kinds of psychological treatment. But to encourage brevity and to encourage clients to arrive at more profound, more elegant, and longer lasting improvement, I usually (not always) avoid the following inefficient and inelegant procedures.

Avoiding Free Association

Free association, favored by psychoanalysis, usually produces much long-winded, irrelevant material—good for writing people's biographies or understanding their "personalities," but *not* for quickly discovering their irrational Beliefs and uprooting them. When used extensively, it tends to impede the active-directive questioning, probing, and teaching of RET and encourages clients to indulge in their misery and to avoid *working* at overcoming it. So I occasionally use it very briefly but often altogether neglect it.

Avoiding Extensive Dream Analysis

Dreams are by no means, as Freud (1965) thought, the royal road to uncovering unconscious thoughts and feelings, which can usually be better revealed by direct RET questioning (Ellis, 1962, 1988). Recent research has shown that dreams are usually related to the activities of the previous day, may serve as "garbage disposal" processes, and may do more harm than good when dwelled on. Although I did extensive and intensive dream analysis when I was a psychoanalyst, I found that I got more useful thoughts and feelings from waking material and that dream material is fascinating but usually vague, inaccurate, subject to dubious interpretations, and wasteful. So I rarely use it, but when I do, I look for the irrational Beliefs that may be included in the dream and then show my clients what these probably are and how to Dispute them.

Avoiding Too Much Therapist's Warmth

I tried Ferenczi's method (1952) of giving clients considerable warmth and support in the early 1950s and found that they loved it, wanted *more* sessions per week, stayed longer in therapy, and sometimes collaborated more with the therapy procedures. But a great many of them became more (instead of less) dependent on me, increased their dire needs for love and their low frustration tolerance, and became more instead of less disturbed. So for a quick and elegant use of RET, I advise great caution in giving considerable warmth except to a few special (usually borderline and psychotic) clients. Empathic listening and reflective feedback to virtually all clients is fine, but watch your oozing warmth!

Avoiding Great Details of Activating Events

Many clients, particularly those with prior psychoanalytic experience, love to describe the unfortunate Activating Events of their lives in long and gory detail. Sometimes this has a catharctic effect that helps them temporarily *feel* but not *get* better (Ellis, 1972b). Usually, it wastes time and encourages them to indulge in their miserable feelings. So for briefer and more effective RET, I try to help them to *summarize* their Activating Events and focus more on their irrational Beliefs and their emotional and behavioral Consequences.

Avoiding Compulsive Talking about Feelings

Many clients, some of them trained to do so by previous therapy, longwindedly and compulsively talk about their feelings, their feelings, their feelings. Although they had better fully *acknowledge* these feelings and freely *express* them in therapy, endlessly obsessing about them and whining about them will do little good and sometimes much harm. I usually say, after a few minutes of feeling talk, "I fully understand that you feel very deeply about what's happening in your life, and I think that some of your strong feelings are quite appropriate and useful. But let's try to focus on your inappropriate and harmful feelings and what you're thinking and doing to create and maintain them. Let's get back to what you are irrationally thinking when you make yourself feel panicked, depressed, and self-hating."

Avoiding Too Much Positive Thinking

From the start, I have used positive thinking and visualizing (Coué, 1923; Peale, 1952; Zibergeld & Lazarus, 1987) in RET in the form of practical coping statements, such as, "I *can* do better if I really try," "I won't *always* get rejected but will *sometimes* get accepted if I keep approaching people," and "Slow and steady wins the race!"

But this kind of positive thinking has several disadvantages: (1) it is often false and utopian and will lead to later disillusionment (e.g., Coué's familiar "Day by day in every way I'm getting better and better"); (2) it often helps achievement, but it implies that one *must* succeed and be approved or else one is worthless; and (3) it is usually practical rather than philosophical. Thus, "I *can* do better" is practical and helps clients' achievement, but "Even when I don't do well, I am determined only to rate my performance and never to berate myself!" is philosophical and healthier. So rather than emphasize the usual kind of practical and success-oriented positive thinking and visualization that Coué and his successors tend to use, and frequently overuse, I more often help clients to employ rational, philosophical, positive thoughts and images. They then can more quickly and effectively acquire a set of profound self-helping attitudes.

Avoiding Overstressing Practical Changes

As RET has always emphasized, people come to therapy with (1) practical problems of how to get more of what they want and less of what they don't want in life and (2) emotional-behavioral problems *about* their practical problems. Thus, they needlessly disturb themselves about (a) how poorly they are solving their practical problems; about (b) how badly disturbed they are; and about (c) how difficult therapy is and how little they are getting from it. Therapists, especially those who practice strategic therapy (Haley, 1976), skill training (Guerney, 1977), and problem-solving therapy (D'Zurilla & Goldfriend, 1971; Spivack & Shure, 1974), largely help clients to solve their practical problems, and hence not to be so emotionally disturbed about having them. Fine! RET also uses a number of practical, problem-solving, and skill-training techniques (Ellis, 1976, 1977b, 1979a, 1988; Ellis & Abrahms, 1978; Ellis & Dryden, 1987; Ellis & Whiteley, 1979).

But RET is a double systems therapy that usually first tries to help people change when they are in a dysfunctional relationship and then *also* helps them change the relationship (Ellis, 1985, 1987, 1988; Ellis & Dryden, 1987; Ellis, Sichel, Yeager, DiMattia, & DiGiuseppe, 1989; Ellis & Yeager, 1989). It assumes that if people change their Activating Events and thereby improve their life situations, they will quickly *feel* better but make few further attempts to *get* better (by changing their basic irrational Beliefs about unfortunate Activating Events). So I help my clients to zero in quickly on their iBs (irrational Beliefs) about their undesirable Activating Events (As), *as well as* to start planning to change those As. But I often avoid too much practical problem-solving and skill-training until they start working to give up their iBs; otherwise, they may never get around to doing so. Or they may do well at changing their As—but then creatively bring about new obnoxious As (especially poor relationships with others) because they still think irrationally, feel disturbed, and act dysfunctionally.

How RET Can Be Effectively Elegant and Long-Lasting

As I have just noted, effective RET is designed to be briefer than other psychotherapies (although with severely disturbed, resistant, borderline, and psychotic individuals it may sometimes continue for several years; Ellis, 1985). But RET especially tries, in most cases, to help bring about an elegant, long-lasting state of improvement whereby clients, first, give up their presenting symptoms (e.g., social anxiety); second, diminish or eliminate other dysfunctional symptoms (e.g., work or sports anxiety); third, maintain their therapeutic progress; fourth, become less likely, by using RET over the years, to seriously disturb themselves again; fifth, when they occasionally fall back to emotional and behavioral problems use RET again to quickly overcome their recurring or newly created difficulties; and sixth, keep seeking and finding maximally enjoyable, but nondefeating, paths to personal enjoyment.

Some of the main procedures that I use and that other RET practitioners can use to effectively help clients achieve elegant and long-lasting solutions to their difficulties include the following.

Achieving a Profound Philosophical Change

RET is not only cognitive but also highly philosophical and I probably never would have created it in 1955 had I not been convinced for about 20 years before that time that, if people had a truly sound philosophy, they could ward off practically all neurotic thinking, feeling, and behaving and could arrange their lives so that they would rarely, if ever, be self-defeating and antisocial. This idea was confirmed by my early years of practicing RET. I saw that psychotics and borderline personalities were usually biologically programmed to act aberrantly but that even they could often save themselves considerable emotional turmoil if they profoundly changed their attitudes toward themselves, others, and their life conditions. I also saw that neurotics could much more easily undisturb themselves, even when afflicted with poor life situations, and could make themselves much less neurotic if they really—and I mean *really*—gave up their dogmatic, absolutist, antiempirical, and illogical thinking and *truly* stayed with their strong preferences and the alternative roads to happiness that these almost always present when they are unrigidly held.

To help my clients make a profound philosophical, mental (and often physical) health-producing change, I started to show them how to achieve these RET-inspired attitudes:

1. Fully acknowledge that they mainly disturb themselves and rarely *get* disturbed by other people or external events.

2. Strongly believe that they *can* refuse to inappropriately upset themselves about virtually anything that happens or that they make happen; and that if they do needlessly make themselves disturbed, they have the ability to soon *un*disturb themselves again.

3. Acknowledge that it is not their desires, goals, values, and standards that really disturb them but largely their absolutist, rigid, irrational must's, demands, and commands *about* these desires and standards.

4. Acknowledge that they will most probably have to work and keep working like hell to change their irrational Beliefs, inappropriate feelings, and dysfunctional behaviors, which create, maintain, and exacerbate rigid demandingness and its accompanying disturbances. See that magic most probably does not exist and that they had better work on their *own* power to heal themselves.

5. Force themselves to steadily do the continual work and practice required to bring about change.

6. Acknowledge that they probably have other dysfunctional symptoms in addition to the ones for which they first sought therapy and, if so, assume that these additional symptoms are mainly created by irrational Beliefs (iBs) and that these can also be changed by thinking, feeling, and acting against them. Work at doing this changing, using regular RET methods.

7. Have the attitude that if they keep thinking and working against disturbed feelings and behaviors just as soon as they are aware of them, they usually are able to quickly change them and become habituated to doing so more easily. Quite importantly, too, see that if they do this steadily for a period of time, they frequently will achieve a basically new antimusturbatory outlook that they thereafter will *bring* to present and future

unpleasant Activating Events, so that they hardly ever disturb themselves (that is, produce *in*appropriate feelings and behaviors) about them. This is what I have seen in thousands of my RET clients. Where, before therapy, they easily and often seriously upset themselves when they or others acted "badly," after therapy they had a definite antidisturbing attitude about the same "bad" situations. Some of them achieved a thoroughgoing anti-neurotic philosophy and rarely seriously upset themselves about virtually *anything*. But, alas, these hard-working and straight-thinking individuals constitute less than 5% of those who have considerably benefited from RET.

8. Clearly understand that one is always prone to making oneself disturbed again, although less often than before therapy, but that when one makes this happen, one has the ability to work hard and quickly at overcoming this new disturbance. One also has the ability—with work!—to keep making oneself less and less disturb*able*.

9. Realize that to exist and be free of misery does not necessarily mean to be happy and fulfilled and that therefore one had better, while working to undisturb oneself, also keep seeking more enjoyable, fulfilling, and self-actualizing pursuits. Give up unrealistically *insisting* on perfect or even great happiness, but keep trying—and experimenting—to be as joyful as they can personally be (Bernard, 1986; Ellis & Dryden, 1987, 1990, 1991; Ellis & Bernard, 1985; Yankura & Ellis, 1990).

Persistent Work and Practice

As I have noted for many years, the power in people's "willpower" consists of their strong *determination* to change themselves *plus* persistent *work and practice* to carry out this determination (Ellis, 1962, 1973, 1988). Similarly, all the rational-emotive attitudes outlined in the previous section will not help clients to change, to maintain their changes, and to keep making themselves more self-helping and self-actualizing unless they persistently work at RET. They had better abandon all hope of magical, miraculous solutions and keep working hard for nonmagical, imperfect ones. I try to help them see this and to nondamningly monitor their own persistent homework.

Acquiring a Vital Absorbing Interest

As Robert A. Harper and I said in our original *Guide to Rational Living* (Ellis & Harper, 1961) and reaffirmed in *A New Guide to Rational Living* (Ellis & Harper, 1975), people are helped to acquire the elegant and long-lasting RET solution when they acquire a vital, absorbing interest in some long-range goal, project, cause, or ideal. Thus, I frequently encourage them to devote themselves to building a family, a business, or a career, or to working for a political, social, economic, or religious cause that they can pursue for a number of years. The advantages of doing so include the following:

1. Clients distract themselves, often, from their disturbed feelings and self-defeating behaviors and do so strongly, for a long period of time. Other kinds of cognitive distraction—such as relaxation techniques, meditation, and Yoga—are much more short-lasting.

2. Clients see that their life has real meaning and that they will probably be vitally absorbed forever. This eliminates their disturbed feelings of meaninglessness and their suicidal tendencies and gives them something important to live for.

3. People usually get so much pleasure from their vital, absorbing interests that they are able to accept the hassles and pains of the rest of their lives and to upset themselves minimally about them.

4. People with a vital, absorbing interest usually enjoy themselves so much in pursuing it that they feel self-actualized and do not have to seek out other or greater enjoyments.

5. Clients who devote themselves to big, ongoing interest often become disciplined, long-range hedonists who can more easily avoid destructive, short-range pleasures (e.g., addiction to alcohol and drugs). They may also, in dedicating themselves to their interest, force themselves to uncomplainingly take on many hassles and may thereby achieve higher frustration tolerance.

6. People may wrongly see themselves as "good" or "worthy" individuals because they are vitally absorbed in a "good" or "worthy" cause. This is a dangerous kind of self-rating, because they will then tend to devaluate themselves again if their cause fails or they stop working for it. But they can legitimately take great pleasure in working for *it*, their cause, instead of glorifying their *selves* for doing so, and this pleasure can add considerably and legitimately to their lives.

INTERVIEW

Editor's Note: The following interview took place in the autumn of 1988 at the Institute for Rational-Emotive Therapy. Across a 4-hour time period on a Saturday and Sunday, Albert Ellis spoke spontaneously with Michael Bernard on a variety of issues related to using RET effectively. The interview questions were preplanned to cover the following three areas deemed to influence RET's effectiveness: "client characteristics," "therapist characteristics," and "therapy characteristics."

Client Characteristics

Sex of Client

BERNARD: When practicing RET, how important is it to take into account the sex of the client? Does client sex influence anything that you might do to make RET more efficient and effective? For example, males might find it less easy to talk about their feelings. Is there anything that RET practitioners would need to remind themselves when working with a male or a female or is it not an important characteristic?

ELLIS: Probably, but I think it is more a matter of the individual person than sex. Although I am fairly sure that, on the whole, we could find some characteristics of "average" males and females that are important in therapy, there are many individual differences within each sex. For example, I— and most therapists, probably, incidentally, who are direct and active— assume that females are more vulnerable and that they are likely to take more things amiss about their relationship, about therapy, and about the therapist. Females in our culture may have a tendency to feel more upset about confrontation in therapy, and therefore, I tend to be more tactful, to test them out to see how they react. I tend to jump in more and be more active and hard-headed with the males, and then, if that does not work, I can always withdraw. When I do find some differences between the two sexes, which is often not the case, I modify my approach to try to take them into account.

Also, the goals and values of females in our culture are sometimes different from those of males. Females are often more interested in relating, mating, and having children than males are. Of course, some males are very interested in having children. But usually, it is the female who is more prone to it, especially as she gets above the age of 35. Females usually have more interest in relating than in driving ahead in business or even a profession, but not all of them. Many today are very concerned—and some are overconcerned—with their professional *and* their mating life.

I don't consciously tend to take the sex of a client much into account. I let people just go ahead and talk about their emotional problems, which are hardly unique to either sex! Unconsciously, I may talk in a different kind of voice, or in a less forceful manner, to females than to males, and so I sound them out. Then I might talk more so, to some females than males, but I make no real effort to do so. You might say that I have an androgynous attitude to begin with and that I then modify it through my experiences with my individual clients. Although RET in general, like most therapies, follows certain general theories and emphasizes certain things rather than other things, humans are always individually different, and I make an effort to see and relate to their individual—and their sexual— differences. I (and presumably other RET-ers) take into account the particular human I am talking to, that is, his or her personality and also, of course, the seriousness of her or his disturbance. Sometimes, for example, with more resistant and more disturbed clients of both sexes, I am tougher and more forceful because I conclude that less toughness just will not work. Or I may be milder with a client of either sex who I think is too vulnerable to be treated very firmly. A good deal of my approach involves risk taking. I first risk what I *guess* is the best approach, and then I modify it, as the responses of the client might suggest.

Age of Client

B: How about the age of the client? When faced with a client who might be older versus one who is younger, is there any aspect of their age that might influence your assessment or your approach when using RET?

E: First of all, when clients are adolescents, from about 13 to 19, I just assume that they know less about therapy and less about the world and that they are probably more suggestible than older people. Therefore, at the beginning, I'm much more often teaching, corrective, and forceful, hoping that I will get through to them, and, I think, I frequently do. If the same person were 25 and 30 years, I would still be didactic but not that much so; they would have much more experience, and I have more of a dialogue, whereas with the young ones I often do more teaching at the beginning, often quite forceful, vigorous teaching.

With the middle range, from 20 to 60 years—most of the clients I see are in that range—I use the general RET approach, showing them how to do their own disputing of self-defeating beliefs. But I do it quite individualistically, according to how bright, how impressionable, how disturbed, and how willing to learn they are and how they do their homework. I don't think their age matters much. But as soon as they become over 60 and especially over 70, I assume that they'll frequently resist changing. Especially with older rigid people, I often go back to very forceful teaching. Just as I use strong coping statements with young children, I often use them with rigid older adults. I insist that they *can* overcome their anxiety and depression, and I help them to strongly repeat to themselves, "I *can* conquer my depression!" "I am worthwhile *whether or not* I perform well!" And lots of times I use less real RET, more teaching and suggestion, less getting them to dispute, because I don't think they're going to do much elegant disputing. But I think that they often follow sensible, rational directives, self-actualizing teachings. Sometimes, older people can be helped only by very strong reassurances that they can get better, they can sleep, or they can get over the loss of a loved one and still enjoy themselves. Especially with disturbed people over 70, when they are bright and sharp, regular RET can greatly help. But those who are not sharp and who are rigid and very upset will rarely do good disputing and can be helped with strong coping self-statements.

I have one client, for example, who is close to 78, and she has the problem of not being able to walk very far without being afraid. When she gets to the city, she's afraid to walk, horrified about tripping and falling. She's a pretty bright woman and can see she has a real phobia. So I very strongly tell her that she *can* walk, she *can* walk and that nothing's going to happen to her. I also say, "And if you do fall, its *not* going to be the end of the world! You'll bruise yourself. But you can get up, the bruise will heal, and you can go back to walking again! It will only be a damned inconvenience!" So I strongly teach her RET; and now, after a few weeks, she is walking in the city—and often enjoying it. I think it's partly the result of my *strong* reassurances and her *vigorous* rational self-statements. She voluntarily ends the session after 20 minutes. She says we don't need the whole half hour because the RET is repetitive, and very strong; "I *can* do it and not fall. And if I do, I do!" she smilingly says as she leaves. So with people over 70 and over 80— yes, I see a number in their 80s—I often do this kind of thing.

B: Does client age guide you to what their values, needs, and concerns might be? Whereas an older person might be somewhat concerned about death and dying, at some point being left alone, a younger person might be more concerned about having children, and the still younger one might be more concerned about identity issues.

E: Right. The older ones are rarely very concerned about achievement. They may be retired or they have gone as far as they can go. Some of them are still artists, writers, or other kinds of poets. I then encourage them to risk performances and surrender their fears of failing, but older people are often not especially concerned about family matters, as long as their children and grandchildren visit them enough. So you're right. Their concerns are different. But they are often more anxious about illness, death, and loneliness. So we work on those problems.

Intelligence of Client

B: How much does the intelligence level of your clients influence the way you go about practicing RET?

E: Well, on one level it doesn't influence me *too* much. Because I give them practically all standard RET: "You largely feel the way you think and you can change your thinking and thereby change your feeling." But, of course, with the intelligent people, I do it on a much higher level. I'm much more philosophical with them and show them that, just because they are intelligent, they can challenge their thinking better and go into aspects of life that we would hardly mention with the person of intelligence that is average or somewhat below normal. It does affect the therapy, especially the finer nuances. I really get the very intelligent people to work much harder not to rate themselves at all, whereas to the others, I will say, forcefully and over and over, "You're a good person because you exist." So high IQs tend more often to reach the "elegant" solution in RET, whereas people with lower IQs can significantly improve, but often less elegantly.

Socioeconomic Status of Client

B: Let's examine the variable of socioeconomic status. If you have someone who you know is from a working-class urban background, would that influence what you do in therapy as opposed to if you're working with someone who comes from an upper-middle-class suburban background?

E: Well, socioeconomic class does often correlate with intelligence. Sometimes, not always, the people from the lower-class, blue-collar background are not as bright, educated, and sophisticated as upper-middle-class individuals. Again, in terms of goals and values, I assume that the people from the blue-collar and lower-class background often have their own conventions and standards and frequently ask for more limited therapeutic goals. But I sometimes teach these clients RET in the way I work with youngsters. I am very forceful and vigorous, show them how to tell themselves that they're OK, that they don't have to damn themselves for anything, and that they can do well, they can change. I omit some of the deeper philosophical levels that I more often use with more sophisticated people, and I often have fewer sessions with them. But one of the virtues of RET is that it is not only useful for YAVIS-type clients but can be successfully used as well with less educated ones, too.

B: Is there any difference in what their expectation is of you as a therapist or of therapy, or in the language you use with them, when you work with a working-class versus a very "well-off" person?

E: Well, I always tell the story of what happened to my personal physician years ago. He had an office on Fifth Avenue at 98th Street, and he had two kinds of clients: a Fifth Avenue clientele, well-to-do and highly educated people, and working-class people who lived only a few blocks away. And he told me that, with the working-class people, he could very forcefully in one or two sessions reassure them and use low-level RET to help them with their psychosomatic problems. In an hour or two, he showed what to do to change their thinking, such as I do with the young people I see, and that worked very well. With the upper-class people, he couldn't do as well. He had to have a whole series of sessions, and the client didn't consistently follow his rational suggestions.

So many blue-collar people look on a physician, or a psychologist, or a teacher, as an authority figure. Sometimes, they listen more respectfully and carefully than do sophisticated clients. They still may have low frustration tolerance and not carry out their homework assignments, but they often do not resist therapy, as do some of the very bright people, who would rather discuss than act. In fact, by discussing and "understanding" RET, they may delude themselves that they've really "got" it—and therefore don't have to work at implementing it!

Cultural Background of Client

B: What about cultural background, such as Hispanic or Israeli? Does that determine at all how you might proceed with what you're doing?

E: Yes, I definitely consider clients' cultural views. In New York City, of course, people come from many different backgrounds. In their standards, rules, and goals, they often vary considerably. In sexual areas, for example, they may be very much against premarital sex or sometimes for it. It depends on what culture and what socioeconomic level they come from. The ones who have particular cultural views I don't try to change very much, or try to get them to have other views, unless they hold those views rigidly and self-defeatingly.

I am seeing a woman right now who is a Mormon, semidevout, but she is also pregnant and has a lover who is an Orthodox Jew whom she might well decide not to marry. So her problem is whether to get an abortion, because if she does, her church and her Mormon family will probably excommunicate her. So I deal with her differently than I would with somebody who comes from a less rigid family and religion. I know that she is going to have a hard time among her cultural group if she does get an abortion, and therefore, in her particular case, it might even be better to have the child and see another man who might want to marry her and become a Mormon.

So when people have strong religious and cultural values, I accept their values but also show them how they may be defeating themselves in terms of their own standards. They can, using RET, choose to stick with their cultural values or decide to change them without damning themselves. Thus, if my Mormon client did decide to go through with an abortion, I would help her to accept herself, in spite of her "wrong" act, and then to plan on becoming pregnant again after she marries. So there are some "samenesses" about RET theory and practice for most people and most cultures. But clients can also keep their cultural values and then not needlessly upset themselves when they lead to frustration and/or are not perfectly followed.

B: Do you treat many Oriental people?

E: I have a number of Chinese and other Asian clients. I treat some of them who come from abroad, such as students, but also those who have been here quite awhile. One woman in one of my therapy groups speaks English quite well. She's of Chinese background but was mainly raised in the United States. My Oriental clients have many American values, but they also have some of the old, strong family values of the mainland

Orientals. My Indian clients are similar. I've had a number of clients who were raised in India. When they live here for a while they have several American values, but they are often very much attached to their families in India. They listen to their parents about whom they should marry and what they should do in life more than Americans tend to do. But my Indian and Oriental clients find RET useful. I try to get them to stop putting themselves down, which is pretty much what I do with my clients from other cultures. I also try to get them to stop damning themselves and to raise their low frustration tolerance. I have several Indians, in particular, who have general low frustration tolerance and who procrastinate mightily. RET helps them to overcome these problems in pretty much the same way that it helps my American clients.

B: So if people are from a different background, it helps to be alert to what the rules are that might be adversely effecting them.

E: That's right. Their must's about the rules tend to be the same; not the rules. That's why I disagree with cognitive-behavioral therapists, who think that people upset themselves when they fail to follow their personal or social rules of living. I assert that they upset themselves with their rigid must's *about* these rules rather than by their nonadherence to the rules themselves.

Religious Background of Client

B: You could probably spend all day talking about the role of religion in your clients, but related to culture is religion and the devoutness with which people hold their religious principles. I'm wondering if when dealing with a Catholic versus a Protestant versus a Jew, each of them fairly devout, will their religion influence the way you proceed in therapy with them.

E: There again, we have the same thing. If they want to believe some religion because they find it helpful, that's OK. Right now I see a Jewish atheist who doesn't believe in God at all but goes to a little church on the way to our sessions and prays. He finds praying useful. He's not even clear what he's praying to, but he just prays and enjoys it. But if people rigidly hold religious views, are scrupulously addicted to dogmatic rules, and punitively damn themselves and others for the slightest infringement of these rules, I may use RET to help them overcome their scrupulosity and their destructive self-damnation and their damnation of others. RET, like some forms of Christianity, always shows people how to give themselves unconditional grace and to accept and forgive human sinners (though not their sins).

These days, I see many people who describe themselves as spiritual but not religious. Most of them are humanists who believe in some central energy or force in the universe and who may help themselves with their "spiritual" or "transpersonal" views. But others are devout believers in antiscientific disciplines like astrology, psychic surgery, exorcism, astral projections, and shamanism. These beliefs may be relatively harmless but also reflect a dire need for certainty and an inflexible refusal to accept inevitable human frustration and failure. New-age philosophy includes some sensible Eastern ideas and cognitive-emotional techniques. But it is often taken to cultish extremes and may then do much more harm than good—as I and Raymond Yeager show in our book *Why Some Therapies Don't Work: The Dangers of Transpersonal Psychology* (1989). Devout religionists and cultists rarely come to see me for psychotherapy. When they do, I try to help them change their rigid demands on themselves and others, which defeat their own goals and values, including some of their religious values. What I call rigid religiosity—that is, imperatively and absolutistically holding either theistic or secular views—tends to get people into emotional and behavioral trouble. But undogmatic, flexible religious views are not necessarily incompatible with emotional health.

B: Do you think it's important for therapists to be alert to the strong values that the client might be holding?

E: Yes, I think it's important to bring them out and to be alert to them and see how they interact with clients' disturbances. People's values, including strong ones, stem from and in turn influence their desires and feelings. Without values, they would lead a bland, nonfeeling existence and might very well perish. So RET encourages clients to have strong values, preferences, and feelings, as long as clients do not absolutize and rigidify them and thereby use them in self-defeating and society-defeating ways.

Client Expectations

B: Can I ask you about client expectations? When clients walk in here, they have certain expectations about what they're going to do to get better and what you are going to do to help them get better. I'm wondering if it's important for the RET therapist to find out what the client's expectations might be and to modify a little bit what they do in terms of those expectations.

E: Yes, to determine their expectations about therapy and about where they would like to get with its help. But I often try to change their expectations about therapy, especially when I see that they have had previous non-RET sessions. So I point out right from the start that RET is distinctly different from psychoanalysis and most other systems and that we're not going to go very much into the client's past. If we do go into the early life, it will be mainly to show the client how she or he constructed (rather than just picked up) self-defeating philosophies—and how the client still clings to them and thereby disturbs herself or himself today. Many clients come to RET knowing that it's a brand of cognitive-behavioral therapy. Others soon learn this and usually are happy about staying in the present, disputing their self-destructive beliefs. I also encourage many of them to quickly start to solve their practical life problems. Some clients expect to talk, talk, talk, and endlessly express their feelings. But I soon slow them down and explain that RET is much more than a "talking cure," and that, to improve, they'd better prepare to *do* more than that.

I sometimes let my clients talk and emote lengthily, but I also manage to get in some solid RET questioning, dialoguing, and teaching. I also push the incessant talkers to do some rational-emotive reading but I can put up with their talking if that's the way they are. I get them to listen to cassettes and to do a fair amount of thinking, feeling, and behavioral homework. At the moment, I have one client who can talk for the whole hour if I let him, hardly allowing me to get a word in edgewise. But I always manage to interrupt sufficiently and challenge him; and I get him to do considerable RET reading. After eight sessions, he quite agrees—and demonstrates—that he has significantly changed some of his self-sabotaging philosophy.

B: So you are flexible in terms of what the client's expectations might be.

E: Yes. But I also actively *direct* most sessions, to educate and encourage clients to use RET techniques on their own. My standard homework assignment, which I give right at the start to almost all clients, and often repeat, is that, when anything bothers them during the week, they had better write down the A (activating event), and the C (consequence), and just bring for discussion into the session a few of these As and Cs. If they do that, we have some current problems to work on together, so they get trained very quickly not to ramble on and on. If they describe A or C in too great detail, I remind them of our time limitations, and I urge them to look at their Bs and dispute their irrational beliefs. If something really unusual happens in their life, they may spend much of the session narrating. But I still push them to go on to their feelings and beliefs about this eventful occurrence. So I am flexible, but at the same time, I encourage my clients not to waste their therapy time and to raise the issues that will be most productive and will also lead to effective homework.

B: So if their expectation is to talk, talk, talk, you take that into account, and then you try to get them to change their expectation as quickly as possible?

E: Yes, right. But in those cases where they won't curb their incessant talking, I tend to live with it and still interpolate a good amount of RET.

"Diagnosis" of Client

B: The final category of client characteristics is the formal diagnosis of your client. Do you take into account the diagnosis—personality disorders or other sorts of diagnoses—in terms of your initial approach, your expectations. How important is the formal diagnosis itself?

E: Well, I think it's very important with psychotic or near psychotic individuals. If I see, as I often do in the first sessions, that the person has paranoid schizophrenia or a severe borderline personality disorder, I usually assume that he or she has a strong tendency to behave and to stay this way and is going to have great trouble changing. I said before that with youngsters and rigid oldsters, I tend to be stronger and more persuasive. I do more teaching and I'm more repetitive because I assume that, even with my talents and with effective RET, they're going to have great difficulty changing. I also check to see whether they're on medication, and if not, I often try to get them on it. Some of them I won't see without medication because I think we're going to waste our time. I told one woman recently that, unless she gets back on her medication, I think we're going to get nowhere. She got huffy, felt insulted, and refused to pay for her session with me. But I think she intended not to pay anyway. Psychotics will often ignore our Institute rules, and even though we say that they have to pay for all sessions in advance, they avoid doing so.

With psychotics, especially paranoids, I try to get them to admit how disturbed they are, to see that they probably have a biochemical disorder, and to try medication. I am quite firm with many of them because I figure they're not really listening and not allowing regular RET to sink in. I often train them to be more practical and to get along better in their everyday life, and I focus on skill training rather than on rational disputing. I often help them to improve significantly and to stop damning themselves for being psychotic; that is, I help them overcome their neurosis *about* their psychosis. But I don't pretend that RET, or any other kind of psychotherapy, will make them unpsychotic.

Now the borderlines, whom I see by the hundreds, and especially the serious ones whom I diagnose as "borderline plus," I assume are semipsychotic and that, once again, this has little to do with their early upbringing (as the object relations psychoanalysts wrongly claim) but that their disturbances are largely biological but can be exacerbated by many environmental factors. They *can* be reached by RET, but therapy takes a long time and will probably lead to limited gains. They often improve significantly but not as much as the light borderlines and neurotics.

What I call the "light borderline personalities" I also see as somewhat (though differently) biologically predisposed to be the way they are, as quite prone to easily upsetting themselves, and as usually requiring longer therapy and harder work on my part, before they will use RET effectively. But I think they can be helped significantly and become practically neurotic or "normal," though perhaps never completely "cured."

With my other clients—the nice neurotics and the few "normals" that I see—I find little resistance. Often, I see them for from 1 to 10 sessions and make good headway with regular, run-of-the-mill RET. Some come with only one real problem—such as a sex or a job problem—and are not very self-denigrating. Others put themselves down about one or two issues—such as for not being good enough parents or not making enough money—but are not general self-downers. These clients are often a delight to work with, learn and apply RET quickly, do their homework regularly, and especially learn to help themselves by using RET bibliographical and audiovisual materials. One of the reasons, in fact, why I see so many seriously disturbed and so few less disturbed people these days is because, in the New York area, the reasonably bright mild neurotics have learned a great deal by reading my books and other self-help books derived from RET (like Dyer's *Your Erroneous Zones* and Burns's *Feeling Good*), and they often help themselves with these books *without* coming to therapy.

You see that I do consider clients' diagnoses and assume that, the more disturbed they are, the longer and harder I and they will probably have to work to get good RET results. But I rarely give up on psychotic and severely borderline individuals. A few, as I said before, I won't see unless they are on medication. And those whom I do see, I think can be distinctly helped, but usually with long-term RET.

B: Do you take into account different mental personality diagnoses, such as the narcissistic personality versus the compulsive one?

E: Yes, I often do. For example, let's take the real narcissists. They're very usually in my "borderline plus" category because of their grandiosity, pollyannaism, run-on-at-the-mouthness, and refusal to listen to my realistic disputing or to do any of their own. So I strongly get after them while expecting relatively few gains. The obsessive–compulsives, I think, are clearly biological. They are wired wrongly, as it were, and frequently have deficient neurotransmitters (especially serotonin), which sometimes can be partially corrected by medication. They often demand absolute, perfect certainty, which I quite strongly show them does not exist and sometimes (not always!) help them forgo.

I see one now who has both the need for certainty and also awfulizes about her child being switched for another child right after she gave birth. She demands a 100% guarantee that her child wasn't switched, which, of course, she can't have. Although I show her that there's no evidence that the child was switched and only a one-in-a-billion chance that it was, and although the child looks just like her, she still insists that it may have been switched and is panicked about the "horror" of such a possibility.

I then try elegant RET and show her that, even if the child had been switched, it would not be so bad, because she has OCD (obsessive-compulsive disorder), her mother is schizophrenic, and several of her other close relatives are borderline personalities. So if she got the wrong baby, it might well turn out to be *less* disturbed than if she got the right one! Finally, after weeks of strongly using RET with her, I am getting her to accept uncertainty, and she is becoming much less obsessed about the highly unlikely baby switching.

Another of my severe OCD clients almost miraculously recovered after 14 sessions. He was one of those who, when he drove a car and hit a bump, always had to stop and get out of the car to be absolutely positive that he had not hit somebody. He would be compulsively forced to stop and get out of the car so many times that he gave up driving. I strongly used RET first to show him the small probability of his unknowingly hitting anybody, and I gave him the anticompulsive assignment of *never* getting out of his car, no matter how many people he "killed" on the road. After he uncomfortably carried out this assignment only three times while powerfully convincing himself that certainty doesn't exist and the laws of probability are clearly on his side, he completely overcame his compulsion to keep getting out of his car.

So I work hard with the OCDs and I get some of them better. But others just give up one major compulsion or obsession and later on go back to it or create others. But I persist. I keep plugging away with my OCDs. Sometimes, I help them take medication and make some progress. A well-known therapist visited me recently and said, "Al, how do you do with obsessive-compulsives? I rarely get anywhere with them." I replied, "Yes, they are very difficult—most probably because of their biochemical anomalies. But with a combination of RET and suitable medication you can often make some progress."

As for the schizoid clients, they, too, I often diagnose as "borderline plus," as being semischizophrenic. So I work hard, and often long, with them. I help them surrender their horror of social disapproval, show them how to improve their interpersonal relations, give them some skill training, and often achieve considerable improvement. But though they function much better, they usually still have underlying schizoid qualities and rarely become truly healthy personalities. Though significantly improved, they still have a few important buttons missing.

Practitioner Characteristics

Practitioner Knowledge of RET Theory

B: Let's move over to therapist characteristics as opposed to client characteristics. In terms of what would make RET more efficient, how important is it for the therapist to know RET practice or RET theory?

E: I think it quite important because I get reports back from my clients who have seen other RET therapists and have benefited from them. But some of the things they were taught by RET-ers are definitely not RET and are often palliative. Some RET-ers heavily emphasize relaxation, biofeedback, positive visualization, meditation, body work, and other therapy methods that help people to feel better but hardly get better. They ignore some of the RET methods that are more likely to help people achieve the profound philosophic change that elegant RET favors.

B: My experience is that a lot of so-called RET therapists don't really understand the fundamental theory. They don't conceptualize people's problems from an RET point of view. Some of the techniques they use are RET, but they don't really understand the theory well enough to analyze the problem from an RET point of view even though they might dispute. But they never pick up the discomfort anxiety or they fail to distinguish between an inference and an evaluation difficulty. Or they don't really understand which irrational beliefs are underlying the particular problem. And so, when they actually do the assessment, they miss the mark because they pick up the wrong thing. I find a lot of errors, and when I train people, I find that, because they haven't really taken the time to digest the theory, they think they're doing proper RET. They use some of the techniques, but they lack the insights that the theory gives them. And I think that it's as important to be able to understand the theory as it is to apply the techniques.

E: Right. Maxie Maultsby's trainees use some RET, but they often do it by rote, somewhat mechanically, and miss some of the subtle points of RET. Other RET-ers use a great deal of Beck's, Meichenbaum's, or Bandura's theory, all of which overlap with RET but again miss some of its finer nuances. Some water down RET theory and practice it with other therapies—such as psychoanalysis—that probably detract from its efficacy and profundity.

Practitioner Values and Attitudes

B: How important is it for the RET practitioner to share the RET value system—for example, to be a risk taker or to use a long-term hedonism to act in a self-interested way?

E: I think it important though not absolutely necessary. If RET therapists really use RET on themselves, they act as good models and have a better chance of persuading their clients to use it. But I confess that I know several RET therapists who are pretty nutty, who don't use RET on themselves, and who still definitely help others. So RET, even when done by a therapist who doesn't use it, *can* be effective. In fact, the client may sometimes learn it and use it better than the therapist!

B: How important is practitioner low frustration tolerance [LFT]?

E: Very important, for several reasons. First, severe disturbance stems from biological as well as environmental influences and can be considerably improved. But clients often fall back to old levels of disturbance and also have low frustration tolerance about working at therapy. Therefore, therapy can be discouraging, and unless you have high frustration tolerance and can easily stand clients who don't improve at all, those who improve a little, those who fall back after improvement, and those who don't work at therapy, you'd better not be a therapist. You can teach it and write about it, but preferably not practice it. I've known a few RET-ers who've given up individual therapy and now do workshops, teaching, or writing partly because of their own LFT. So I think that high frustration tolerance is good for any therapist, including RET-ers.

Therapist's Style of Confrontation

B: How about the therapist's ability to be direct and confront clients forcefully?

E: I think that's two things. One is the ability to do it, the therapist's competence. Second, direct and forceful therapists had better have little need for the client's approval. If you really *need* your client's approval and upset yourself about their opposing you or about their quitting you and telling people that you're not helping them, then you won't confront them. You'll indulge them, you'll pat them on the head, you'll get along with them very nicely, but you won't be direct and forceful. Therefore, I think it's important to be able to confront them but of course not always to do it. Some people you'd better not confront, some psychotics and borderlines. But when it would be desirable to confront a client and you can't because of your own fear of rejection, watch out.

B: So you think it is important for therapists to be able to confront clients and be direct as part of RET. And they're going to be ineffective if they're not able to communicate a certain value system, a point of view, and keep after people. If they're not able to do that for some of the reasons you just mentioned, then they're not going to be as effective?

E: That's right, they're not going to be as effective as they could be; but even with nonconfrontive RET, therapists can often achieve good results.

B: How about the degree of warmth, empathy, and unconditional positive regard that a practitioner has as a person and as a way of relating to a client. Will these qualities help to make him or her an effective RET practitioner?

E: It's very important that you not be moralistic and condemnatory, especially when clients act stupidly or immorally. As a therapist, try to *really* believe that clients' *acts* are foolish but that *they* are OK. Using RET, you can always accept *people* and show them by your tone and your manner—as well as your words—that both you and they can fully accept *them*, but not necessarily their *behavior*. So I think that's quite important again for therapists. And I think that many therapists who practice other theories, such as psychoanalysis, often give RET-type acceptance. Thus, they listen to clients telling them that they hate their mother, lied to their mates, or otherwise acted badly and still *accept* these clients. So I think that many clients improve because of therapeutic acceptance, even when it isn't explicit in the therapeutic theory.

B: How important is it to be a warm person?

E: Well, warmth helps clients remain in therapy. If you're nice, warm, and friendly, it helps them come back. But on the other hand, it has some disadvantages. Did I ever tell you the story of how I used Ferenczi's technique years ago?

B: No.

E: Well, when I was a psychoanalyst, before I started RET, I read Ferenczi, who wrote that the reason people are disturbed is because their parents didn't really love them enough and that the purpose of analysis is to give them that love. And so he did what he called *active psychoanalysis* and gave them real warmth. Freud was scandalized and said Ferenczi would soon have his female clients with him on the sofa! But Ferenczi didn't really mean that. He meant warmth, love to make up missing parental love. So I said that seemed a better theory than the sex theories of Freud. I was never hooked on the Oedipus complex. I always looked for it and never found it. So I first thought that Ferenczi was OK. As a matter of fact, the object relations analysts today are partly following him. They're saying that, during the first and second year, if a child senses lack of parental love, it cannot be an individual in its own right and thus loses its identity. I doubt that, because only *certain* children are that vulnerable to potential neglect and decide that they absolutely *need* warmth to develop a sense of self.

So anyway, for about 10 months, I was very warm to my clients and went out of my way to tell them how lovely they were, and how I liked them. I was doing psychoanalytically oriented therapy, but added Ferenczi's warmth. My clients immediately loved it, adored me, asked for extra sessions, and recommended many of their friends to me. But then I noticed many of them becoming sicker. They become *more* dependent, *more* needy, so I abandoned Ferenczi! But to keep clients coming, warmth will work, so you can use it for rapport building and to encourage collaboration, as long as you also give clients regular RET. But giving much warmth does have its Achilles' heel.

Now, empathy means different things and you have to watch how you define it. Mainly, it means that you actively listen to clients and see things in *their* frame of reference. You show them that you're truly understanding them and their feelings, which is fine for any kind of therapist, including the RET-er. There is another form of empathy that is indigenous to RET, where you empathize with what clients are telling themselves.

B: I believe you've called it "advanced accurate empathy": you anticipate what they're thinking.

E: Yes, by empathically listening to what clients are telling themselves and showing that you really understand them much better than they do *themselves,* and by helping them listen to and comprehend their *self-*statements, both you and they *fully* understand what is going on inside them. As I do this, even though I do most of the talking during our first sessions, I find that many of my clients voluntarily say, at the session's end, "I've never felt so understood in all my life."

B: That's why knowing the theory is so important for therapists. If they don't really know the theory, they are unable to show clients how to really understand themselves.

E: That's right, that's a very good point you are making there. That kind of empathy with your client's thoughts, as well as with his or her feelings, is very important. It also includes unconditional acceptance because you are undamningly listening to what the client thinks, feels, and does. Carl Rogers did this very well, and in RET, we not only do it but also teach clients how to give nonjudgmental acceptance to themselves.

Therapy Characteristics

Presenting the RET Model

B: I want to move into aspects of the practice of RET that make it effective. It seems to me that there's an educational way of teaching RET and that there's more of an implicit, clinical way. By educational, I mean that, for all your clients, you clearly teach them the ABCs and explain quite didactically the basic theory of emotional upset. Or you can teach that implicitly by just analyzing a particular emotion and showing the relationship between thoughts and feelings. I'm wondering from your own experience, first of all, if it is legitimate to contrast the two styles and, second, if one style is better than another style, or if you can do both.

E: Well, in the first session or two, I do a good deal of the educational. I don't usually call it the ABCs, but I show clients that *they* upset themselves. As a great American philosopher, Pogo, said, "We have met the enemy and it is *us*." And I give clients my famous irrational thinking model of going out in the street, first, *wanting* a minimum of 10 dollars and feeling *disappointed* when they have only 9, and the *needing* a minimum of 10 and feeling *panicked* when they still have only 9. So, I am quite educational in my first session. But even during that session, I get into some *specific* disordered feelings and behaviors and show them the ABCs of *that* problem and how to dispute the irrational beliefs that they have personally constructed to create that disturbance. I not only reveal one or more of their *own* dysfunctions but try to give them some practice in changing it and a homework assignment to keep undoing it.

Elegant versus Inelegant RET

B: If the goal of RET is to bring about generalized changes so that clients experience fewer emotional disturbances in a variety of different present and future situations as a consequence of fundamental changes in philosophy and thinking, are RET practitioners really doing enough to bring about the elegant solution?

E: No. Sometimes RET practitioners are very good about showing clients how to overcome specific feelings of anxiety, depression, and self-downing but could do better at helping them acquire a *more general* philosophy of nondisturbance—as I emphasize in my book *How to Stubbornly Refuse to Make Yourself Miserable About Anything—Yes, Anything!* (1988).

B: I would have thought that by teaching clients rational values as distinct from or in addition to disputing the irrational beliefs—the rational values being self-acceptance, other acceptance, long-term hedonism, risk taking, and shame attacking—the clients would acquire more generalized changes. Russ Grieger discussed with me teaching clients the philosophy of happiness as an important basis for thorough change.

E: When did he discuss it with you?

B: When I spoke to him, earlier this year. But my belief is that, to bring about the elegant solution, we should use a combination of teaching rational values and using the disputational method of posing the right questions and knowing how to answer them. That would result in the profound changes that are necessary to bring about general emotional well-being.

E: Right. And what we'd better not forget, and sometimes do, is that RET *first* tries to help people overcome their emotional and behavioral difficulties and then *also* to actualize themselves and, as Russ Grieger says, to lead a happier life.

B: Isn't that your goal; to give people a new way of thinking and philosophy so whenever they come up with a negative activating event they no longer disturb themselves?

E: Yes, because we're helping them acquire a philosophy that nothing is terrible and that they virtually *never* need be utterly miserable. But what we also would like them to see is that there are many enjoyable aspects of living and that if they actively look for these aspects, and often *work* at achieving them, they can lead more fulfilling existences.

B: What I think we might want to consider—and I think again this is what Russ Grieger is saying—is teaching people the RET philosophy of life. Most self-help books are more problem-focused, and they don't teach people the philosophy of happiness. A lot of your work that appeared in *Humanistic Psychotherapy* (1973) and even in *Reason and Emotion in Psychotherapy* (1962) provides the philosophical underpinnings of the therapy. And it's just those philosophical underpinnings that I think will bring about the longer term changes. The therapy brings about the short-term changes, but it's the philosophy that brings about the longer term, more general changes.

E: I think you're right. Some clients we can show only how to stop defeating themselves, and that is of great value. But other clients we can also teach a *generalized* antidisturbance and prohappiness outlook, and you are rightly emphasizing this. But let's face the fact that, though most people can be taught how *not* to be miserable, the *specifics* of making each individual happy or happier are much more difficult to teach!

B: Yes, but we can use adjunct RET material, too, to help people make long-term changes and think about their personal happiness. They can read your self-help books to get over their immediate problems, but at the same time, you help them to become more philosophical and rational in their lives, generally speaking. It's a bit as if you can't be a good therapist unless you know the theory of RET fully, and you can't make enduring changes unless you've got the philosophy that underlies the self-help techniques. That's how I would see it.

E: I agree. I have always said that a main goal of RET is to go beyond symptom removal and to help people make *profound philosophical changes.* We want to be efficient therapists and to help people acquire better skill training. But it would be nice if RET therapists were also effective philosophers.

Use of Medication

B: What about the use of drugs as a facilitator of RET therapy for people who are depressed?

E: I think that, with some people, such as many endogenous depressives and certainly psychotics, drugs stop some of the acute pain and help them think and feel better, so that they're more likely to benefit from the RET. Now, for some clients, the drugs don't seem to help at all. So drugs are no panacea. But if people's neurotransmitters are really off, it's sometimes almost impossible to get them to think straight by using RET. So RET in conjunction with the drugs is often a good idea.

Therapist's Mistakes

B: Finally, I'd just like to talk briefly about the common mistakes a therapist can make in using RET. Are there specific mistakes an RET practitioner can make in the assessment of a client problem that might make RET less efficient or, in fact, just not effective at all? For example, one might be ignoring secondary symptom stress.

E: Yes, that's right. Therapists can ignore secondary symptoms and work only on clients' primary symptoms. In agoraphobia, clients usually have panic about their panic, so if that is ignored and therapists deal only with the primary panic, the clients often make little progress. In RET, we usually help clients overcome their symptom stress first—and then work at overcoming the original symptom.

B: Would there be a tendency not to assess the full range of emotional disturbances, just to stop on the first one and start to work on that without adequately assessing all the different emotions that might be involved in a particular problem?

E: Yes. Clients may come for sex problems, such as sexual anxiety. So I can help them with that. But, then, as they usually have other forms of anxiety, I always ask them what else they are anxious about now that they are overcoming the sex problem. They may say, "nothing," or they may say, "school" or "work." So we work on their *other* anxieties. Or if they're doing well and are rarely anxious, I may ask, "How about rage? Or depression? Or procrastination?" So RET doesn't necessarily deal only with a presenting symptom, but with others as well. Also, if clients are socially avoidant, I may first deal with their fears of rejection but may well also bring up their low frustration tolerance—their unwillingness to socialize because of their belief that they should not have to *work* at finding and keeping friends.

B: What about assessment in other areas like practical skills? Is that an important oversight that an RET therapist might make? Might they for- get about the importance of practical skills and concentrate just on the emotions?

E: True! Therapists may assume that, because they help clients become less socially anxious, they now know how to relate well. Well, they might not! So in RET, we also investigate these clients' social skills, get them to record details of their social interactions, and go over them to see whether they are still acting unskillfully. Merely assessing what people are telling themselves often does not bring out their practical difficulties. And I often tell therapists that RET assesses and treats several levels:

(1) clients' practical problems; (2) their problems *about* these practical problems, which we call their "neurotic problems"; (3) their problems about their neurotic or emotional problems, which we call the "secondary symptoms"; and (4) their problems about being in therapy and about not improving fast enough or well enough. RET assesses and deals with all four of these levels of dysfunctioning.

B: Can you expand on clients' therapy problems?

E: Yes. Many clients have several problems about therapy, such as finding their homework too hard, hating or loving their therapist, and self-downing, often expressed as "I shouldn't have to have therapy and am an incompetent person if I do go for it."

B: So you're suggesting, perhaps, the assessment of ongoing intratherapeutic problems that might interfere with effectiveness. Normally we don't tend to do that?

E: Well, we often do it as the therapeutic problems arise, but we might better do it more systematically.

B: Can you anticipate what those problems might be?

E: Yes. With dependent clients, we might anticipate that they will get over-attached to their therapist; and with hostile and frustration-intolerant clients, we might anticipate that they will resist homework and hate therapists who push them to do it.

B: What are some of the common mistakes in disputing—for example, making sure that you identify and dispute the main should's rather than the conditional ones or the less important ones? Is there anything else in the disputing area that is a common problem? Is it common for inexperienced RET practitioners to dispute inferences rather than evaluations?

E: Yes. They often dispute clients' faulty inferences and not their commanding must's and they mainly use antiempirical instead of deeper philosophical disputing.

B: So even RET practitioners sometimes largely fall back into disputing inferences and not the must's from which they're usually derived?

E: There's nothing wrong with that if they don't stop there. I often first dispute clients' inferences. Somebody comes to see me and says, "George wouldn't go to a concert with me. That means he doesn't like me. I must have done something wrong, and I'm unlovable." So I may first dispute these inferences and show how unrealistic and false they are. But I go on and ask, "But what's your underlying *must* that leads you to make such inaccurate inferences?" So they then see that they are bringing to the incident with George the philosophy, "At all times, when I invite George (or others) to a concert, they *must* like me and rush to accept my invitation; *otherwise*, they don't like me, I must have something wrong, and I'm unlovable!" So I get to the inferences *and* the must's, whereas practitioners who use RET inelegantly might only get at the inferences and empirically dispute them and still leave their clients with their basic underlying explicit, or tacit, must's. Elegant RET is realistic *as well as* antimusturbatory.

B: When you are disputing, is there an error that can be made in making the disputing too abstract for a person who needs to have it concrete?

E: Yes. That's why, again, the "clinical" form of RET would be better often than the "educational" form of RET. If I teach a woman that even Hitler wasn't *a shit* because he was a fallible human who merely did *shitty acts,* she may "see" that but still hate herself when *she* acts badly. So I'd better show her more specifically why she can accept *herself* even when she hates what she *does.*

B: But even in the clinical form, sometimes you can get into an abstract philosophical dispute, and the client can't see how that applies to a particular situation.

E: Yes. For example, if I say to John, "There's no reason why anyone *must* succeed, though it's highly desirable that they do," that sounds fine. But I still had better show him concretely why he doesn't *have to* succeed at sports, job, etc., or at whatever *he* desires.

B: Would abstract disputation lead to the client's having intellectual but not emotional insight? Before emotional changes occur, would he or she need to be able to use those general disputes in specific situations?

E: Right. So we try to get clients to tailor their disputing to the usual specific situations that they're upsetting themselves about. And we want them to do *strong* disputing; otherwise, they often *lightly* believe, "Yes, I don't have to succeed to be a good person" (which is intellectual insight) but they still *strongly* believe, "But I really *must* succeed or I'm no good!" (which is their emotional reaction).

B: And I guess other common mistakes in therapy involve advice giving and practical problem solving.

E: Yes, rather than getting to the basic differences between rational and irrational thinking. If I help Mary get a good job, that's great. But I still had better help her change her thinking if she irrationally believes, "Now that I've got this good job, I am *therefore* a good person!"

B: A common mistake I have found is to reduce emotional reactions by saying, "Look, if someone's upset with you, that's his or her problem so you don't have to worry yourself about it." The person feels better because all of a sudden he or she no longer sees that as a problem, and the therapist thinks that he or she is doing RET, because the client is no longer upset.

E: Yes, because if someone is enraged at you that *is* his or her problem. But you still may have acted badly to him or her, and that's *your* problem. Also, someone may be very displeased, but not enraged, at you for treating him or her badly, and you'd better not *define* his or her displeasure as his or her "problem," had better not gloss over it, and had better correct *your* behavior.

REFERENCES

Bernard, M. E. (1986). *Staying alive in an irrational world*. Melbourne: Carlson/MacMillan.

Burns, D. (1980). *Feeling good*. New York: Morrow.

Coué, E. (1923). *My method*. New York: Doubleday.

Dyer, W. (1977). *Your erroneous zones*. New York: Funk and Wagnalls.

D'Zurilla, T. J., & Goldfriend, M. R. (1971). Problem solving and behavior modification. *Journal of Abnormal Psychology, 78*, 107–126.

Ellis, A. (1950). Towards the improvement of psychoanalytic research. *Psychoanalytic Review, 36*, 123–143.

Ellis, A. (1955a). *New approaches to psychotherapy techniques*. Brandon, VT: Journal of Clinical Psychology Monograph Supplement, Vol. 11.

Ellis, A. (1955b). Psychotherapy techniques for use with psychotics. *American Journal of Psychotherapy, 9*, 452–476.

Ellis, A. (1957a). *How to live with a neurotic: At home and at work*. New York: Crown. (Rev. ed. Hollywood, CA: Wilshire Books, 1975.)

Ellis, A. (1957b). Outcome of employing three techniques of psychotherapy. *Journal of Clinical Psychology, 13*, 344–350.

Ellis, A. (1958). Rational psychotherapy. *Journal of General Psychology, 59*, 35–49. (Reprinted: New York: Institute for Rational-Emotive Therapy.)

Ellis, A. (1962). *Reason and emotion in psychotherapy*. Secaucus, NJ: Citadel.

Ellis, A. (1969). A weekend of rational encounter. In A. Burton (Ed.), *Encounter* (pp. 112–127). San Francisco: Jossey-Bass.

Ellis, A. (1971). *Growth through reason*. North Hollywood, CA: Wilshire Books.

Ellis, A. (1972a). *Executive leadership: The rational-emotive approach*. New York: Institute for Rational-Emotive Therapy.

Ellis, A. (1972b). Helping people get better: Rather than merely feel better. *Rational Living, 7*(2), 2–9.

Ellis, A. (1972c). Psychotherapy without tears. In A. Burton (Ed.), *Twelve therapists* (pp. 103–126). San Francisco: Jossey-Bass.

Ellis, A. (1973). *Humanistic psychotherapy: The rational-emotive approach*. New York: McGraw-Hill.

Ellis, A. (1974). Rational-emotive therapy in groups. *Rational Living, 9*(1), 15–22(b).

Ellis, A. (1976). *Sex and the liberated man*. Secaucus, NJ: Lyle Stuart.

Ellis, A. (1977a). *Anger—How to live with and without it*. Secaucus, NJ: Citadel Press.

Ellis, A. (1977b). Skill training in counseling and psychotherapy. *Canadian Counsellor, 12*(1), 30–35.

Ellis, A. (1979a). *The intelligent woman's guide to dating and mating*. Secaucus, NJ: Lyle Stuart.

Ellis, A. (1979b). The issue of force and energy in behavioral change. *Journal of Contemporary Psychotherapy, 10*(2), 83–97.

Ellis, A. (1985). *Overcoming re-resistance: Rational-emotive therapy with difficult clients*. New York: Springer.

Ellis, A. (1987). The evolution of rational-emotive therapy (RET) and cognitive behavior therapy (CBT). In J. K. Zeig (Ed.), *The evolution of psychotherapy* (pp. 107–133). New York: Brunner/Mazel.

Ellis, A. (1988). *How to stubbornly refuse to make yourself miserable about anything—Yes, anything!* New York: Lyle Stuart.

Ellis, A. (1990). Rational-emotive therapy. In I. L. Kutash & A. Wolf (Eds.), *Group psychotherapist's handbook* (pp. 298–315). New York: Columbia.

Ellis, A., & Abrahms, E. (1978). *Brief psychotherapy in medical and health practice.* New York: Springer.

Ellis, A., & Becker, I. (1982). *A guide to personal happiness.* North Hollywood, CA: Wilshire Books.

Ellis, A., & Bernard, M. E. (Eds.). *Clinical applications of rational-emotive therapy.* New York: Plenum.

Ellis, A., & Dryden, W. (1987). *The practice of rational-emotive therapy.* New York: Springer.

Ellis, A., & Dryden, W. (1990). *The essential Albert Ellis.* New York: Springer.

Ellis, A. & Dryden, W. (1991). *Therapeutically speaking: Albert Ellis in a dialogue with Windy Dryden.* Stony Stratford, England: Open University.

Ellis, A., & Harper, R. A. (1961). *A guide to rational living.* Englewood Cliffs, NJ: Prentice-Hall.

Ellis, A., & Harper, R. A. (1975). *A new guide to rational living.* North Hollywood, CA: Wilshire Books.

Ellis, A., & Whiteley, J. M. (1979). *Theoretical and empirical foundations of rational-emotive therapy.* Monterey, CA: Brooks/Cole.

Ellis, A., & Yeager, R. (1989). *Why some therapies don't work: The dangers of transpersonal psychology.* Buffalo, NY: Prometheus.

Ellis, A., Sichel, J., DiMattia, D., Yeager, R., & DiGiuseppe, R. (1989). *Rational-emotive couple therapy.* New York: Pergamon Press.

Eysenck, H. J. (1952). *Journal of Consulting Psychology, 16,* 319–424.

Ferenczi, S. (1952). *Further contributions to the theory and technique of psychoanalysis.* New York: Basic Books.

Guerney, B. G., Jr. (1977). *Relationship enhancement: Skill-training programs for therapy, problem-prevention and enrichment.* San Francisco: Jossey-Bass.

Haley, J. (1976). *Problem solving therapy.* San Francisco: Jossey-Bass.

Maultsby, M. C., Jr. (1971). Rational emotive imagery. *Rational Living, 6*(1), 24–27.

Maultsby, M. C., Jr., & Ellis, A. (1974). *Technique for using rational-emotive imagery.* New York: Institute for Rational-Emotive Therapy.

Peale, N. V. (1952). *The power of positive thinking.* New York: Fawcett.

Phillips, E. L. (1956). *Psychotherapy.* Englewood Cliffs, NJ: Prentice-Hall.

Spivack, G., & Shure, M. (1974). *Social adjustment in young children.* San Francisco: Jossey-Bass.

Wolpe, J. (1983). *The practice of behavior therapy* (3rd ed.). New York: Pergamon.

Yankura, V., & Dryden, W. (1990). *Doing RET: Albert Ellis in action.* New York: Springer.

Zilbergeld, B., & Lazarus, A. A. (1987). *Mind power.* Boston: Little, Brown.

Keys to Effective RET

Russell M. Grieger

Let me begin this chapter by stating that I practice rational-emotive therapy (RET). I am thoroughly convinced of the primary importance of human thinking and conceptualization in feeling and acting; I incessantly conceptualize my clients' problems in ABC terms; I assume that emotional and behavioral disturbances result from a person's endorsing and living by perfectionistic demanding, awfulizing, and/or self-rating philosophies; I believe that profound, elegant change follows when humans give up these philosophies and alternatively endorse preferring, antiawfulizing, and self-accepting ones; I practice RET in an energetic, active, directive way; I see my therapeutic role as being more of a teacher and coach than a doctor; I attempt to blanket my clients with emotive and behavioral as well as cognitive techniques; I see cognitive disputation as the major tool of change; and, assuming that people will inevitably slip back to their former pathologies unless they continue to work on themselves the rest of their lives, I emphasize the importance of their learning both the theory and the techniques of RET for future use so that they do not have to rely on me in the future. I attempt to practice all this with individuals, with couples, with parents, with families, and in groups (including workshops and seminars).

There are many excellent texts that tell how to do what may be called classical RET (Ellis, 1962, 1971, 1973, 1977; Ellis & Dryden, 1987; Ellis & Grieger, 1977, 1986; Grieger & Boyd, 1980; Walen, DiGiuseppe, & Wessler, 1980). I recommend all of these to the reader to absorb, for there can be no more important tools for doing RET effectively than a thorough understanding of RET's theory and philosophy and a grasp of RET's process and techniques.

What I will share with the reader are *some* of the ideas and tools I have learned from reading about, thinking about, and especially practicing RET

Russell M. Grieger • 818 East High Street, Charlottesville, Virginia 22901.

during the last 17 years. In the first section, "Organizing and Guiding the Client," I argue that educating the client in a structured way about the theory and practice of RET tremendously enhances most clients' ability to use their therapy effectively. In knowing what to expect of their therapist and of themselves, and in understanding why they and their therapist do what they do, they most often conclude that the RET process makes sense, has direction and purpose, and will lead to the desired results. It can be both motivating and comforting. The second section, "Helping Clients Take Responsibility," suggests that, for RET to be maximally effective and for people to thoroughly use and profit from the RET process, they "need" a thorough "indoctrination" in the value and potential of "personal re- sponsibility." And finally, in the third section, titled "Therapist Checklist for RET Effectiveness," I provide six points for the therapist to check with each client to make sure their RET is maximally effective.

I again hasten to emphasize that what I discuss in this chapter I inte- grate into the practice of classical RET and do not substitute for the tradi- tional process. What is new or different are "add-ons," not changes. I have found that the combination of the classical with what is contained in this chapter helps me to be more effective in the RET I do.

ORGANIZING AND GUIDING THE CLIENT

We RET-ers are delighted when a bright, cooperative client walks into our office and diligently applies himself or herself to therapy. This person will easily understand RET's theory and structure, quickly gain the neces- sary insights, and forcefully use its tools to make a personal difference. Our job is easy.

Unfortunately, a good many clients are ill equipped to participate so effectively. Because of both a biological predisposition to irrationality (Ellis, 1976) and years of practice (Grieger & Boyd, 1980; Maultsby, 1984), most clients have the worst of two worlds: They are talented at being disturbed, yet poor at bringing about change.

There are many reasons why this is so. Some clients simply do not know what to do to change: they are ignorant. Some are very poor thinkers, being either cognitively scattered or unschooled in how to think logically. Others, experiencing a great deal of emotional turmoil, find it next to impossible to organize themselves to problem-solve. Still others are very helpless and dependent; they rely on others to tell them what to do. Others are lazy, having low frustration tolerance and being committed pleasure seekers, and therefore working in therapy sporadically at best. And others hold erroneous beliefs that block them from participating (for instance, believing that they are too hopelessly disturbed to get better, thinking that they are morally obligated to be upset when things go wrong, or perceiving that being upset in some way is in their best interest).

Because of all this, I have always appreciated Ellis's point (1976, 1978) that therapists who are active, directive, forceful, commanding, scientific, and psychoeducational tend to be more effective than those who are not. Similarly, I also have come to appreciate that the more organized, enlightened, and structured the client is, the more she or he can participate in a collaborative, responsible, and thorough manner, thereby lessening the possibility that she or he will passively drift, depend on the therapist, get lost or confused, and act irresponsibly.

It is with this in mind that I put together a booklet, *A Client's Guide to Rational-Emotive Therapy* (Grieger, 1986a),* which I give to each client as part of their RET. The "guide" is not a self-help book like *A New Guide to Rational Living* (Ellis & Harper, 1975). Rather, it is a book that literally guides clients through their psychotherapy. It outlines the sequential *steps* for them in therapy and, for each step, the rationale and goals, what the therapist will do, and what are the client's responsibilities. With the message being, "I want you to be knowledgeable about and appreciative of what goes on here so that you can participate fully in bringing about the changes you want," it is both a road map and an attempt to foster the client's taking of responsibility for change.

The clients are given the "guide" in either the first or the second session, after I have completed educating myself about why they came to see me and what is the basis of the problem. I explain that the book will literally guide them through their therapy process, help them know what's going on and why, and direct them to do certain homework assignments that will complement what goes on in my office. After a general overview, I ask them to read it over, and I specifically assign them "Step One" as their first homework assignment for the next session. Then, I move the client through the guide bit by bit to parallel where they are in therapy. Clients are to bring the book with them to each session, as the homework assignments are a part of each session.

My experience is that most clients find the "guide" helpful. They like its structure and are comforted that there is an organized process that they can follow. Those who have trouble using it are usually those who find difficulty following through on any homework assignments and are treated in the usual manner.

The "guide" is now presented in the same form as it is given to clients.

---

*Along with my colleague Dr. Paul Woods, I am currently revising and expanding *A Client's Guide to Rational-Emotive Therapy* (1986a). Its new title will be *The Rational-Emotive Therapy Companion*.

THE GUIDE

Dear Client:

The reason you entered psychotherapy is to resolve problems you are having in your life. I will do my best to help you in this. Together we want to work as efficiently as we can to get you to feel better, to function more effectively in your job or at school, and to relate better with others.

So that we may make the quickest possible progress, I have prepared this booklet to guide you through your psychotherapy. While all of us are unique, and while no one's therapy is exactly like anyone else's, you will find this step-by-step guide helpful in understanding what we are doing and knowing what are your responsibilities. This book will also suggest things for you to do to make the most of your therapy. These will include the following:

1. Doing periodic reading. The readings will be particularly relevant to understanding and overcoming the problems or concerns on which you wish to work.
2. Doing written and behavioral homework. These will help you efficiently work against and overcome your problems.
3. Listening to tapes of our sessions. A great deal often happens in psychotherapy. Some of it can be remembered, while some cannot. To get the most out of our sessions, I will audiotape them and give the tape to you to listen to before the next one. Please do so and bring the tape to our next appointment. We can then discuss things from it, save it for future reference, or record over it.

Please feel free to discuss any or all of this with me. I look forward to working with you. I want you to know that I am committed to helping you achieve a quick and thorough resolution of your concerns.

Sincerely,

Step One: Committing Oneself to Change

> Commitment is what transforms a promise into reality.
> It is the words that speak boldly of your intentions. And the actions that speak louder than the words.
> It is making time when there is none. Coming through time after time, year after year.
> Commitment is the stuff character is made of; the power to change the face of things.
> It is the daily triumph of integrity over skepticism.
>
> Shearson Lehman,
> American Express advertisement

By the time you decided to enter psychotherapy you had most likely spent a great deal of time innocently and unwittingly engraining the ways of acting and reacting that you now find painful and self-defeating. It is understandable that, with all this "practice," you find it easy to think, feel, and act as you do.

While I will certainly do my best to help you undo these self-defeating patterns, I and many others have found that people change to the extent to which they themselves work in psychotherapy—that is, when they *do* what is necessary to change. This depends on a full, personal, and responsible commitment to solving their problems and to bringing about their own growth and change.

It follows, then, that the first, crucial step in your psychotherapy is to commit yourself to doing the work necessary to bring about the changes you want. Without this commitment, your efforts may very well be sporadic and half-hearted, and your gains will be slow, accidental, and incomplete. So, to facilitate your commitment, take some time (about half an hour) to read, reflect upon, and complete Assignment 1, which immediately follows. Bring it to your next session so that I can help you refine it and so that we can both be clear about and agree upon the directions you are heading in.

ASSIGNMENT 1: COMMITMENT CONTRACT (PLEASE COMPLETE)

I commit myself to and take full responsibility for doing whatever is necessary to overcome the following painful and/or self-defeating feelings and actions.

1. _____

2. _____

3. _____

4. _____

5. _____

I commit myself to and take full responsibility for doing whatever is necessary to develop the following pleasurable and/or self-enhancing feelings and actions.

1. _____

2. _____

3. _____

4. _____

5. _____

I will continue to keep my commitment to doing whatever is necessary to eliminate my self-defeating patterns and to promoting my well-being for the duration of this therapy and for the rest of my life.

Signed _____

Date _____

Good! Congratulations! You have now taken the first major step toward solving your problems. So that you will keep your commitment alive, I suggest you read this commitment contract at least once a day and perhaps even tape it in a prominent place or copy it and carry it in your pocket, so that you can frequently look at it.

Step Two: Understanding Emotional Disturbance and Its Treatment

> People are disturbed not by things but by the views they take of them.
> Epictetus, 1st century A.D.

The world-famous clinical psychologist and psychotherapist Albert Ellis (1971) once said, "I have long been convinced that people become and remain emotionally disturbed largely because they do not clearly define what their 'disturbance' is and what they can do to minimize it." I wholeheartedly agree with Dr. Ellis. The more you know about your emotional disturbance and how to overcome it, the more focused will be your efforts and the more efficient will be your change.

The second step in your psychotherapy, then, is to become educated about the nature of emotional problems and their treatment. Your responsibility now is to complete reading assignments that will give you this knowledge. These assignments will, in addition to being interesting, help you understand what your problems are and what we will do to overcome them. Perhaps most important, they will help you to see your role in creating and maintaining the problems that you so much want to be rid of. Bring anything that you do not understand or agree with to my attention, and we will discuss it fully.

Now, complete Assignment 2, which follows.

ASSIGNMENT 2: READING ASSIGNMENT

I will assign some items from the list below for you to read. Read these items carefully at least twice. Underline what you find important, take notes (space is provided following the reading list), and do anything else that will help you understand the concepts and relate them to your problems. Remember! Be *vitally interested* in your own well-being, as if you are the most important person in the world to you! Take this reading *seriously*, as it can lay the foundation for effective and long-lasting change! Be *committed* to the promises you made in Assignment 1, for your commitment will make a difference!

PAMPHLETS AND ARTICLES

Burns, David D. (1980). The perfectionist's script for self-defeat. *Psychology Today,* November, 34–35.

Ellis, Albert. (1971). Emotional disturbance and its treatment in a nutshell. *Canadian Counselor,* 5 **(3),** 168–71.

Ellis, Albert. (1973). The no cop-out theory. *Psychology Today,* July, 13–23.

Ellis, Albert. (1973). Unhealthy love: Its causes and treatment. In Mary Ellen Curtin (Ed.), *Symposium on Love.* New York: Behavioral Publications.

Ellis, Albert. (1975). *RET abolishes most of the human ego.* Paper delivered at the American Psychological Association National Convention, September.

BOOKS

Burns, David D. (1980). *Feeling good: The new mood therapy.* New York: William Morrow.

Burns, David D. (1985). *Intimate connections.* New York: William Morrow.

Ellis, Albert. (1975). *How to live with a neurotic.* North Hollywood, Calif.: Wilshire.

Ellis, Albert, and Becker, Irving. (1982). *A guide to personal happiness.* North Hollywood, Calif.: Wilshire.

Ellis, Albert, and Harper, Robert A. (1975). *A new guide to rational living.* North Hollywood, Calif.: Wilshire.

Maultsby, Maxie C. Jr. (1975). *Help yourself to happiness.* New York: Institute for Rational Living.

Miller, Tom. (1983). *So, you secretly suspect you're worthless! Well . . .* Skaneateles, N.Y.: Lakeside Printing.

Notes about the Reading Material

Step Three: Uncovering and Appreciating Your Irrational Thinking

> Until an individual accepts the fact that he is responsible for what he does, there can be no treatment. It is not up to therapists to advance explanations for irresponsibility. Individual responsibility is the goal of treatment and unhappiness is the result and not the cause of irresponsibility.
>
> William Glasser, M.D.

I have summarized below some of the crucial insights you learned in your reading assignment. Read this summary and refer back to the readings if you need to do so. Some people find these insights bitter pills to swallow; they resist them. Nonetheless, they are true. I cannot emphasize enough how important it is to your getting better for you to understand and accept them. If you have any questions, concerns, or disagreements about any of these insights, please raise them with me now since what we will do in psychotherapy follows from them.

INSIGHT 1

How you feel and behave is largely determined *by the way you think*, not by the things that happen to you or by the actions of others. That is, your *moment-by-moment thoughts*, which usually represent deeply believed attitudes or philosophies, *"cause"* you to feel and act as you do. We represent this in terms of the ABC theory, whereby A stands for the activating event, or what happened; B stands for your beliefs, or what you thought and believed when it happened; and C stands for your emotional and behavioral reactions, or how you felt and acted *by thinking what you did* when it happened.

INSIGHT 2

Regardless of what happened to you in the past (for example, whether your parents loved you or not), you first became disturbed *when you adopted, endorsed, or bought into your irrational beliefs* (your Bs). In other words, no matter how badly you were treated or how irrational was the thinking of significant people in your life, it was when *you* decided to *believe* what you do, or when *you agreed with* the nutty ideas that others held, that your troubles began. And you get upset and are disturbed today because you continue to indoctrinate yourself with the same irrational beliefs that you learned in the past.

INSIGHT 3

Although you are responsible for creating and maintaining your own irrational thinking, it is important not to judge or condemn yourself. Humans find it very easy to think irrationally and self-defeatingly. First, we come into this world with a strong capacity to err and to think crookedly; second, we are bombarded in our society with irrational, neurotic ideas. Therefore, it is important to be gentle with yourself. Realize that you share with the vast majority of people the problems you have, and forgive and accept yourself even though you have created and maintained your own problems. This is Insight 3. Please heed and practice it.

INSIGHT 4

Insight 4 follows from the fact that by the time you entered therapy you had so propagandized yourself to believe what you do that you probably simply accept what you believe as truth. You most likely think and believe what you do without much awareness and certainly without question. It follows, then, that *an energetic and sustained effort*, first, to become aware of your irrational thoughts and beliefs and, second, to assault them is necessary to give them up. This insight, then, says that you "must" work long and hard to give up your current, self-defeating way of thinking if you are to get over your emotional problems.

Now with these insights firmly in place, you are ready for Step Three in your psychotherapy. Your job here is twofold: one, to find out specifically what are your irrational thoughts and beliefs; two, to appreciate how these beliefs cause your painful feelings and your self-defeating actions. Both the discovery of these beliefs and their appreciation are extremely important, for knowledge without appreciation does little good.

To help you uncover and appreciate your irrational thinking, Step Three involves both taking a brief, self-administered and self-scored test and also doing written homework.

Testing for Your Irrational Thinking. There are several irrational belief tests now on the market. The two that I find most useful are the Dysfunctional Attitude Scale (DAS)[1] and the Irrational Beliefs Test (IBT).[2] I will select one of these for you to take. Each one asks you to mark the degree to which you agree or disagree with a series of statements. Each also gives you scoring instructions and helps you interpret what the scores mean. Taking the test can be fun, and the results should prove both interesting and helpful.

ASSIGNMENT 3: TAKING THE TEST

Please be serious about this. Bring both the test itself and your questions and insights to our next session. It may be a good idea to insert the test and the results in this book for frequent reference.

Written Homework. It not only is important to know what general irrational beliefs you hold, but it also is important to become skilled at "hearing" your irrational thoughts on a moment-by-moment basis. In learning to spot what you are thinking to upset yourself at any given moment (and recognizing the irrational beliefs behind these thoughts), you are well positioned to do the things necessary to change your self-defeating thinking. Without this skill, you will probably go on reacting to your own thinking without any power to act and feel as you want.

Assignment 4, which immediately follows, is designed to help you learn to track down and recognize your irrational thinking. With this skill, you will be ready to move to Step Four, the change process.

ASSIGNMENT 4: THE IRRATIONAL THINKING LOG

Your assignment now is a daily one. Your instructions are to devote from 15 to 30 minutes each day to filling out one of the thinking logs that follow. I

---

[1]The Dysfunctional Attitude Scale (DAS) was developed by Dr. Arlene Weissman. A brief version of this scale is presented by David Burns, M.D., in his book *Feeling Good: The New Mood Therapy* (see reference for this in Step Two).
[2]The Irrational Beliefs Test (IBT) was developed in 1969 as part of R. G. Jones's doctoral dissertation.

have provided 14 of these to last you two weeks, but I will give you more if you want to do more than one per day or if you need to continue this for more than two weeks. Remember! The purpose of this homework is to help you become very conscious of your own irrational, self-defeating thinking. The more aware you become of your irrational thinking, the more you will be able to overcome it.

The irrational thinking log is very simple to follow and do, although you may initially have trouble identifying your irrational thinking. Don't worry if you find this difficult. You will become quite skilled at this in a very short time if you persistently do the homework. I will coach you so bring your sheets to each session. Instructions are as follows:

1. Each day, take a time when you become upset over something. Use getting upset as a cue to do your log. Then, either as soon after the event as possible or at some designated later time, begin by *briefly writing down what happened*—the activating event, or the A. Do not belabor this by describing it endlessly, as the real cause of your problems is your thinking (at B) about the event, not the event itself.
2. Briefly describe *how you felt* and *what you did* in relation to the event. This is the C, or the consequence of your thinking about the event. A mistake people often make here is to confuse what they thought with how they felt. For example, people often write, "I felt he should not have done that." In fact, this is a thought ("I *thought* he should not have done that!"). This thought caused the emotions. Feelings refer to anger, guilt, depression, anxiety, and the like and are to be reported here.
3. As a last step in this homework assignment, write down in sentence form *what you thought*, at B, to make you feel and act at C as you did about the event. Two hints here. First, to help you discover the thoughts, ask yourself, "What was going through my head when I first started feeling/acting as I did?" Second, listen very carefully for your *demands* (expressed with words like *should, ought, must*, and *need*), your *catastrophizing* (expressed as *awful, horrible, terrible*, and *tragic*), and your *self-downing* (as in, "I'm a failure" or "I'm bad"). After you've written your thoughts, double-check to see if one of these themes is hidden there; if so, rewrite the thought to include it.

Again, ask any questions of me to help you become skilled at uncovering your irrational thinking. Becoming good at this is important. Happy hunting!

A caution. Your goal in doing written homework is to become quite sensitive to your irrational thinking. In doing so, you may be surprised how frequently you think these thoughts and how deeply you believe what you do. Some people are shocked at this and conclude that they are worse off than they really are and that there is too much in their heads to conquer. Do not fall into this trap. Rather than taking this attitude, remember that getting better requires awareness of your thinking. The more you become tuned in to these thoughts, the better positioned you will be to bring about the changes you want.

Irrational Thinking Log

A	B	C
Activating event →	Irrational thoughts/ beliefs	→ Emotional and/or behavioral consequences

1. Briefly describe the activating event.
2. Briefly record the painful emotion(s) (e.g., anxiety, guilt, depression, anger) you experienced in relation to A.

   Briefly record your self-defeating behavior(s) in relation to A.
3. Write down the thoughts you had which caused your painful emotions and self-defeating behaviors. Write them in sentence form. Number them consecutively.

   1.

   2.

   3.

   4.

   5.

Step Four: Changing Your Irrational Thinking

If we do not change our direction, we are likely to end up where we are headed.

Chinese proverb

We cannot solve life's problems except by solving them. This statement may seem idiotically tautological or self-evident, yet it is seemingly beyond the comprehension of much of the human race. This is because we must accept responsibility for a problem before we can solve it. We cannot solve a problem by hoping that someone else will solve it for us. I can solve a problem only when I say, "This is *my* problem and it's up to me to solve it." But many, so many, seek to avoid the pain of their problems by saying to themselves, "This problem was caused me by other people, or by social circumstances beyond my control, and therefore it is up to other people or society to solve this problem for me. It is not really my personal problem."

M. Scott Peck, M.D.

So far you have committed yourself to change, learned about the nature of your emotional problems, and become familiar with the specific irrational beliefs that cause your problems. You are now well-positioned to bring about the changes you want—to break the habit of responding to situations with your automatic irrational thoughts, *and* to give up the deeply held, harmful ideas or beliefs that create your painful feelings and self-defeating behaviors.

A word to the wise is important here! In order to change it will be necessary for you to work hard—to devote time and energy to doing the work necessary to change. After all, you have believed these irrational ideas for years and have thought about and dealt with scores of situations with them. In effect, they have become habitual, deeply endorsed, "second nature." Furthermore, you may never have learned, or perhaps have got rusty at, the critical thinking skills important for change, and you may therefore have to bone up on these skills.

So, some hard work is now in order. But you can do the work, and it is worth it! All you have to do is be willing to spend the time and energy. Rather than seeing this work as a burden or chore, I encourage you to think of it as an adventure. After all, you are working to change some extremely important things about yourself that will lead to all sorts of benefits, clearly a project worthy of effort and excitement.

To bring about the changes in your thinking, acting, and feeling, I will give you assignments in each of three areas. I will describe each in turn, but you will be doing all three concurrently.

1. READING ASSIGNMENT

Yes, more reading! This time, your reading is designed to help you clearly understand what is illogical, false, and self-defeating about the ideas or beliefs (at B) that underpin your problems. These readings will also serve to teach you new, alternative ideas that are contrary to your irrational ones and that both make more sense and pay off for you. The goal is for you to acquire a new knowledge base that you can learn, endorse, and eventually adopt, thereby bringing about better results for yourself.

ASSIGNMENT 5: READING ASSIGNMENT

From the list of readings in Step 2, and possibly from other sources, I will now assign you readings. Again, please read the material carefully, digest it, and discuss it with me at the next session. A couple of blank sheets follow on which to take notes.

Notes about the Reading Material

2. BEHAVIORAL ASSIGNMENTS

It has been found that one of the most effective methods of destroying irrational beliefs is to act contrary to them. Doing this not only serves to call up our irrational thinking, which we can then combat with written homework (see 3, below) and other methods, but it also serves to help us see that our irrational beliefs are nonsense—that, for example, we do not need to act perfectly, that we won't perish if we are rejected, that the world doesn't end if we are in some way frustrated.

Thus, I will assign you things to do each day to help you give up your irrational thinking. Probably these will be one or more of the following, which I will fully explain in our sessions:

Pleasurable pursuits—committing yourself to activities.

Rational-emotive imagery—vividly picturing difficult events and practicing thinking rationally about them.

Shame-attacking exercises—performing "silly" or "embarrassing" acts in public to show yourself that you do not need *ever* to feel ashamed.

Courting discomfort—deliberately doing things you find uncomfortable, or staying in uncomfortable situations a little longer.

Risk taking—doing things you fear.

Behavioral rehearsal—practicing doing things at which you are unskilled or that you are fearful of doing.

Rewarding and penalizing—pleasuring or punishing yourself for doing or not doing something.

Sometimes people react with fear to undertaking behavioral assignments. Other people resent doing them. Still others find them boring. These are all typical reactions, yet reactions to be ignored. It is important to follow through on these behavioral assignments as they are important techniques for ridding yourself of your irrational beliefs.

ASSIGNMENT 6: BEHAVIORAL ASSIGNMENT

I will assign you things to do between now and our next session. These assignments are designed to help you see that your beliefs are both irrational and self-defeating and to encourage you to give them up. If you find yourself reluctant to do this assignment, because of anxiety, resentment, or boredom, ignore these feelings and do the assignment anyway. We can talk about these feelings and what is behind them in our sessions. The long-range benefits will far outweigh the short-term or brief (and irrelevant) discomfort that you may feel. On the sheet provided, keep a log of *your behavioral assignment* and *any* thoughts you had about doing it.

Weekly Behavioral Assignment Log

Assigned activity: _____
_____
_____

Reward: _____

Punishment: _____

Date	Completed: Yes/No	Irrational thoughts
_____	_____	_____
_____	_____	_____
_____	_____	_____
_____	_____	_____
_____	_____	_____
_____	_____	_____
_____	_____	_____
_____	_____	_____

3. WRITTEN HOMEWORK

Written homework is designed for you to destroy your irrational thoughts and beliefs by a direct, active, energetic assault on them. In this homework you will employ the logicoempirical method of *repeated and persistent scientific questioning and disputing*. The idea is to take your long-held beliefs and, instead of automatically believing them as you have done for so long, to hold them up to scrutiny. You want to identify what is wrong with them, why they are nonsense, how they hurt you, and what evidence there is to refute them. In other words, you will want to *debate against* them, perhaps for the first time in your life, instead of automatically endorsing and acting on them as you have done for so long. This task will probably be difficult for you at first, but you will soon become quite good at it.

We are fortunate to have many different written "disputation" forms from which to choose. Some of these come from Dr. David Burns's book *Feeling Good;* others derive from Dr. Albert Ellis's work at the Institute for Rational-Emotive Therapy in New York City; and still others have been developed by psychotherapists around the world. I will chose the one that best suits your particular problems.

ASSIGNMENT 7: WRITTEN DISPUTATION OF YOUR IRRATIONAL BELIEFS

This assignment is absolutely crucial to your change. You are to reserve from 15 to 30 minutes per day for at least one month to do your written homework. You may do more than this, but this is an absolute minimum. During this time you are to complete at least one homework sheet. I will supply you with a month's supply to get you started.

Take this assignment very seriously. This is as important as anything else in your life right now. Remember that you have spent a lifetime practicing and rehearsing the way you now think and believe; you have the nonsense down pat. It only follows that strong, persistent effort against this habit, and these beliefs, is necessary for change to take place. *Bring your written homework* to our sessions so that I can go over it with you. I want to coach you in getting better and better at doing it. In becoming skilled at this, you, in effect, learn to be your own psychotherapist for future problems you may have in your life.

Step Five: Combating and Overcoming Resistance

> Any real change implies the breakup of the world as one has already known it. The loss of all that gave one an identity, the end of safety. And at such a moment, unable to see and not daring to imagine what the future will now bring forth, one clings to what one knew, or thought one knew; to what one possessed or dreamed that one possessed. Yet it is only when persons are able, without bitterness or self-pity, to surrender a dream they have long cherished or a privilege they have long possessed that they are set free—they have set themselves free—for higher dreams, for greater privileges. All people have gone through this; go through it, each according to their degrees, throughout their lives. It is one of the irreducible facts of life.
>
> Author unknown

The fact that you are now reading this suggests that you have come a long way in your psychotherapy. Your progress has been tremendous, and your level of self-awareness is much beyond that of most people.

Nevertheless, you may to your own surprise find yourself fighting against me, against your therapy, or even against yourself. You may, for example, start denying that you have problems; you may not want to attend your sessions or to bring up important difficulties; you may be tempted to argue against some of my observations and messages; and you may at first agree but later refuse to carry out your homework assignments.

All of this is a fairly typical stage in the psychotherapy process, a stage recognized by almost all people who do psychotherapy. It is called *resistance* and, in fact, is so typical that whole books have been written to guide people like myself in helping people work through it. The *danger* is that you will allow your resistance to interfere with your progress and even cause you to stop your psychotherapy entirely.

In order to guard against this and to continue to get better, your task now is to understand what resistance is and what you can do about it so as not to let it undermine both what you've already accomplished and what you can further accomplish. So, now your goal is to understand and overcome your resistance.

First, resistance often comes about from confusion or a lack of understanding. You may, for example, not fully understand what I am saying, or what are your tasks, or how to execute your assignments, or how your tasks relate to your goals. If you find any of these true, please bring them to my attention. I can then help to clarify things for you and get you back on track.

A second, perhaps more serious, form of resistance often comes about from unrealistic fears and irrational misconceptions on your part. These fears and misconceptions, while unfounded, may appear entirely reasonable to you. I assure you, however, that they are entirely untrue. Once you let go of them, or ignore them, and continue your therapeutic working through, you will find that your fears are groundless and that your life will indeed be much better without your symptoms.

Dr. Albert Ellis, the founder of rational-emotive therapy, has written an excellent book titled *Overcoming Resistance*. In his book he has listed many resistances that clients can hold, all of which result from false logic, including the following:

1. Fear of discomfort—believing that the effort to change is too difficult, that you cannot tolerate the discomfort and hassle of doing your homework, that it's easier to drift along with your problems than to make the effort to change them.
2. Fear of disclosure and shame—believing that you should not feel, think, or act the way you do; that you are stupid, bad, or awful for all that; and that it would be terrible if I or anyone else knew how you really felt or thought.
3. Feelings of powerlessness and hopelessness—believing that you are unable to change, that your problems are too big to overcome, that you are too weak and small to conquer your problems.
4. Fear of change—believing that you must have safety and certainty and, therefore, that you have to keep your symptoms, even though they are uncomfortable, because you are used to them.
5. Fear of failure and disapproval—believing that you must always succeed; you may fear that your symptoms may lead you to risk subsequent failure and disapproval (for example, overcoming a public-speaking anxiety may prompt you to talk in public, do poorly, and get disapproval).
6. Self-punishment—in believing that you are a bad person, you may believe you must continue to suffer for your "badness."
7. Rebelliousness—believing you have to completely control your destiny and have absolutely perfect freedom to do what you like, you may rebel against me or your psychotherapy because you see it as an impingement on your freedom or power.
8. Secondary gain—having received payoffs for your symptoms, you may not want to give up your symptoms for fear of losing these payoffs (for example, you may get attention and sympathy for acting depressed or helpless).

In addition to the resistances mentioned above, I have observed that some people also hold the following ones:

9. Discouragement—believing that, since you don't feel better immediately after identifying your irrational beliefs or after disputing them a time or two, you can never overcome your disturbance.
10. Fear of loss of identity—believing that you are your feelings, you may incorrectly conclude you won't be you anymore if you change the way you feel.
11. Fear of loss of feelings—believing that thinking rationally will lead to no emotions at all, you may resist changing your beliefs for fear you'll become cold, unemotional, mechanized, or dull.

12. Fear of mediocrity—believing that you must be perfect, you may not want to give up your perfectionist demands for fear this will lead to less than ideal behavior and thus condemn you to mediocrity and worthlessness.

13. Righteousness—believing that other people should act perfectly, particularly toward you, you may refuse to give up your anger-producing beliefs because this lets them off the hook. You may not want to admit that they, as fallible human beings, have the right to make mistakes, that they are not condemnable because of their bad behavior, and that it is not correct for you to set out to make them suffer.

Like the irrational beliefs we are working to overcome, these phony ideas "should" be seen for what they are—irrational and self-defeating!—and "should" be worked against. As with your main irrational beliefs, use the ABC theory to organize your assault against them, as in the diagram that immediately follows.

A→	B→	C→
The prospect of thinking, feeling, and acting differently	Irrational, resistant thoughts	Resistant feelings and behaviors

ASSIGNMENT 8: OVERCOMING YOUR RESISTANCES

In overcoming your resistance, I will instruct you to do many of the things you were to do for Step Four, changing your irrational thinking. This time, though, you are to use these techniques to do violence to your resistant thoughts. So, for this assignment, you are to do two things. One, you are to ignore your resistance and do the assignments previously given you for Step Four. In other words, have your resistances (your fears, your doubts) if you like, but force yourself to continue your Step Four work anyway.

In order to combat your resistant ideas directly, I will now also assign you both behavioral and written homework to search out and destroy these ideas. Be sure to do this work, as it would be a shame to come this far and stop yourself from completing your change. Be willing to take the risk of working against your irrational beliefs. After all, if you do not like the results, you can always go back to thinking, acting, and feeling the way you did before.

Step Six: Going Forward

Life shrinks or expands in proportion to one's courage.

Anaïs Nin

Responsibility is a unique concept. It can only reside and inhere in a single individual. You may share it with others, but your portion is not diminished. You may delegate it, but it is still with you. You may disclaim it, but you cannot divest yourself of it.

Admiral Hyman Rickover

Life is either a daring adventure or nothing.

Helen Keller

Congratulations! You have come a long, long way from where you started. You have, with your own efforts, made fundamental changes in yourself and in the quality of your life. You have every right to be proud of what you have done.

But a word of caution is in order. Remember the insights you have already learned, especially (1) that it is exceptionally easy to think irrationally, and (2) that hard work against your irrational thinking is necessary to change. The bad news now is that it is easy to backslide—to get lazy and to stop working on your thinking. You will, at times, still think and act irrationally (after all, that is human nature); *and*, if you are not careful, you will stop working altogether and drift back into your old way of doing things.

The good news, though, is that you are in the driver's seat. You have the choice whether to drift or whether to continue to devote regular time, each day, to your ongoing well-being and happiness. I encourage you to think of the long-range benefits of the brief and sometimes inconvenient efforts you would be wise to make each day. I encourage you to think of doing daily psychological workouts for your mental health much as you would do daily physical workouts for your physical health.

To finish your therapy, then, I will share with you ways to maintain your gains and strategies for dealing with backsliding. Fortunately, Dr. Albert Ellis has written a pamphlet, titled "How to Use Rational-Emotive Therapy (RET) to Maintain and Enhance Your Therapy Gains," that we can use as a guideline in this. I urge you to adopt many of those strategies as part of your daily routine.

Finally, and ultimately, your life is *your* responsibility. Whether you go forward with what you have learned or whether you backslide depends on your keeping alive your commitment to your own well-being. While I will always be available to you as a resource in case you find yourself in serious difficulties or in case you simply want a tuneup, it would be wonderful if my services became irrelevant to you in the future. Therefore, your final assignment is to renew the commitments you made in the first part of your therapy, in Assignment 9.

ASSIGNMENT 9: LIFETIME COMMITMENT CONTRACT

I commit myself to, and take full responsibility for, doing whatever is necessary to maintain and enhance the following thoughts/beliefs, feelings, and behaviors.

1. _____
   _____
2. _____
   _____
3. _____
   _____

4. _____

5. _____

I commit myself to, and take full responsibility for, doing the following things to maintain and enhance my therapy gains (be sure to indicate the frequency for each).

1. _____

2. _____

3. _____

4. _____

5. _____

Bibliography

Ellis, A. (1976). The biological basis of human irrationality. *Journal of Individual Psychology*, **32**, 145–68.

Ellis, A. (1978). Family therapy: A phenomenological and active-directive approach. *Journal of Marriage and Family Counseling*, **4(2)**, 43–50.

Ellis, A. (1985). *Overcoming resistance: Rational-emotive therapy with difficult clients*. New York: Springer.

Ellis, A. (1987). The impossibility of achieving consistently good mental health. *American Psychologist*, **42(4)**, 364–375.

Ellis, A., & Harper, R. (1975). *A new guide to rational living*. North Hollywood, Calif.: Wilshire.

Grieger, R., & Boyd, J. (1980). *Rational-emotive therapy: A skills-based approach*. New York: Van Nostrand Reinhold.

Maultsby, M. C., Jr. (1975). *Help yourself to happiness: Through rational self-counseling*. New York: Institute for Rational-Emotive Therapy.

Maultsby, M. C., Jr. (1984). *Rational behavior therapy*. Englewood, Cliffs, N.J.: Prentice-Hall.

HELPING CLIENTS TAKE RESPONSIBILITY

In their excellent text *The Practice of Rational-Emotive Therapy*, Ellis and Dryden (1987) listed 13 criteria of psychological health, including self-interest, social interest, high frustration tolerance, flexibility, acceptance of uncertainty, commitment to creative pursuits, scientific thinking, nonutopianism, self-responsibility for one's own emotional disturbance, and self-direction. Of these 13, I believe that self-direction, defined by Ellis and

Dryden as the assumption of personal *responsibility* for one's own life, may arguably be more important than any of the others. Taking the stance that one is responsible for one's own life allows a person to energetically and purposely pursue most of the others (e.g., self-interest, social interest, and commitment to creative pursuits). On the other hand, not to take personal responsibility means to lose (or at least lessen) such things as self-interest, a commitment to creative pursuits, and risk taking.

Accordingly, doing RET effectively, to me, in addition to mastering RET's basic theory and techniques, includes paying special attention to the client's attitudes toward personal responsibility. In this section, I first address the issue of responsibility as an attitude, belief, or philosophical posture, and I then note how and where responsibility can be integrated into the RET process.

The Philosophy of Responsibility

In a 1985 paper titled "From a Linear to a Contextual Model of the ABC's of RET" (Grieger, 1985a), I proposed that human cognition can be differentiated by a number of different categories arranged from the more general and philosophical to the more specific. I also proposed that the more general the cognition, (1) the more likely the cognition is to be beyond awareness; (2) the more pervasively the cognition is likely to influence the person's life; and (3) the more the cognition directs how a person will respond in any given situation. I further listed three cognitive categories, which, starting from the most general and philosophical, are life positions, values, and interpretational habits.

The concept of *life positions* is most relevant to this discussion:

> These positions, probably adopted when we are young, determine both the scope and boundaries of how we experience the world and how we act in it. These positions are not what we think, do, or feel on a moment-by-moment basis; rather, they are generalizations or abstractions, often unrecognized and unarticulated, that guide and set the boundaries of our thinking, doing and feeling. They are the most basic assumptions, the context that most fundamentally guides our lives. (Earle & Regin, 1980; Grieger, 1985a, pp. 79–80)

Albert Ellis has on hundreds of occasions brilliantly educated us about the power of certain irrational life positions, if I may use that term, in creating and sustaining emotional disturbance. These include *demandingness, catastrophizing, low frustration tolerance* ("I Can't-Stand-It-Itis"), and *self-rating*. To these, I add the life position of responsibility, which, although it may not lead directly to emotional disturbance, does profoundly affect one's effectiveness in both life and therapy and is probably a part of most disturbances. If removal of the irrational beliefs (e.g., demandingness) reduces or eradicates emotional disturbance, thereby getting a person out of a hole, then teaching a person to take the attitude of personal responsibility helps him or her both to remove the disturbance and to take charge of life in an upward, forward manner after the disturbance's removal.

Understanding the concept of *responsibility* can be aided by understanding the dichotomy between "being at effect" and "being at cause" (Rhinehard, 1976). *Being at effect* is the position in which one believes that the circumstances in one's life, be they environmental or psychological, dictate one's destiny, well-being, and behavior. If articulated, it would sound something like "What happens to me in life, my happiness, my goals' being met, even what I do, are dependent on the circumstances of my life by chance working out. If the outside world cooperates, and if my mood holds up, but only if, I can stick to a course of action, act responsibly, and then, hopefully, have things turn out." With such a philosophy, it is easy to imagine this person feeling helpless and inept, being rather passive and dependent, and having a great deal of anxiety, depression, and bitterness when circumstances are or may be adverse. It is also easy to predict how this person would behave in the role of therapy client.

Being at cause equals personal responsibility. It embodies the position that one is personally responsible for her or his well-being, for the choices one makes in life, and for how one responds to events. It embodies the ABCs of RET and, if articulated, would sound something like the following: "No one or no thing is put on this earth to make my life work. Although circumstances do sometimes thwart me and overwhelm me, I accept the responsibility for and commit myself to giving myself the best life I can, regardless of the circumstances. Furthermore, I can make choices about my emotional reaction to the situations I face even if I can't change the situations themselves. I refuse to see myself as a victim of circumstances even though, now or in the future, I may be victimized." It is easy to see that a person who holds this life position would find it hard to be, or at least to sustain, depression, helplessness, rage, or bitterness. On the contrary, one can easily envision this person moving forward in life despite adverse circumstances and certainly participating actively in therapy.

It can be argued, of course, as Dryden (1988) and Ellis (1988a) correctly did in critiquing my 1985 paper, that circumstances do indeed constrain people and do indeed "have an important influence on one's well-being." I acknowledge this. But when I talk about the life position of responsibility, I refer not to the fact of a particular circumstance, but to the global and non-situation-specific generalization that a person carries into each day. It is this abstraction that I "assess" and attend to as I move each client through the stages of RET.

Integrating Responsibility into RET

Rational-emotive therapy can be conceptualized as a series of rather sequential, though overlapping, stages, including (1) psychodiagnosis and goal setting; (2) developing client insight; and (3) working through (Grieger, 1985b; Grieger & Boyd, 1980). The issue of responsibility is relevant to each of these stages.

Psychodiagnosis and Goal Setting

In addition to separating practical from emotional problems, detecting irrational beliefs, and uncovering secondary emotional problems about emotional problems, I typically tune my ear to client thinking or statements that reflect whether the client takes the "effect" or "cause-responsibility" attitude. I also typically make direct inquiries about a number of matters that reflect on where the client stands vis-à-vis personal responsibility:

1. Who or what do you think is making you so unhappy or making you act so bad? Most people lay the responsibility for how they feel and act directly on someone or something else—the A, or the activating event—and some go further, either angrily blaming the A or feeling sorry for themselves for experiencing the C. They see themselves as "victims of circumstances." The more convinced a person is that the A causes his or her misery, and especially the more bitter of self-pitying the person is about it, the less willing this person will be to participate responsibly in therapy, and the more necessary it is to attend the issue of responsibility in the insight stage.

2. Do you know of other people who respond differently to this same situation? Do you believe you have only one choice and have to feel or act this way? Again, the person who replies that there is only one way to respond and that she or he has to respond this way is "at effect," and I assume that extra effort will be needed to turn this position around later.

3. Who is responsible for your happiness in general? Most people say, "Well, I am." But when pressed, they reveal that they really hold the circumstances in their lives responsible. What they really believe is "Well, I am responsible for my happiness, but after all, how can I really be responsible if he or she puts roadblocks in my way!" I note this response and either then or later engage the client in a discussion about the "philosophy of happiness" (see the next section "Rational-Emotive Insight"). In a nutshell, this philosophy states that, given there are no guardian angels or designated human beings assigned to take care of us, we had better decide that our happiness is our own job, our total responsibility.

Goal setting may be the first point in RET where there is an opportunity to directly teach the attitude of responsibility, for in the last analysis, RET has to do with promoting personal freedom and with the ability to make *choices* in life, such as between thinking rationally or irrationally, between acting for short- or long-range pleasure, and between remaining in or leaving a relationship.* And in setting a goal, a person is required to take a stand, to state where she or he *intends* to go.

So, the issue of goal setting in RET is no small matter. Not only does it give direction to the change effort, but it also provides salient information about a person's sense of person responsibility. Does this person set goals easily? To what degree is the person committed (i.e., "I hope I can change" vs. "I will change")? In general, what does the goal setting say about the person's stance regarding responsibility? If the client reveals himself or herself to be "at effect," there is the opportunity to address directly the responsibility issue, to discriminate between "at effect" and "at cause," to delineate the drawbacks to being "at effect," and, in general, to deal with this issue as a preliminary to actively (and hopefully cooperatively) beginning RET.

Rational-Emotive Insight

I believe this is a most crucial stage in RET. It is at this stage that the person learns what is at the root of the presenting problems and what needs to be done to bring about change. Without this information, change is at best haphazard and accidental.

The insight stage is also rich for teaching responsibility. In this stage, the therapist has the job not only of providing basic information but also of helping the client both to appreciate the profound importance of the information and to develop the commitment to do something with the information. As I look back, it is when I have failed at this stage that I have had the most difficulty in helping people.

1. *Teaching the ABCs.* The ABC theory both explains the scientific causality of emotional disturbance and communicates the responsibility that a person has for his or her own disturbance. With this knowledge, the person can shift from simply, "I'm upset" or "He upsets me," both of which entail no responsibility, to "I upset *myself* when he does that by the thinking *I* do and the attitudes *I* hold." This is a profound shift and embodies responsibility.

What I suggest here is that the therapist really has three insights to impart through the ABC theory, all of which the client would be wise to get. One is a basic *understanding* of the ABC theory, which most people easily gain. The second is both an understanding of the ABC theory and an *appreciation* of the personal responsibility that it embodies. Quite a few people are either unable or unwilling to appreciate the responsibility part.

---

*In RET, we usually do not promote specific choices; rather, we help people rid themselves of irrational beliefs and emotional disturbance in order to be free to see and make self-enhancing choices.

The third is an understanding of both the theory and the responsibility message, plus the *commitment* to use the understanding of the ABCs to make changes in one's life.

For RET to be effective, the therapist would do well to appreciate how difficult it is for many people to accept and use the second and third insights that the ABCs offer, particularly those who have been wronged or deprived and feel angry and/or sorry for themselves. All experienced RET-ers can recall hearing a statement like the following: "Sure I'm depressing myself about being alone, but I still wouldn't be depressed if I had somebody." Note that this person understands the ABC theory yet is unwilling to incorporate responsibility into this understanding.

I pretty much didactically teach the ABCs to all of my clients in a rather organized manner. I also spend a great deal of time emphasizing the responsibility messages in the ABCs, and I keep confronting people with this issue throughout the therapy process whenever they communicate that they are not responsible.

2. *Responsibility for awareness and reasoning.* Humans are unique in their ability to think abstractly—to conceptualize, reason, use judgment, and theorize. Yet, although they are blessed with this distinctive faculty, it is neither instinctive nor automatic for humans to think appropriately in any given situation. Although humans instinctively think, they are not "thrown" to choose awareness over unconsciousness, fact over fiction, or rationality over irrationality. The exercise of the mind is therefore volitional, and this means that thinking effectively is each person's responsibility (Brandon, 1983).

In exercising the mind, a first choice has to do with *awareness*. Because of a blind endorsement of beliefs, years of habituating practice, and allergies to thinking (Ellis, 1962), many people pay little attention to what goes through their heads, including their deeply held, profoundly influential beliefs. One of the early RET chores is to teach clients how to track down their irrational thoughts by using such common tools as written ABC homework. Becoming aware of these thoughts and the beliefs they represent allows the working-through stage of RET to proceed. An equally important chore is imparting to the client an appreciation of the importance of developing the habit of purposefully, *mindfully* thinking about thinking, and thus choosing *awareness* over blindness as a way of life. Again, I didactically and repeatedly discuss this with all of my clients.

A second chore has to do with *reasoning*. Because people are bombarded by so many forces, both outside pressures and inner habits, relinquishing irrational beliefs requires them to develop a healthy respect for reasoning. This means at least (1) realizing that merely holding a thought does not make it true; (2) honoring fact above reverie, clarity over vagueness, congruence over contradiction, and logic over illogic; and (3) committing oneself to consistently using reasoning in dealing with life.

In RET we use disputation as a major weapon for change. We teach clients to challenge their irrational beliefs socratically and to take a scientific point of view in which the quest is to falsify their own ideas. However, we would be remiss, in my opinion, if we did not also take the time to enlighten them about the importance of (and power in) their *responsibly* and *volitionally* choosing *reason* as a guiding posture in their dealing with daily life. And going further, we would be remiss if we did not take the time to teach people both the rules of logic and the scientific methodology. I was very heartened to see Ellis (1988b) do the latter in his latest self-help book.

3. *Responsibility for happiness.* Observation shows us that it is very difficult for us humans to be and remain happy. Many factors in life certainly challenge us and make the experience of happiness difficult to attain. At least three factors are (1) the many hassles and tragedies that occur (all the way from traffic jams to cancer); (2) the fact that we live among other people, none of whom are angels and all of whom at times act stupidly, selfishly, and disturbed emotionally; and (3) our own proclivity to think and act in self-defeating, misery-producing ways.

Yet, all too frequently, people believe that happiness is their birthright and that it will descend on them because they simply deserve it. Others believe that they are powerless to make an impact on their lives and that whether they are happy or sad is a matter of luck or fate. Still others, believing they are bad or worthless, are convinced that they do not deserve happiness.

I have found it important to help people see not only that happiness can be acquired, but that they are personally responsible for attaining their own happiness. The issue is whether they are willing to take this attitude and specifically engage in the actions necessary to get the love or success they want in life and to achieve their psychological goal of happiness.

The issue of personal responsibility for happiness arises at this stage or in the working-through stage. Regardless of when it arises, it is best to treat it as an insight that the client "needs" to acquire and/or as an issue that the client "needs" to work through.

Let me offer a brief transcript that shows how this issue intertwines with irrational thinking (in this instance, with low frustration tolerance). The client in question initially came to therapy to conquer agoraphobiclike anxieties following passing out in a shopping center. After overcoming her anxieties, she wanted help in overcoming depression about the end of her marriage. Finally, she turned her attention to her reluctance to take the initiative to find somebody to date and perhaps to mate:

CLIENT: I resent having to go out to find somebody.
THERAPIST: Sounds like you're saying that circumstances should work out because you want them to without your making an effort. [Note both the demand (should) and the "being at effect."]

CLIENT: Of course!

THERAPIST: So, what will happen in your life if you take that attitude?

CLIENT: Nothing! Absolutely nothing!

THERAPIST: Right! So, how does that help you?

CLIENT: It doesn't. But it's difficult.

THERAPIST: Of course, it is. But are you saying that it shouldn't be difficult? Remember the should's?

CLIENT: Yes.

[Note: We spent time on her disputing this demand.]

THERAPIST: Good. Now, as in your fears and depression before, if you take charge and dispute these ideas, you'll be less frustrated and freer to go out and find somebody. But there's more to the battle. I also hear another attitude: "My life is not really my responsibility. It's the job of fate to direct somebody to come to my door and inquire if there is an attractive woman living here who wants a mate."

CLIENT: That sounds pretty good.

THERAPIST: Let me share with you a fairly important distinction. It's between being a victim and being responsible. [Note: I took time to explain "being at cause" vs. "being at effect" at this point.] Now, in addition to ridding yourself of your iBs, which we will continue to work on, you might also develop some awareness of which of these responsibility positions you take each day and then make some choices. I want you not only to get out of the hole of low frustration tolerance, but also to take charge of your life and move ahead. If you keep this victim, "at effect" stance, you'll be lucky to end up with someone. You may not be depressed when you're alone, but you'll still be alone. Why don't you both rid yourself of your depression and LFT *and also* develop a position of self-responsibility.

Rational-Emotive Working Through

The issue of responsibility plays a very important role in this stage of RET, the stage where, through cognitive disputation and other methods, efforts are made to weaken irrational beliefs and strengthen rational ones. The client who either relies on the therapist to do all the work or works only during the therapy session will be inefficient at best and ineffective at worst in bringing about the desired results.

It is best for clients to view their RET as being a 24-hour-a-day, seven-day-a-week thing. To this end, I repeatedly tell them this and also emphasize homework between each and every session. Additionally, I extract promises, sometimes in writing, from them about what they will do between sessions. Their waffling about making a promise provides an opportunity both to check for cognitive resistances and to pursue discussions about their responsibility. Making a promise and failing to comply provides the same opportunity.

One of the more common waffling responses when a person is asked to do homework is "I'll try." Notice how little personal responsibility this response communicates. I have learned a very effective intervention when this response is offered. Taking a pencil in the palm of my hand, I tell the person to try to take the pencil from my hand. Invariably, the person takes the pencil. I say, "No, I said try to take it, not take it. I want you to try, not actually take it. Give back the pencil and try." Usually, the client will make dramatic efforts, grimacing and bringing their fingers close to the pencil in my palm with hand quivering, but not taking it. I then make the point: "See, trying gets no results, and it shows no responsibility. The only thing that gets results and shows that you're being responsible is actually to take the pencil. You either take it or you don't. Now, will you promise to do the homework, and will you stand responsibly behind your promise, or not?" By this time, most people get the point, and the door to both the homework and the responsibility is opened.

To sum up, the process of RET provides multiple opportunities to promote the attitude of personal responsibility. What I have tried to do is to show some of the obvious places in RET where the therapist can do so. I emphasize again, however, that none of these efforts replaces classical RET. Rather, they are additive.

Applications to Relationship Therapy

Rational-emotive couples therapy (RECT) distinguishes between *relationship dissatisfaction* and *relationship disturbance* (DiGiuseppe & Zee, 1986; Ellis & Dryden, 1987; Walen *et al.*, 1980). Relationship dissatisfaction exists when one or both partners dislike some aspect of their relationship life and rationally prefer it to be different. For example, partners may be dissatisfied over sex, affection, in-laws, or the amount of intimacy, but they may not be angry and may still relate to each other appropriately. Relationship disturbance exists when one or both partners become emotionally disturbed— angry, anxious, guilty, jealous, and depressed—about some dissatisfaction. In RECT, we usually first treat the relationship disturbance by typical RET means and then deal with the relationship dissatisfaction.

Along with relationship disturbances, the issue of responsibility plays a significant role in the success or failure of a relationship. The RECT therapist would be wise to pay special attention to this issue as well. In a 1986 paper, I listed four areas of personal responsibility that influence a relationship (Grieger, 1986b). Briefly, they are:

1. Do the partners take responsibility for their emotional reactions to dislikable or dissatisfying relationship events? It is probably true that members of most dysfunctional relationships not only feel victimized and blame their mates for real or imagined sins but also hold their mates responsible for how they react—their unhappiness, anger, and obnoxious behaviors— to the sins. Blaming the mate for how they feel certainly complicates the relationship crisis and, as Ellis (1977) observed, blocks dispassionate attempts to deal with the original issue.

2. Do the partners take responsibility for their own well-being, or does

each hold the other responsible? All too frequently, personal responsibility for happiness is woefully lacking in troubled relationships. When one or both partners feel dissatisfied with life in general, or when the partners fail to provide the happiness and excitement wanted in life, they often blame each other and feel victimized, self-pitying, depressed, and/or alienated. What they fail to realize is that each has surrendered his or her responsibility for making life work to the other.

3. Does each partner take responsibility for making the relationship work? In many troubled relationships, one or both partners are not fully committed to the relationship. They ride along waiting to see how it will turn out, "being at cause." A client of mine who happens to be in a solid marital relationship recently commented, "Our marriage is based more on commitment than love. We are fully committed to each other even when we are not feeling loving." Also, people in troubled relationships often fail to go beyond the myth that a relationship is a 50–50 proposition. They weakly give it their best shot, but only *if* the other party gives first or meets them halfway. Notice how weak the responsibility is here. Imagine the reactions these people will have when the road gets rocky. By contrast, imagine how the person who takes 100% responsibility for the relationship's working responds when difficulties arise.

4. Are the partners trustworthy? Do they keep their commitments and promises to each other? Do they act loyally, putting the other above all others, as they vowed? In a good many troubled relationships, the people involved are very distrusting because each has demonstrated little trustworthiness. They take their commitment very lightly; they do not take responsibility for what they say they will or will not do. They take the attitude "I will do what I say unless, of course, it is difficult." I have found trust to be ruined because of failed promises over smaller issues (e.g., taking out the trash) as well as over larger ones (e.g., sexual fidelity).

As in individual RET, I do fairly classical RECT. The difference is that I also carefully assess the degree of responsibility in each partner in these four areas, and I am willing to make responsibility a major topic of discussion. Usually, this topic becomes a part of dealing with relationship dissatisfactions after relationship disturbances are handled, except in the case of blaming the other for one's own emotional reactions (see Item 1 above).

THERAPIST CHECKLIST FOR RET EFFECTIVENESS

In the final section of this chapter, I briefly address a few issues that I think influence RET's effectiveness.

Don't Forget the Client's History

RET generally ignores where, when, and how the client became disturbed. Connections between the client's past experiences and current disturbances are usually discounted. When clients wonder what happened historically to cause their problems, the therapist tells them that the past is a useless place to work and that the reason they are disturbed is because they are currently repeating irrational beliefs previously learned. This approach serves to force the client into the here and now and, parenthetically, fosters self-responsibility.

Nevertheless, there are times when it is important to delve into the client's past. Not doing so at these times may cause a superficial or even failed RET outcome. Three instances that prompt me to work historically are the following.

One is when a client's irrational beliefs were learned under very dramatic circumstances. Examples are when a person was sexually, physically, or severely verbally abused as a child. I find it essential to know about these events and to assist the client to track down and dispute both her or his prior and current irrational beliefs about these events.

A second instance is when a client supports negative judgments about the self with events in the past. For instance, a client may conclude that he is worthless because his father did not show him love. In addition to disputing the logic of making this self-judgment, based on the historical fact, it is also often effective, in disputing the irrational beliefs, to explore the circumstances surrounding the past so that the client can see it should or had to happen exactly as it did with no personal blameworthiness.

A third instance in which I work on past events is when a client is still currently upset about something that happened in the past. It is one thing to dispute currently held beliefs about these events and another to vividly re-create these events through imaging and to dispute them as if one were right there.

Because of the possibility that past-history issues are present in any client, I regularly require each client to fill out what I call a *psychobiography*. This written assignment asks clients first to describe the significant people in their lives (specifically their parents, siblings, mates, and friends), how these people have acted toward the client, how they have contributed to the presenting problems, and what the client has concluded irrationally from these experiences. I also have clients describe their school, work, religious, sexual, and any other experiences that have contributed to their current problems, along with how they reacted to the events and what they concluded from them. The information acquired is not always used but often proves quite valuable.

Be Flexible

In RET, we advocate that the therapist be active, directive, verbal, and forceful. We tend to downplay the importance of the therapeutic relationship, opting rather to present ourselves in a more didactic, problem-solving manner. We tend to teach the ABCs to clients somewhat dispassionately and to help them learn the skills of discovering and destroying irrational beliefs and behaviors.

Although this approach is generally most effective, I caution the reader neither to adhere rigidly to all this nor to forget that, in the last analysis, what RET boils down to is a conversation between two human beings. Thus, don't forget to attend to and acknowledge the client's feelings, as some clients are unaware of or confused about how they feel, some are ashamed or embarrassed about and/or deny how they feel, some "need" their feelings acknowledged, and some are obsessed with how they feel and, in fact, feelings themselves. Moreover, feeling states are wonderful diagnostic clues to the client's irrational thinking. So, remember that the ABC theory contains the C; it, too, is appropriate grist for the mill at times. Be sure to determine how much feeling attention each client requires.

Similarly, don't forget that a relationship exists between client and therapist whether it is nurtured or not. You have a relationship with each client; the only question is about its quality. Clients act differently with a therapist they like and respect and who they perceive likes and respects them. I will never forget the time I coconducted an RET workshop with Albert Ellis in which he demonstrated RET with a volunteer from the audience. This "client" sat between Ellis and me, so that I looked over the volunteer's shoulders directly into Ellis's eyes, almost as if I were the client. I vividly remember having the sense that I was the one in conversation with Ellis. I felt as if his attention were totally on me, and that a great deal of warmth and respect was coming from him. I remember how rewarding that feeling was. It taught me how motivating it is for a client to experience unconditional acceptance and caring from the therapist. Don't forget this point and become too inflexibly businesslike.

Also, don't forget to watch for client resistance. Ellis (1985) and Grieger and Boyd (1980) have delineated a number of irrational beliefs that cause people to resist working to change. Their resistances come from fears of discomfort, shame, feelings of hopelessness, guilt, fear of change and success, rebelliousness, and other sources (Ellis, 1985). When resistance is encountered, stop what you're doing with the client and do RET on the irrational beliefs behind the resistance.

And don't forget that the words we use in RET are not sacred. The client has not read our professional texts and may not use the same vocabulary we do. Do not be afraid to throw away RET's buzz words and talk the client's language. It's the meanings that count, not the words.

Make Disputation Powerful

Even with the best of insights, motivation, and responsibility, RET can go awry if the disputation process is not powerful or profound. Getting caught up in inelegant solutions to problems (i.e., either working to change the undesirable situation at A or working to help the client to deny or rationalize the badness of a situation, rather than working to give up irrational beliefs about bad situations) is one way to undercut powerful disputation. To be effective, the therapist would be wise not to get caught up in the drama of activating events (e.g., the death of a child), indulge overzealous desires to please, protect, or help the client, and fall prey to a client's sense of victimization or helplessness. In sidestepping these traps, one can focus the client on disputing the should's, awfuls, and self-judgments.

Powerful disputation also requires clients to go much beyond sloganizing and *really* think through the logic that led to their irrational conclusions. It is very easy to assume that a person really believes, for instance, that he is not a worthless person when he says, "I am not worthless just because she stopped loving me." This statement is certainly true, but you cannot be sure that the client really believes or understands its truth unless you ask, "Can you tell me why that is so?" This type of question often meets with puzzlement or glibness and often leads me to help clients discover the truths behind their glib parroting of rational statements. Be sure to make certain that the client really does understand the conceptual basis of their disputation and can clearly make the relevant distinctions. Be skillful with the range of RET disputation methods, including those offered in this text.

See the iB Package as a Whole

Ellis (Ellis & Dryden, 1987) has often said that demandingness is the key irrational belief, awfulizing, low frustration toleration, and self-rating being derivatives. Although I certainly agree that these three derive from demandingness, demandingness also derives from each of the others as well. For if I am no good or am in danger of being no good for failing this task (self-rating), then, with such dire consequences at stake, it follows that I *must* do well (demandingness). Similarly, if it is awful for you to reject me (awfulizing, low frustration tolerance), I easily conclude that I *have* to have your approval (demandingness).

So, there is circularity or a cybernetic system at work here, so that one irrationality tends to beget another, which tends to beget the original one, and so on. To make disputation most effective, I find it helpful to keep this circularity in mind so that I do not miss any of the irrational beliefs that a client may hold.

Remember the Universality of Self-Esteem

Though RET theory disapproves of it, remember that virtually all human beings self-rate and therefore struggle with their self-worth. People typically worry about whether they are valuable, lovable people or not. Do not lose sight of the fact that self-rating is a part of most every person's emotional disturbance, and do not, therefore, fail to make this a part of virtually every client's RET.

Be Committed and Responsible

It is easy for the therapist who sees clients hour after hour, day after day, to lose energy, get bored, and even burn out. It is therefore extremely important, in order to be an effective RET therapist, I believe, to regularly renew one's commitment to one's clients and to reinvest in one's respect for them as individual, flesh-and-blood human beings. I know of no magic way to do this except through reminders and, more importantly, through a renewal of one's commitment to "being at cause," or personal responsibility. To renew oneself is not only personally satisfying but also energizing and is bound to lead to more effectiveness as an RET therapist.

SUMMARY

In this chapter, I have not gone over the basics of rational-emotive therapy. There are many fine texts and training tapes that do this. What I have done is to communicate some additional ideas and procedures that I have learned through working with my clients and now use as part of my RET. I have not been able to communicate them all because of space limitations. Nevertheless, I hope that the reader will find them thought-provoking and useful.

REFERENCES

Brandon, N. (1983). *Honoring the self: Personal integrity and the heroic potentials of human nature.* Los Angeles: Jeremy P. Tarcher.

DiGiuseppe, R., & Zee, C. (1986). A rational-emotive theory of marital dysfunction and marital therapy. *Journal of Rational-Emotive Therapy.* 4, 22–37.

Dryden, W. (1988). Comments on Grieger's contextual model of the ABC's of RET. In W. Dryden, & P. Trower (Eds.), *Developments in cognitive psychotherapy* (pp. 94–99). London: Sage.

Earle, M., & Regin, N. (1980). *A world that works for everyone.* San Francisco: The EST Enterprise.

Ellis, A. (1962). *Reason and emotion in psychotherapy.* Secaucus, NJ: Lyle Stuart.

Ellis, A. (1971). *Growth through reason.* North Hollywood, CA: Wilshire Books.

Ellis, A. (1973). *Humanistic psychotherapy: The rational-emotive approach.* New York: McGraw-Hill.

Ellis, A. (1976). The biological basis of human irrationality. *Journal of Individual Psychology, 32,* 145–168.

Ellis, A. (1977). Anger: How to live with and without it. Secaucus, NJ: Citadel Press.

Ellis, A. (1978). Personality characteristics of rational-emotive therapists and other kinds of therapist. *Psychotherapy: Theory, research and practice, 15*, 329–332.

Ellis, A. (1985). *Overcoming resistance.* New York: Springer.

Ellis, A. (1988a). Comments on Grieger's contextual model of ABC's of RET. In W. Dryden & P. Tower (Eds.), *Developments in cognitive therapy* (pp. 100–105). London: Sage.

Ellis, A. (1988b). *How to stubbornly refuse to make yourself miserable about anything—Yes anything.* Secaucus, NJ: Lyle Stuart.

Ellis, A., & Dryden, W. (1987). *The practice of rational-emotive therapy.* New York: Springer.

Ellis, A., & Grieger, R. (1977). *Handbook of rational-emotive therapy: Volume I.* New York: Springer.

Ellis, A., & Grieger, R. (1986). *Handbook of rational-emotive therapy: Volume II.* New York: Springer.

Ellis, A., & Harper, R. A. (1975). *A new guide to rational living.* North Hollywood, CA: Wilshire.

Grieger, R. (1985a). From a linear to a contextual model of the ABC's of RET. *Journal of Rational-Emotive Therapy, 3*, 75–99.

Grieger, R. (1985b). The process of rational-emotive therapy. *Journal of Rational-Emotive Therapy, 3*, 138–148.

Grieger, R. (1986a). *A client's guide to rational-emotive therapy.* Charlottesville, VA.

Grieger, R. (1986b). The role and treatment of irresponsibility in dysfunctional relationships. *Journal of Rational-Emotive Therapy, 4*, 50–67.

Grieger, R., & Boyd, J. (1980). *Rational-emotive therapy: A skills-base approach.* New York: Van Nostrand Reinhold.

Maultsby, M. C., Jr. (1984). *Rational behavior therapy.* Englewood Cliffs, NJ: Prentice-Hall.

Rhinehard, L. (1976). *The book of EST.* New York: Holt, Rinehart & Winston.

Walen, S. R., DiGiuseppe, R. A., & Wessler, R. L. (1980). *A practitioner's guide to rational-emotive therapy.* New York: Oxford University Press.

Orthodox RET Taught Effectively with Graphics, Feedback on Irrational Beliefs, a Structured Homework Series, and Models of Disputation

PAUL J. WOODS

As a result of 25 years of teaching experience before I actually began practicing psychotherapy, I structured the early stages of RET therapy with clients along the lines of a teacher structuring a learning experience. During my associate fellow training at the Institute for Rational-Emotive Therapy in New York, I was urged to be more "evocative" and less "didactic." Subsequently, what I have tried to do is combine a lecturing style with an evocative interaction style.

Throughout my work with a client, but especially in the beginning, I am mindful of such things as the basic insights desirable in RET (Grieger & Boyd, 1980, pp. 81–121) and the major theoretical concepts involved (Ellis & Dryden, 1987, pp. 1–27). Opportunities to develop such insights and communicate major concepts are, therefore, reacted to appropriately. But matters such as these and the use of other general RET techniques are not discussed in this chapter. Rather, the focus is on sharing some original

PAUL J. WOODS • Department of Psychology, Hollins College, Roanoke, Virginia 24020.

materials and approaches that I have developed to help with the inculcation and application of basic RET.

One point deserves mention at the outset. My experience has shown that it is very important to audiotape therapy sessions. It is also more effective to provide a high-quality tape recorder than to encourage clients to bring their own recorders. I use two *external* microphones to produce the best recording possible. The tapes are then given to the clients for review after each session and are a valuable therapeutic and learning aid.

INTRODUCTORY MINILECTURES

Usually, in the second session, I introduce some "minilectures" to the client by saying something like

> It would be helpful if I could communicate some basic ideas and concepts to you related to the manner in which we see the human organism functioning. We will be better able to communicate with one another and work on your problems if we share a set of conceptions and use a common language. Hence, I will spend 20 minutes or so of this hour on a "chalk talk" or "minilecture" on some aspects of our understanding of human emotional distress and ways to deal with it. Is this okay with you?

If the client doesn't have something immediately pressing, we go on with the minilecture, starting with a basic ABC presentation and the three-box diagram shown in Figure 1. This is actually put on the board and discussed one step at a time, beginning with the A. I point out that we'll focus on "bad" events in our work because people don't usually become seriously distressed over "good" events. I usually continue as follows:

> When "bad" events occur, and before we react, we must become aware of them. When we do, we "mull them over" or otherwise contemplate and *evaluate* them. At this point we also probably bring preexisting general beliefs about the way things should and should not be.

Some clients can grasp this process as a decision-making stage, and that

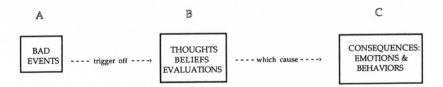

FIG. 1. Basic presentation of the ABCs.

helps them to realize that As can't automatically create Cs. With brighter or more educated clients, I'll say something like

> I don't want you to think we're oversimplifying matters. This is just a beginning. Next, in explaining the theory and therapeutic strategy of RET, I'm going to expand to a 5-box diagram and then, ultimately, to one with 14 boxes.

When the diagram in Figure 1 is clear, I then expand it to the form shown in Figure 2. I put this figure up, again one section at a time, starting with "bad" events at A. But then I often expand a bit more by pointing out that these bad events may occur in the past or in the present or may be anticipated in the future:

> When we are contemplating such events we do so at Point B with either defensible thoughts, beliefs, and evaluations or indefensible ones. Yes, there are really only two categories: a thought, belief, or evaluation can be either reasonable or unreasonable, and we use the terms *rational* and *irrational*.

The two B-level boxes are then drawn and labeled.

> Regardless of which category dominates, there will be consequences. These consequences will be *emotions* and *behaviors;* we will both feel and act.

The two C-level boxes are now added, with only the categories "Emotions" and "Behaviors" at this time.

> If we are thinking basically rationally, then we will argue that the emotional consequences are quite likely to be appropriate to the problem at Point

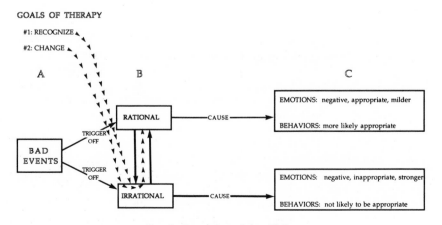

FIG. 2. Expansion of the ABCs.

A. And since we are focusing on bad events at Point A, the appropriate feelings *are* going to be negative. We certainly wouldn't judge positive emotions to be appropriate to a bad event. Not only are the negative feelings created by rational thoughts about the bad event appropriate, they are also *desirable*. That is, these negative feelings provide the *motivation* for you to deal with the problem at Point A by such tactics as changing it, escaping from it, or preventing it in the future. If you are not at all upset by mistreatment, then you are going to continue to be abused or taken advantage of. Such continued mistreatment is not in your own best interests, and if you didn't feel somewhat bad about it, you would, in effect, not be taking very good care of yourself.

I add the words *negative* and *appropriate* in the upper C-level box following "Emotions."

With respect to the behaviors resulting from rational thinking processes, there is no guarantee that they will be appropriate, for you may actually lack certain skills, such as assertiveness. But we can argue that rationally generated behaviors are *more likely* to be appropriate than are the behaviors generated by irrational ways of thinking.

I add "more likely appropriate" in the upper C-level box following "Behaviors."

Moving on to the final lower-level box at point C—these diagrams may make it clear that the consequences developing in this box are hardly likely to be appropriate to reality, resulting as they have from irrational thinking. Can an irrational assessment of things produce good results? Once in a while—maybe accidentally—but certainly not on a regular basis. So we'll argue that the emotional consequences of irrational thinking will be negative and inappropriate. They are also likely to be stronger than the emotions arising from rational thinking.

I add *negative, inappropriate,* and *stronger* following "Emotions" in lower C-level box and *milder* following "Emotions" in upper C-level box.

Note that we are not saying that the emotional reactions to rational thinking are *always* mild, for with really bad events, they will be strong, and appropriately so. We're just saying that they are *relatively milder* than the emotional reactions produced by irrational thinking.

Finally, the behavioral consequences of irrational thinking are "not likely to be appropriate" to the problem at Point A. Here, for example, you are more likely to *kick* the flat tire rather than change it.

I add "not likely to be appropriate" following "Behaviors" in the lower C-level box. Then I ask if the client has any problems with or questions about the diagram and react to any that are raised.

At this point, clients often volunteer that they find themselves in the lower box at Point C. I respond, "Well, let's proceed and show you how you can work at spending less time there."

While we have this diagram on the board there are several points I would like to make. Notice that we can go back and forth between rational and irrational ways of thinking.

I add the arrows going up and down between the two B-level boxes labeled *rational* and *irrational*.

We can even do this within the same sentence: "I don't like what you are doing, therefore you *must* stop." The first part is rational, the second irrational. Thus our thoughts, beliefs, and evaluations can have a rich mixture, and can *also* involve critical assessments of irrational components resulting in their rejection and replacement with rational ones. *But,* I am not going to draw any arrows back and forth between the two C-level boxes. As you probably have observed (*pointing to the lower C level box*), if you are very upset, telling yourself, "Don't be upset" doesn't put you up here (*pointing to the upper C-level box*). Merely saying, "Don't be anxious" doesn't calm you down, does it? Or how about a man who is really angry? If you say to him, "Don't be so mad," what is likely to happen?

Most clients answer, "He'll get more angry."

The point is that you can't go *directly* from inappropriate strong negative feelings and inappropriate behavior to appropriate levels of feelings and appropriate actions. If you are in the lower C-level box and you would rather be in the upper C-level box, then it will be necessary to call a "time-out" for some detective work. Notice your distress and then "go backward in time" to search for the thoughts, beliefs, and evaluations at Point B that *caused* your emotional upset at Point C. We will work at teaching you to be a skeptical critic of your own B-level processes so that you can detect irrational components and *change* them to rational thoughts, beliefs, and evaluations. That is, we'll work at going from the lower B-level box to the upper B-level box. When you get there, you will then *automatically* end up in the upper C-level box, which is where you would like to be!

Most clients understand and accept this analysis. Many, however, express frustration or disbelief that they will ever be able to succeed. Encouragement and a request for patience are then appropriate:

Be patient. We'll go one step at a time, but before we begin, it is important that you generally understand these basics so that you can see where we are heading and why we are doing what we are doing at any particular point along the way.

Any further questions or concerns about the five-box diagram are then answered:

> Finally, while I still have this diagram on the board, there are two points I would like to make regarding the *goals of therapy.*

I add "Goals of Therapy" in the upper left part of the diagram.

> Goal 1 is to teach you how to recognize these.

I add "1: Recognize" under "Goals of Therapy" and draw an arrow from there to the irrational B-level box.

> When we talk about irrational beliefs you'll probably *recognize* them as familiar, for they are a common part of everyday thinking and language, but we will be talking about recognizing them as being *irrational.* Then Goal 2 will be to teach you how to *change* them from irrational to rational.

I add "2: Change" under "Goals of Therapy" and draw an arrow from there down to the irrational B-level box and then up to the rational B-level box.

In actuality, there is much interaction during these presentations, with questions both to and from the client. For most clients, I also try to point out that our knowledge about past and present events at Point A can come to our conscious attention only through various changes in physical energy (sound waves, light waves, etc.) and that there is generally no way such fluctuations in physical energy can *directly* affect our emotional reactions and our behavior. That is, the point is made that events in the world *must be* (using *must*, not as a demand, but to denote a causational relationship) understood, interpreted, and evaluated before we respond to them.

Often, I share a reprint of a paper I wrote entitled "Do You Really Want to Maintain That a Flat Tire Can Upset Your Stomach? Using the Findings of the Psychophysiology of Stress to Bolster the Argument That People Are Not Directly Disturbed by Events" (Woods, 1987a). I introduce it with a question: "Do you really believe that a doughnut-shaped piece of vulcanized rubber that is flat on one side can directly upset the functioning of your gastrointestinal system?"

This is a good place to introduce various B-level alternatives and to ask how they would feel about each:

> Suppose you were to see a flat tire on your car just as you were leaving for work, and you thought or actually said out loud, (1) "Oh, my God! This is the worst thing that could happen this morning! I'll be late for the 9 o'clock meeting and what will they think of me?" How would you feel?

The client usually agrees that she or he would be rather upset. Then,

> Suppose you said, (2) "Oh, darn! This is a problem! I'll have to call and tell them I'll be late and then arrange to have the flat tire fixed." How would you feel now?

Clients generally agree that they wouldn't be as upset. Finally,

> Suppose you said, (3) "Hot dog! Here's a good excuse to miss that damned meeting!" How would you feel in this case?

Clients usually see that they would at least feel relieved and maybe even happy.

It's made clear that I am not advocating any of these particular thought processes at this time, but merely trying to help them see that the flat tire at Point A is *there in all cases* and that their changed feelings at Point C really were caused by the different thoughts at Point B.

(It is important to note that such strategies, aimed at changing the way clients believe, are initiated only *after* the assessment battery, which includes a test of irrational beliefs, has been completed.)

When time and the client's own agenda permit, I suggest we continue the minilectures by working next on Therapy Goal 1, recognizing irrational beliefs. (I cover the 4 basic iBs of demandingness, awfulizing, low frustration tolerance, and condemnation, and then the 10 derivatives assessed by the Jones Irrational Beliefs Test.)

Demands

To introduce and educate clients regarding demands, I have prepared a brochure that opens to a 33-inch flowchart showing what we know and understand to be the consequences of success and failure with demands in contrast to success and failure with preferences. The format of the flowchart is shown in condensed form in Figure 3.* Its horizontal format does not lend itself to book publication, so the basic contents are re-created in a vertical format here (Figure 4).

The following indicates the contents of each of the notes cited. The actual notes are too extensive to reproduce here:

> Note 1. Emphasizes that a choice does, indeed, exist and cautions against "That's the way I have always thought and I can't change now."

*This chart and other RET materials are available commercially. For a descriptive brochure, write The Scholars' Press, Ltd., P.O. Box 7231, Roanoke, VA 24019.

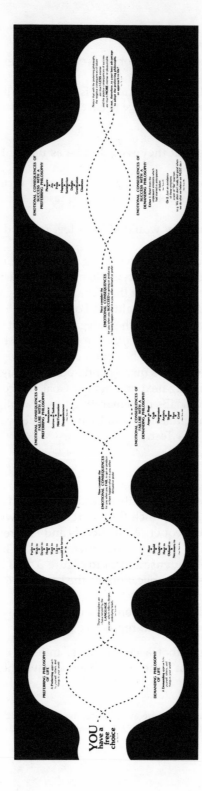

FIG. 3. Flowchart showing the consequences of success and failure with demands in contrast to success and failure with preferences.

Consequences of success and failure with demands and with preferences
••••••••••••••••••••

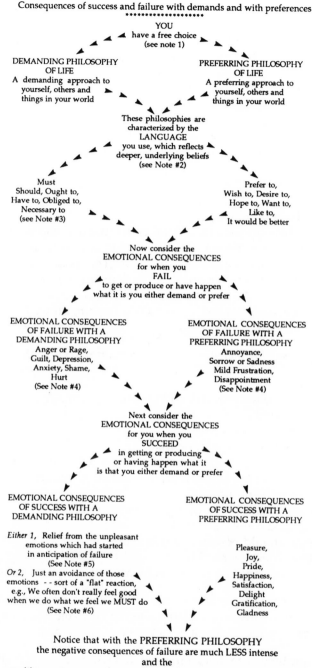

YOU
have a free choice
(see note 1)

DEMANDING PHILOSOPHY
OF LIFE
A demanding approach to
yourself, others and
things in your world

PREFERRING PHILOSOPHY
OF LIFE
A preferring approach to
yourself, others and
things in your world

These philosophies are
characterized by the
LANGUAGE
you use, which reflects
deeper, underlying beliefs
(see Note #2)

Must
Should, Ought to,
Have to, Obliged to,
Necessary to
(see Note #3)

Prefer to,
Wish to, Desire to,
Hope to, Want to,
Like to,
It would be better

Now consider the
EMOTIONAL CONSEQUENCES
for when you
FAIL
to get or produce or have happen
what it is you either demand or prefer

EMOTIONAL CONSEQUENCES
OF FAILURE WITH A
DEMANDING PHILOSOPHY
Anger or Rage,
Guilt, Depression,
Anxiety, Shame,
Hurt
(See Note #4)

EMOTIONAL CONSEQUENCES
OF FAILURE WITH A
PREFERRING PHILOSOPHY
Annoyance,
Sorrow or Sadness
Mild Frustration,
Disappointment
(See Note #4)

Next consider the
EMOTIONAL CONSEQUENCES
for you when you
SUCCEED
in getting or producing
or having happen what it
is that you either demand or prefer

EMOTIONAL CONSEQUENCES
OF SUCCESS WITH A
DEMANDING PHILOSOPHY

EMOTIONAL CONSEQUENCES
OF SUCCESS WITH A
PREFERRING PHILOSOPHY

Either 1, Relief from the unpleasant
emotions which had started
in anticipation of failure
(See Note #5)
Or 2, Just an avoidance of those
emotions - - sort of a "flat" reaction,
e.g., We often don't really feel good
when we do what we feel we MUST do
(See Note #6)

Pleasure,
Joy,
Pride,
Happiness,
Satisfaction,
Delight
Gratification,
Gladness

Notice that with the PREFERRING PHILOSOPHY
the negative consequences of failure are much LESS intense
and the
positive consequences of success are much MORE intense or pleasurable.

Is it not, therefore, to your best advantage to adopt the preferring
philosophy or approach to life
(See note #7)
?

FIG. 4. The basic contents of the flowchart depicted in Figure 3.

Note 2. Deeper, underlying beliefs do not refer to unconscious motives. Illustrates the broadly demanding philosophy of life and a preferring alternative.

Note 3. Differentiates absolute from conditional demands.

Note 4. The particular emotion at any time depends on the conditions in which the preferring or demanding philosophy is applied. Examples are given.

Note 5. Relief is not true happiness, nor is it a *positive* emotional feeling.

Note 6. Not only are you deprived of a positive emotional reaction, but you also deprive others of a reward from you when they have done well.

Note 7. There are also behavioral consequences, and when demands are not satisfied, our behavior is not likely to be in the best interests of ourselves or others. This point is illustrated with how anxiety arising from a demand interferes with performance. It's a real paradox. If you demand to do well, you are *less* likely to. If you merely hope to do well, you are *more* likely to.

Examples of Demanding Statements (these are scattered *below* the flowchart in the brochure).

1. I must behave properly and say the right things so that I will not be criticized.
2. I have to do well.
3. You shouldn't have done that!
4. As something might go wrong, I have to worry about it.
5. I must continue to work on this until it is perfect.
6. I have to be on time.
7. I ought to do this now, and there isn't time!
8. That should not have broken.
9. People should be more considerate.
10. I have to have what I want.
11. It is necessary to have someone around on whom I can depend.

Examples of Preferring Statements (these are scattered *above* the flowchart in the brochure and constitute rational alternatives, corresponding here by number to each of the irrational statements given above).

1. I hope they like what I am going to do. If they don't, that's too bad; I still think it's a good idea.
2. I prefer to do well and I'll try hard to succeed, but I don't absolutely *have* to do well.
3. I wish you hadn't done that.

4. I hope all goes well; worrying about the possibility of something going wrong will not prevent it from doing so.
5. I want to do the best job I can.
6. I hope I make it on time.
7. I would like to be able to do this now, but there isn't time.
8. I wish that had not broken at this time.
9. It would be nice if others were more considerate.
10. I would like to have what I want.
11. I don't really need to have someone around to depend on, although I find it highly preferable.

In the brochure, the demanding sequence of events symbolically follows the "low road" across the bottom of the flowchart, and the preferring sequence follows the "high road."

We go through the flowchart one position at a time, alternating for contrast between the "low road" of demandingness and the "high road" of preferringness. Then, there is one place I like to elaborate on. After we have finished discussing the consequences for failure and pointing out that the negative emotions are much stronger when one has been demanding, I'll say something like

> You might agree that, with demandingness, it's pretty bad when things go wrong, and you might conclude that, if you just make sure things don't go wrong, then everything will be okay in your life. Well, I hope to convince you that, even if things go well, with a demanding philosophy of life you are not likely to experience much in the way of positive feelings. Consider, for example, some challenging event that you would make yourself anxious about, such as making a presentation to a group or having a job interview. You become quite anxious because you are demanding that you *must* do well. Now let's assume that *you do just fine.* Everything goes very well. Do you feel pleased, proud, happy, and satisfied, or do you just feel relieved?

I wipe my hand across my brow, with "Phew! I'm glad that's over!" Most clients admit that they would just feel relieved. In fact, many admit that they have, indeed, experienced something similar to the scenario just described, and that all they *did* feel was relief.

> Now consider another circumstance in which you are demanding but are not anxious in anticipation. Demand, for example, that your spouse had *damned well better* remember your birthday this year or that your kids *must* do better in school. Now, let's assume that, without any reminders, your mate *does* remember your birthday. Do you feel pleased and happy and give him or her a hug, or do you just think, "Well, that's what he or she is supposed to do!" Or if your child comes home with a good report card, do you feel pleased and proud, or do you say, "Well, finally! That's what you should have been doing all along!"

Many agree that they *have* been living with such consequences created by a demanding outlook. I then make one final point to the effect that not only have they been depriving themselves of some good feelings, but they have also been *failing to reinforce* others for doing well.

Thus, we feel that the only way to get positive emotional reactions is to succeed in the context of a preferring outlook on life. You are pleased when you get what you want—not when you get what you demand.

After finishing the entire flowchart one step at a time, I summarize by pointing out:

In contrast to a preferring philosophy, when things go wrong with a demanding philosophy of life, you are more highly stressed and experience stronger negative emotions. When things go right with a demanding philosophy, you do not really experience much in the way of positive emotions. But with a preferring philosophy of life, when things go wrong you are much less distressed. When things go right, you then, and possibly only then, experience positive feelings.

So take your pick. You have the choice. Just pay my bill (*smile*), but take your choice of how you want to run your life.

Somewhere in the presentation of this flowchart, most clients volunteer that they have, indeed, been following the "low road" of demandingness, and that the result is higher levels of misery when things to wrong and no really good feelings when things go right.

Awfulizing

I introduce this iB by referring to the common human tendency to exaggerate the badness of things. We tend to blow things out of proportion. To help clients remember this iB, I often relate the story of the girl who wrote home to her mother from college as follows:

Dear Mom,
    Please go sit down before you read any further.
    A few weeks ago, I got terribly drunk at a fraternity party, fell out of a window, landed in some bushes, and broke my leg. I've been in the hospital ever since. While here, I've fallen in love with this boy who is the orderly on our floor. He's a very nice boy, Mom, but he is of a very, very different religion from us, and he's also of a different race. But I do love him, and we are going to get married because I'm pregnant.
    Now, Mom, forget all of the above because *none of it is true, but I did flunk chemistry, and I just want you to keep it in perspective.*

                                                                    Love,
                                                                    Jan

And that's the issue: keeping things in perspective.

> Rate the bad things in your life in a realistic fashion. Consider a 100-point scale where the upper end involves really major catastrophies and tragedies. Now, where does rejection by a lover or failure at a job really belong?

Sometimes, with "difficult awfulizing customers," I construct a scale, on a roll of paper, of realistic actual or possible bad events, *excluding* at first the one they have been awfulizing. These are rated from 0 to 100 and placed proportionately on the scale, which extends from the ceiling to the floor. In my office this approach becomes very dramatic, for my ceiling is 12 feet high!

After the scale is filled in with a dozen or so events, each rated low, medium, or high, we then go back to the original awfulized one that led to this particular demonstration in the first place. The client is asked where it belongs among all the items on this vertical scale. The result is usually a more reasonable, realistic rating.

Low Frustration Tolerance

I have little to add with respect to this iB except to report that, when asked what is wrong with statements such as "I can't stand this" or "I can't stand that," an encouraging percentage of clients answer, "Well, you really *can* stand it." I respond, "Exactly. You may *not like* something, but you certainly can stand it."

Condemnation

Believing that people, including yourself, deserve to be damned, blamed, condemned, or somehow made to suffer for the errors they have made hardly seems like a decent approach to the problem of misbehavior.

When probing for implicit condemnatory iBs, you may find some of the terms or methods of attack listed below to be of use, for some clients reject "damning" and "condemnation" as too strong.

speak ill of the person	discredit the person
ridicule	disgrace
make a fool of	berate
disparage	belittle
denounce	disapprove
deprecate	reproach
run down	attack
assail	impugn
vilify	curse
find fault	criticize
put down	

For irrational condemnation, these are directed at the person rather than at the act, trait, characteristic, or quality.

Self-Worth

I bring up the invalid idea that the self can be rated as good or bad as a separate issue in order to explicitly and thoroughly deal with this condemnatory belief. I also point out that the reason some regard certain A-level events, such as failure or rejection, as "awful" is that they believe their self-worth has been threatened.

Self-worth and self-esteem are highly valued, but actually or potentially destructive, concepts in our society that are promulgated not only by the popular culture but also by many non-RET therapists and counselors. This thinking is so pervasive that I can't recall ever having a client or a student even remotely approach a statement such as "I believe self-esteem is an invalid concept. I unconditionally *accept* my self without any strings attached." I do find many nonclients who "feel good about themselves," but of course, that idea is also pernicious, for whenever they fail in some important way, they then no longer "feel good about themselves" and become seriously distressed.

When discussing this topic, I have clients take a few minutes to read a short article I wrote entitled "How to determine one's value as a human being" (Woods, 1983). It starts out very seriously, describing the data one must recollect if one is going to determine one's *worth* as a human being:

> If we are going to rate ourselves as good or bad, worthwhile or worthless, then we absolutely must do the job thoroughly and correctly. . . . To really arrive at a valid decision regarding our self-worth we must, therefore, have a complete record of *all* of our actions, deeds, and thoughts since infancy. That is, we must have the kind of thoroughly total record that will be available at the Day of Judgment. . . . It's a big task but very important! Do not shirk at it because it is going to arrive at the most important assessment you have ever made—your net value as a person. . . .
>
> We begin with the Cluster of Attributes Deserving Damnation (CADD) because most people who are feeling badly about themselves are more eager to document these. . . . Even the slightest negative item in thought or deed MUST be included, otherwise your relative value as a human being will not be correctly arrived at. So don't forget or gloss over as unimportant items such as the following:
>
> - The times you got mad at your mother
> - Your vote for a candidate who then won the election and performed badly on the job
> - The times you lied and said you liked something when you really didn't
> - Not returning incorrect change given in your favor
> - Leaving a smaller than accustomed tip
> - Laughing at a dirty joke
> - Taking the largest piece of cake

IF YOU ARE BEGINNING TO RESIST THIS JOB, THEN RECORD YOUR LACK OF ENTHUSIASM AS ANOTHER ENTRY IMMEDIATELY, BECAUSE *YOU SHOULD BE EAGER AND WILLING* TO WORK ON SUCH AN IMPORTANT TASK AS THAT OF DETERMINING YOUR SELF-WORTH.

And good people would certainly not do any of the following, so be sure not to omit them from your CADD list:

- Getting angry
- Feeling impatient with your children
- Feeling lustful toward someone you are not married to
- Turning down an invitation by saying you were busy when you were not
- Burping at a dinner party
- Wishing you never had any children
- Thinking, even briefly, that you should have married your first love
- Hoping a distant relative would die and leave you some money

As one reads through the article (which is merely excerpted above), the entire enterprise becomes more absurd and ridiculous. I point out one final problem:

Even if you were able to generate a fairly extensive and representative listing of all of the negative and positive actions and thoughts from your past, and then even if you were able to validly rate each one, you'd still have the problem of deciding what grand sum of all these items would be necessary to be called a worthwhile person.

I then close with a suggested alternative of unqualified self-acceptance:

We will greet with applause and admiration your decision to abandon the whole project as ridiculous. And we will cheer with a most hearty "RIGHT ON!" your decision to stop rating your SELF entirely! We will further engrave your name on our plaque which is labeled: PTMRITOBI (Persons Thinking More Rationally in Their Own Best Interests) IF you agree to merely accept yourself with no strings attached.

We suggest that you recognize you are like the rest of us humans—fallible. And we suggest you accept *that* human quality without complaining and without demanding that you should be perfect and infallible.

At this point, the minilectures have been completed. (Remember, there have been digressions and client "agenda" items along the way. But I virtually always reenter the above sequence when appropriate and try hard to cover all of it with everyone.)

REPORT BOOKLET ON THE CLIENT'S IRRATIONAL BELIEFS: HOMEWORK

The next item relevant to my general, but flexible, plan is to report on the results of the Jones IBT. I'll point out that among the battery of assessment instruments there was one that sampled some of their beliefs relevant to the areas we've been discussing.

One of the tests you took is an attempt to assess some of your B-level thoughts and beliefs. We have actually assessed 10 areas in which the basic beliefs we've been talking about are applied.

We then go over a report booklet I've prepared to accompany the Jones IBT, entitled "Beliefs That Disturb."* Each of the 10 scales is examined in a consistent fashion that involves:

1. A name or label for the area of concern.
2. A statement of the irrational belief.
3. A scale marked to show how strongly the client apparently accepts the belief.
4. An argument about why we consider the belief irrational.
5. A discussion and supporting arguments for a rational alternative to the irrational belief.

The cover of the booklet states:

> This is based upon the writings of Albert Ellis, Ph.D., Executive Director of The Institute for Rational-Emotive Therapy, with particular reference to *Reason and Emotion in Psychotherapy,* published by Lyle Stuart, New York, and *A New Guide to Rational Living,* published by Prentice-Hall, Englewood Cliffs, NJ, and Wilshire Books, North Hollywood, CA. The ideas and arguments are basically his; only the style and most of the words in this report are mine. The questionnaire estimating your adherence to these beliefs was constructed by Richard G. Jones. Full credit and appreciation for it is hereby acknowledged.

What follows, for illustrative purposes, is the text for the first area, "Demand for Approval."

AREA 1. *APPROVAL FROM OTHERS*

YOU FEEL THE *NEED* TO HAVE THE SUPPORT AND APPROVAL OF EVERYONE YOU KNOW OR CARE ABOUT.	Strength of your belief	
	_____ Very high	8–10
	_____ High	6–7
	_____ Moderately high	5
	_____ Moderate	4
	_____ Low	2–3
	_____ Very low or zero	0–1

This belief can create problems for many reasons. For example, demanding approval causes you to worry and upset yourself about whether or not you will get it. If you do get it then you worry about losing it. Being overly concerned with the approval of others interferes with your doing what you really want to do with your life. Demanding approval from virtually everyone sets an unrealizable goal. No matter what you do some

---

*A complete package of materials based on the Jones Irrational Beliefs Tests (IBT) is available. Write the author for information and ordering instructions: Dr. Paul J. Woods, Department of Psychology, Hollins College, Roanoke, VA 24020.

people will approve and some people will disapprove, but the great majority won't really care.

You can decide to live and run your own life according to your best interests and wishes and desires, and if you do you will find people who will support you and approve of you and like you, even though they may not be the same people whose approval you are now demanding. But basically, for your own happiness and best interest, you will be best advised to regard the approval of others as nice but not necessary. It's important to know that *self-respect does not come from the approval of others* but from your own satisfaction and pride with the way you are running your life. So you can stop demanding respect from others and, more elegantly, even stop demanding that you must have self-respect! Instead of self-respect you can focus on *self-acceptance*. Self-acceptance is nonjudgmental so that even if you don't do well you still do not have to negatively evaluate or reject your SELF. With self-*acceptance* you are more likely to work on improvement of your behavior—with self-*rejection* you are less likely to do so.

I go through this booklet pointing out the client's scores and discussing each area in turn, and then I give the booklet to the client for study.

My students and I have used the Jones IBT extensively and have reported findings relevant to its validity and usefulness in understanding a variety of problems, such as anxiety, anger, anger expression, Type A behavior, psychosomatic disorders, premenstrual syndrome, and suicidal ideation (Bredekin, 1988; Gentilini, 1988; Luttrell, 1987; Oesterle, 1984; Secrist, 1986; Woods, 1983, 1984, 1987b; Woods & Coggin, 1985; Woods & Lyons, 1990; Woods & Muller, 1988). I can also report a less formal indication of its validity from work with clients. Among the hundreds with whom I have discussed the report "Beliefs That Disturb," it has been very rare (2%–3%) to have clients disagree about the strength of their belief in any of the 10 areas. This is especially true in those areas where the test indicates strong acceptance of a given belief. I'll ask, "Does that sound right?" and receive almost uniform acknowledgment that it does.

ANALYZING AN EMOTIONAL EPISODE: HOMEWORK

After the series of basic minilectures and a discussion of the "Beliefs That Disturb" report based on the client's answers to the Jones Irrational Beliefs Test, I indicate that we are now ready to begin systematic homework. I present the RET theory and therapy flowchart shown in Figure 5 and "walk clients through it" one step at a time using a large version laid out in front of us. Although at first glance this flowchart looks overwhelming to many, by taking it one box and arrow at a time (recording it all on audiotape), I have had very little difficulty in getting clients to see the

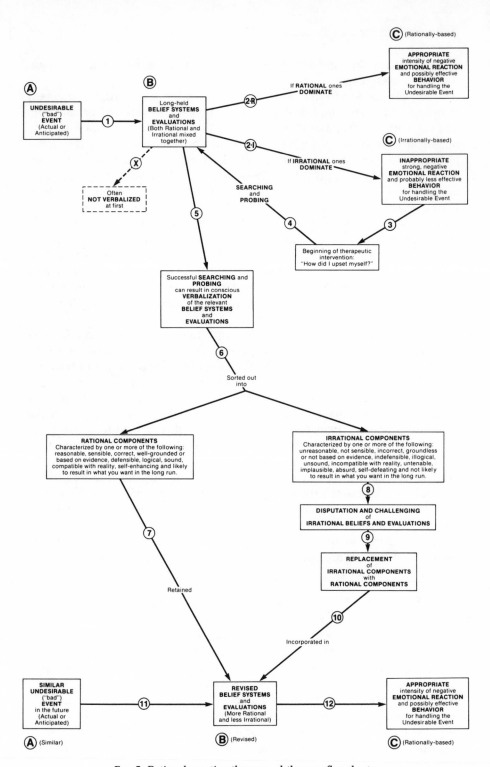

FIG. 5. Rational-emotive theory and therapy flowchart.

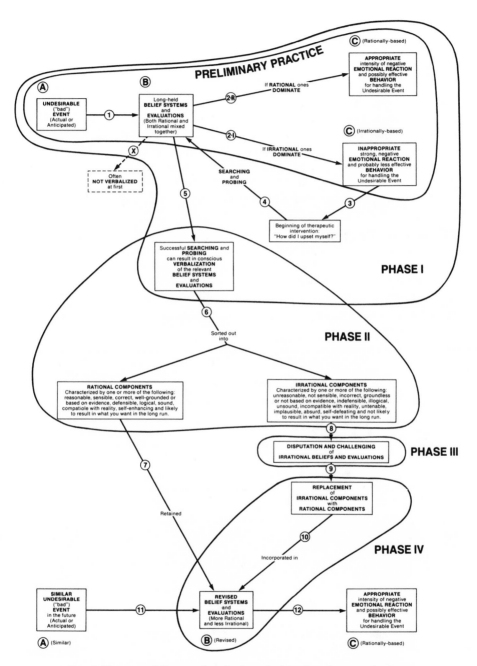

FIG. 6. Theory and therapy flowchart marked to show homework phases.

whole picture and understand the framework in which we are working. A common reaction is something like "It all makes so much sense!"—to which I respond with a reinforcing "Right! That's why we call it *rational-emotive therapy.*"

I then show them how we can work patiently, persistently, and consistently within this complex flowchart by proceeding gradually, one step at a time, with a series of homework assignments. These are presented on the same flowchart, as shown in Figure 6. Each phase of the homework series is explained, and questions are answered. If time permits, we do some of the "preliminary practice" exercises in the office. It time does not permit, the client is assigned to try several for homework.

I now discuss each phase in sequence.

Preliminary Practice

Experience has shown preliminary practice to be an essential clarification step before proceeding any further. The form used is shown in Figure 7. What appears so clear and obvious to RET practitioners, and to more

PRELIMINARY PRACTICE
AT
ANALYZING EMOTIONAL EPISODES

Take some, preferably simple, situation that you distressed yourself over such as misplacing something, getting behind a slow driver, having something break or fall, being ignored by a waitress or salesperson, or having to speak before a group. Try to think in our terms and analyze the episode according to A (what happened?), B (How you thought about it) and C (How you felt and acted).

Do C first because the disturbance you feel is often your first awareness that there is a problem.

- -

C. CONSEQUENCES: How did you _feel_ and what did you do?

A. ACTIVATING EVENT: What happened?

B. THOUGHTS   What went through your mind when
   AND   this event happened?
   EVALUATIONS:

FIG. 7. Homework form for preliminary practice (see Figure 6).

experienced clients, is just not very clear to the beginner. I think I have probably seen all possible confusions among As, Bs, and Cs with "simple" problems such as "I got mad because my car wouldn't start" or "The job interview made me anxious" or "She shouldn't have treated me like that." (At this stage, it is therefore usually not appropriate to point out that the As *can virtually be anything that the person is contemplating*, which includes Bs, Cs, AB connections, BC connections, and ABC sequences, i.e., the factors that with further Bs lead to *higher order* C-level problems.)

It is important to recognize that we are introducing clients to a new way of analyzing and understanding emotional and behavioral problems and that we are imposing *separations* in an ABC sequence, which has for them previously been a unitary, undifferentiated whole.

It usually requires no more than part of a session with a few, preferably client-generated, episodes to make significant progress in teaching the basic ABC classification scheme. (Note: Watch for and politely correct "I feel" statements when it is thoughts or beliefs that are being referred to.)

It is frustrating to both the therapist and the client to proceed further before the client is comfortable and skilled at this basic level.

Phase I

The homework form for this phase is shown in Figures 8 and 9. Following completion of the preliminary practice phase, I go over these forms with the client and then assign them for homework. The client may continue with an episode started in preliminary practice or may pick a new one, but I point out that, from here on, the same episode will be followed through all phases. For the first episode, something relatively uncomplicated is most effective, but of course, that is *not* a requirement. Also, more than one episode can be started at this time, and these multiple episodes can be followed together, one phase at a time, in subsequent sessions.

The client returns at the next session with a first attempt at Phase I. It may or may not still contain ABC confusions, but it almost always has serious B-level omissions. The omissions often involve, as is to be expected, failures to recognize nonverbalized but implied components: "He didn't call when he knew he was going to be late" (implied: *"as he should have!"*). When the therapist suspects, on the basis of knowledge of what thoughts or beliefs are likely to be causing, say, anger, as in this example, the strategy of prompting is used: "He didn't call as he . . . ?" Or if more is needed, "He didn't call as he ssssssssh . . . ." Most of the time, the client who has been brought to this stage finishes with "as he *should* have." Other omissions involve the total absence of components that RET theory indicates are quite likely to be present. For example, if there are no condemnatory thoughts or beliefs listed in an anger episode, the therapist can probe: "Well, what do you think he deserves for such a failure?" Such

ANALYZING AN EMOTIONAL EPISODE

PHASE I - CLARIFYING THE A B C 's

Episode name or code letter: _____ Date: _____
- -

A - - - triggers off - - → B - - - which causes - - → C

| Activating Event | Beliefs
About & Evaluations
of the Activating Event | Consequences:
Emotional Reaction &
Behavioral Response |

- -
PROBABLY THE FIRST ASPECT YOU WILL NOTICE IS THAT YOU ARE
EMOTIONALLY UPSET. TAKE THIS UPSET AS A SIGNAL FOR THE
APPROPRIATENESS OF THIS ANALYSIS AND AT YOUR EARLIEST
OPPORTUNITY, FILL OUT THE FOLLOWING AS COMPLETELY AS YOU CAN.
- -
C. EMOTIONAL & BEHAVIORAL CONSEQUENCES:
How did you feel - i.e., what was the nature of your disturbed emotional reaction?
And what did you do?

A. THE ACTIVATING EVENT:
This is the focus of your attention. It is often something that actually happened.
And what happened can include your own behavior or your own emotional
reaction over some previous episode. It can also be something in the future that
you were thinking might happen. In any case, it is usually a negative event that is
being contemplated.

FIG. 8. First part of homework form for Phase I (see Figure 6).

probing often elicits the suspected damning, blaming, or punitive thought. Thus, we proceed to flush out all the Bs for the Phase I stage of the "Analysis of an Emotional Episode."

Often, B-2 either is not filled in or is a restatement of items in B-1. In the first episode being worked on, I often let this part go. In subsequent episodes, however, it is often useful to probe for more general beliefs, such as "People shouldn't treat me in ways I don't like."

After discussion and agreement from the client, all additions and corrections are made in color on the homework form. It is handed back to the client for further checking and review. When we are both satisfied that we have a fairly thorough description of all aspects of the particular emotional episode, we then move to Phase II and focus on all the Bs.

Phase II

It's helpful to be able to get to this point in the same session in which Phase I is critiqued. The form for Phase II is shown in Figure 10. The client

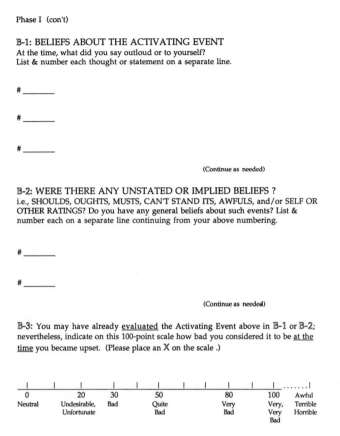

Phase I (con't)

B-1: BELIEFS ABOUT THE ACTIVATING EVENT
At the time, what did you say outloud or to yourself?
List & number each thought or statement on a separate line.

_____

_____

_____

(Continue as needed)

B-2: WERE THERE ANY UNSTATED OR IMPLIED BELIEFS ?
i.e., SHOULDS, OUGHTS, MUSTS, CAN'T STAND ITS, AWFULS, and/or SELF OR
OTHER RATINGS? Do you have any general beliefs about such events? List &
number each on a separate line continuing from your above numbering.

_____

_____

(Continue as needed)

B-3: You may have already evaluated the Activating Event above in B-1 or B-2;
nevertheless, indicate on this 100-point scale how bad you considered it to be at the
time you became upset. (Please place an X on the scale .)

0	20	30	50	80	100	Awful
Neutral	Undesirable, Unfortunate	Bad	Quite Bad	Very Bad	Very, Very Bad	Terrible Horrible

FIG. 9. Second part of homework form for Phase I (see Figure 6).

is asked to review the Phase II form and is then questioned about his or her understanding of the definitions of *rational* and *irrational*. Then, I read the numbered Bs one at a time, and the client is asked to classify each. Decisions about "rational" or "irrational" are verbalized by the client. If there is any disagreement, the decision is challenged and discussion ensues until we are both satisfied with the classification of each B-level component. (Challenges and discussions at this point usually serve to introduce and illustrate the next two phases of disputing and the creation of rational alternatives.) The form of Phase III is then reviewed and assigned for homework.

Phase III

The Phase III form shown in Figure 11 involves a systematic disputation of each of the B-level components designated as irrational in Phase II.

ANALYZING AN EMOTIONAL EPISODE

PHASE II - CLASSIFYING THE $\mathbb{B}$'s

Episode name or code letter: _____ Date: _____

- -

REFER BACK TO PHASE I FOR THIS EPISODE AND AFTER LOOKING AT WHAT
YOU ACTUALLY SAID OR THOUGHT TO YOURSELF ($\mathbb{B}$-1) AND ALSO WHAT
YOU BELIEVE ABOUT SUCH $\mathbb{A}$ - LEVEL EVENTS ($\mathbb{B}$-2) , SEE IF YOU CAN
DECIDE FOR EACH NUMBERED THOUGHT, STATEMENT OR BELIEF
WHETHER IT IS RATIONAL OR IRRATIONAL.

Write the numbers of each thought, statement or belief under Rational or Irrational

- -

Your thoughts statements and beliefs can be characterized by being either:

RATIONAL	OR	IRRATIONAL
reasonable, sensible, based on evidence, defensible, compatible with reality, self-enhancing, and likely to result in what you want in the long run?		unreasonable, not sensible, not based on evidence, indefensible, incompatible with reality, implausible, self-defeating, and not likely to result in what you want in the long run?

Rational $\mathbb{B}$-level items (rBs)   Irrational $\mathbb{B}$-level items (iBs)

  # _____   # _____

  # _____   # _____

  # _____   # _____

(Continue as needed)

FIG. 10. Homework form for Phase II (see Figure 6).

If all goes according to plan, the client returns to the next session with a disputation for each iB. I have the client *read* each disputation to me, and I play the role of a supportive drama coach as well as a helpful critic. Initially, most clients are not very good at disputing what they have formerly held with conviction. Hence, the strategy is to reinforce successive approximations to a thorough and convincing disputation. (The tape recording of this session is, I feel, particularly valuable.) I encourage clients to be enthusiastic and dramatic, and I model such responses for them.*

In the beginning, I don't expect very much from clients. They may produce nothing more than "That's irrational because I used the word

*Vigorous, dramatic, and enthusiastic disputation is what Ellis calls "emotive-evocative" disputation. Most clients do not do this well, and modeling by the therapist is very appropriate. Even if the content of the client's disputation is sound, we don't just want the words to be correct—we want voice volume, tone, pitch, and emphasis to be appropriate as well.

ANALYZING AN EMOTIONAL EPISODE

PHASE III - DISPUTING IRRATIONAL BELIEFS

Episode name or code letter: _____ Date: _____

- -

REFER TO THE <u>IRRATIONAL</u> LISTING IN PHASE II OF THE B-LEVEL
THOUGHTS, STATEMENTS AND BELIEFS FROM PHASE I. <u>COPY</u> EACH
IRRATIONAL BELIEF (iB) BELOW WITH ITS NUMBER. THEN ARGUE WHY IT
IS IRRATIONAL. THAT IS, CRITICALLY ATTACK OR DISPUTE EACH ONE.
GIVE AS MANY ARGUMENTS AS YOU CAN AGAINST EACH AND STATE
YOUR ARGUMENTS WITH PASSION.

- -

_____

_____

_____

_____

(Continue as needed)

- -

In the light of your above disputations, go back to the evaluation you made of the
Activating Event at the time you got upset (B-3 in Phase I).

Now, at this point in time, how would you evaluate that event?

0	20	30	50	80	100	Awful
Neutral	Undesirable, Unfortunate	Bad	Quite Bad	Very Bad	Very, Very Bad	Terrible Horrible

FIG. 11. Homework form for Phase III (see Figure 6).

should." I get them to really *attack* their demands, not just admit that they
made them.

It is also important to be sensitive to A-level disputations, for they
leave the Bs intact. For example, if the iB is "He shouldn't have insulted
me!" an inadequate A-level disputation would be "He really wasn't insulting me; he was just in a hurry." The client merely changed the A and left
the *should* intact. It is essential not to let clients get away with such an
"inelegant" argument: "You may be right that he really wasn't insulting
you, and it's good to have a realistic appraisal of things that go on. But let's
assume that his intention really *was* to insult you. Now, how can you attack
your belief that he *must not* talk to you that way?"[+]

[+]There is, of course, an important discussion between errors of inference and irrational beliefs, although one could argue that errors of inference are irrational because they are stress-
producing or self-defeating. At this stage in therapy, however, most clients have enough new
material to assimilate without being further burdened with more subtle distinctions.

After each disputation is critiqued and completed, I usually ask, "Does that convince you?" or, "Are you satisfied with your argument that the original statement was, indeed, irrational?"

Often, a review of Phase III with the probing, challenging, and modeling takes more than one session because digressions and further discussions develop along the way. When the review is completed, however, we move to Phase IV, the replacement of each irrational belief or statement with a rational alternative.

Phase IV

The form is shown in Figure 12, and I go over it with the client before assigning it as homework. We may even illustrate one or two rational alternatives. Initially, I thought this might be an easy assignment, es-

ANALYZING AN EMOTIONAL EPISODE

PHASE IV - CREATING RATIONAL ALTERNATIVES

Episode name or code letter: _____ Date: _____
- -
REFER TO EACH NUMBERED IRRATIONAL BELIEF (iB) THAT WAS DISPUTED IN PHASE III. NOW CONSTRUCT A RATIONAL ALTERNATIVE (rB) FOR EACH ONE.

IT WOULD BE BEST IF YOU WOULD AGAIN COPY EACH iB SO THAT YOU CAN COMPARE AND CONTRAST IT WITH THE RATIONAL ALTERNATIVE YOU CREATE.
- -

   iB # _____

   Alternative rB

   iB # _____

   Alternative rB

                                   (Continue as needed)
- -
As you disputed your irrational beliefs and changed them to rational ones, what feelings did you notice?

NOW GO BACK AND READ ALL OF YOUR ORIGINAL STATEMENTS FROM PHASE I THAT WERE CLASSIFIED AS RATIONAL IN PHASE II AND THEN ALL OF THE ABOVE RATIONAL ALTERNATIVES WITHOUT LOOKING AT ANYTHING ELSE. IF YOU CAN LEARN TO THINK THIS WAY, WHAT DO YOU PREDICT YOUR EMOTIONAL AND BEHAVIORAL REACTIONS CAN BE TO SIMILIAR ACTIVATING EVENTS IN THE FUTURE?

FIG. 12. Homework form for Phase IV (see Figure 6).

pecially compared to I and III, but for some, it is very difficult. I have had people draw a complete blank when asked to generate a rational alternative! "He really *shouldn't* have given me so much work to do!" was, for example, *all* one client could say regarding the fact that her boss had piled more work on her than she could manage.

It is important to monitor rational alternatives for sincerity and conviction. Again, the tape recording of the session is valuable to the client, especially in hearing that *very strong* preferential statements can be made as alternatives. Initially, client attempts may take the form of "I would *prefer* that he didn't talk to me that way," which just doesn't have the emotional intensity appropriate to the situation and therefore may degenerate to the original demanding belief: "He *shouldn't* have talked to me that way!" I may model with dramatic emphasis, "I would *very much prefer* that he didn't talk to me that way," or "It would be a *helluva lot better* if I were shown some respect!" In this manner, you can reinforce the RET point that it *is* appropriate to be annoyed or irritated when you are mistreated, but it is (1) *not* appropriate to be hostile or enraged and (2) *not* appropriate to be complacent or accepting of mistreatment either.

Conclusion

This systematic and persistent analysis of a given emotional episode through all phases has proved to be a very effective therapeutic and learning experience. It is rare that we do more than three or four episodes because the effects *generalize* and clients become able to carry out very rapid, condensed versions of the whole process. You know you are succeeding when clients call or come in and say with pride, "Let me tell you how I handled such and so this week."

Examples of Irrational Beliefs (iBs) with Disputational Responses and Rational Alternatives: Homework

The actual modeling of specific rational alternatives to specific irrational beliefs can be, I believe, a valuable adjunct to RET work. I have prepared a sampling of irrational thoughts and beliefs accompanied by rational alternatives for each of the following emotional problems: anxiety, depression, guilt, self-downing, anger, intimidation, and jealousy.

With a particular client, I have so far used only the sections that are directly relevant. (We are hoping to publish the entire set eventually.) Each section opens with a discussion of the emotional problem and a description of its cognitive origins. Then there is a page with only the illustrative listing of irrational beliefs, and the client is asked to check the ones she or he believes, at least some of the time. The remaining pages in the section repeat each iB followed by a disputational model of an alternative way of thinking.

I illustrate with two iBs selected from each section.

Anxiety

iB: I simply must perform well, and if I don't it will be terrible.

What I can think instead:

I have quite probably fallen back on the unsupportable notion that my performance will reflect negatively on my value as a person. That is, if I don't do well, that means I'm no good. I can become determined to accept myself nonjudgmentally as a human being, no matter how well or how poorly I do something. Then, my self-worth will not be placed on the line every time I have to perform, and it will no longer be terrible if I don't perform as well as I am capable of performing or as well as someone else is capable of performing.

I can merely try to do my best, within the constraints imposed by time and energy, then profit from my experience to help me perform better in the future. And I certainly do not have to rate or judge my *self* on the basis of my performance.

iB: What if he/she/they don't like me?

What I can think instead:

Well, what if he, she, or they don't like me? What does that mean? It certainly doesn't mean that there is automatically something wrong with me. After all, do I like everyone I meet? It may be that I have some characteristics of which these other people aren't fond. If they then decide that, because of those characteristics, they don't like me, they are the ones making a mistake: they are judging me rather than my behavior or characteristics, and that is their problem. And, after all, there are other people who *do* like me, aren't there? We may just be different or incompatible; I may not be wrong at all. Anyway, wouldn't it be a dull world if there were no differences among people?

At worst, they may have valid reasons for disliking my characteristics or behavior (i.e., if I chronically lie or am truly lazy). In that case, I can think, "Well here are some things I need to work on to change," and I can begin to take concrete steps to improve my behavior. But even if my behavior is not what I or others would like it to be, I am no less a worthwhile person. No one is perfect or ever will be. We all have room for improvement.

Depression

iB: If only I had been treated better when I was younger, I wouldn't be where I am now. But as I was treated badly, I am what I am, and there is very little I can do to change myself.

What I can think instead:

Where in the world did I get the idea that I can develop and change only up to a certain magical point in my life, and that then, after that point, I am finished and can never do anything or have any experience that will make a difference? People are changing and improving their lives every day, even into old age. There is only one point in my life at which it is too late for me to change, and that is death. Until then, I can, and will, work at improving matters and changing myself. And I can work at this task even though I was treated badly and even though that bad treatment may have contributed to my current situation and status in life. That was then; this is now. What I do from this point is what counts.

iB: It seems that no matter how hard I try, I can never succeed.

What I can think instead:

Of course there are some things at which I have not succeeded, but it is totally incorrect to tell myself that I have never succeeded. I wouldn't be alive now if that were true. What is probably going on is that there are some things I consider important at which I have not succeeded. That's disappointing, it's true. But just because it *seems* as if no matter how hard I try I never succeed, that doesn't mean it is really the case. My thinking has become distorted on this subject. And anyway, almost all people fail at some things they consider important. The thing for me to do is to evaluate my strengths and weaknesses objectively (perhaps with help from others who know me) and then to try for success at things that match my strengths.

(I can also try things that do not match my talents, just for the sheer pleasure of challenging myself in new areas, even though I know I may not succeed. After all, success isn't everything!)

I have also very likely been telling myself that success shouldn't be so hard. Nonsense. Most things worth having take a great deal of effort to obtain, and I *can* continue to try harder, and harder, and harder to get and achieve what I want.

Guilt

iB: I have done some really bad things, and that means that I am basically no good.

What I can think instead:

I have done some really bad things, and what that means is that "I have done some really bad things." And that's all that means! It doesn't mean that I am basically no good. If I were, then that would mean that everything I have ever done or possibly could do would be bad. A "no-good" person could really never do anything worthwhile, or correct, or good. Therefore, obviously, no one in the world, including me, can correctly be labeled as "no good."

I can decide that I am sorry, or regretful, over the "bad" things I did, and I can try to consider whether there is anything I can do now to help reduce the badness of my past mistakes. I can, for example, apologize to those who have been affected by my "bad" behavior, and I can try to assure them that I plan to reduce my "bad" actions in the future. I can also see if there is anything I can work on to undo any harm or damage I may have done.

But most important, I can gain motivation to work on improving my behavior in the future by giving up the self-damning, guilt- and depression-producing notion that I am "no good."

iB: I can never forgive myself for the things that I have done.

What I can think instead:

I had darned well better accept the fact that I am a mistake-making, nonperfect human being just like everyone else. I don't have to forgive myself any more than I have to condemn myself. I can work hard at changing my thinking, toward the goal of just plain accepting myself. If I make progress in moving toward such a goal I will markedly reduce my guilt and depression. If I reduce my guilt and depression, then I will be more motivated and more effective in my program to improve my behavior from now on.

Self-Downing

iB: I can never do anything right!

What I can think instead:

I may do some things wrong or poorly, but that certainly doesn't mean that I can never do anything right. I probably think this way because I, like most other people, seem to remember the bad things better. Then, when I again do something unfortunate, undesirable, or unwise, I actively search my memory so as to recall previous errors. I don't have to do this. I don't have to keep focusing on my weak points and mistakes.

In all fairness I can just as well "balance the picture out" and remember that I have, indeed, done a few things right. (There was that time in ninth-grade algebra when I solved an equation at the blackboard. And then that time in high school when I passed that test when I didn't think I would. And so forth.) If my memory and patience held out, I could, indeed, list thousands of things that I have done right in my life. So I had better stop being negative. When I feel better, after recognizing that I have succeeded many times, I can see that if I can learn something from my mistakes, I can decrease their frequency.

iB: I am not the person I should be.

What I can think instead:

Does that mean I shouldn't be the person I am, that I should be somebody else? That makes no sense at all.

Instead of making a global rating of myself as a person, I can focus on some particular skills or abilities that I would like to change or improve on. Instead of saying, "I am not the person I should be," I can say, "I am a person who has some characteristics or skill deficits that I would like to change."

Then, after this major change in outlook, from downing myself totally to merely examining some of my qualities critically, I had better consider whether it is feasible to change those that I don't like. And at this point, it's important for me to differentiate what I can change from what I can't, and then to accept the latter while I focus on how I can deal with the former. In any case, whatever I decide to do, I can focus on trying to accept myself just as I had better accept the rest of reality. Actually, things should be the way they are, and I should be the way I am. But because I am able to influence some aspects of the future, I can work on those things that can be changed and stop focusing on the past and downing myself for being the way I am.

Anger

iB: I must always have what I want without any trouble.

What I can think instead:

On the surface, it appears as if it would be nice to get everything I want without any trouble, but then I would be less likely to appreciate what I did get. Further, there is no reason why I must always have what I want. No one else always gets what they want. What makes me so special?

iB: People should always be nice to me, and I have the right to be deeply hurt when they are not.

What I can think instead:

I don't particularly like it when people are not nice to me, but I surely can stand it. People are often not nice for reasons that have nothing to do with me anyway. They may themselves be disturbed or have problems about which they are upsetting themselves and may be taking out their upset on me. Therefore, I shouldn't take their behavior to heart. Actually, people are nice to me sometimes, and if I reduce my anger by changing my attitudes and ideas, then more people will be nice to me more often.

Further, I have the right to be deeply hurt, but that's a right it would be better for me not to exercise. If I replace the wrong belief that people should be nice to me with the alternatives above, I won't experience the pain that comes from this wrong thinking.

Intimidation

iB: Power is all that counts. Pushing people around shows that I've got power, and that makes me someone.

What I can think instead:

First of all, I don't have to "be someone." I don't have to be big, important, or powerful to accept and like myself. I can just be me.

Pushing people around doesn't even show that I've got power or importance to start with. "Power" to deal with people and challenges in life comes from skill and knowledge, not from pushing others around. People who deserve power or prestige or respect deserve it because of knowledge or skills or abilities they possess to achieve things in life (as long as they exercise these things), not because they are merely bullies who push others around.

iB: The only thing that matters is what I want, and it doesn't matter who has to get pushed around for me to get what I want.

What I can think instead:

If everyone believed this, then no one would be safe, including me! What I want is important, but it is not the only thing that matters. Other people have rights, and their rights deserve to be honored. If they are not honored, then my rights will not be honored either. If no one's rights are honored, then we are all in danger. I can work for what I want and try to get it as long as the rights of others are not violated.

Jealousy

iB: I can't stand it when my partner pays attention to someone else.

What I can think instead:

I can recognize that it is *probably not* a threat to our relationship. I can hope that my partner may even feel better about me or appreciate me even more after having paid attention to others. But no matter what, I had better stop telling myself, "I can't stand it." I may not like it, but I darn well can stand it. In fact, I could even try *liking* the fact that my partner at times attends to others who appear to appreciate it and enjoy it. After all, would I want a partner no one else liked or thought attractive?

iB: There may be something wrong with me if someone I care about pays too much attention to others.

What I can think instead:

I don't *have to* automatically assume that there is something "wrong" with me just because someone I care about pays attention to someone else. If my partner or friend or child happens to enjoy a particular movie star or a particular popular musician, I doubt if I would think that there was something "wrong" with me. Just as there is nothing "wrong" with me if I am not a popular star of some sort, there is nothing "wrong" with me if someone I care about attends to others at times. Of course I am *different* from these others, but that's all—just different, not inferior or bad or "wrong." In fact, it's partly because of my particular characteristics or differences that many of the people I care about also attend to and care about me—at least once in a while.

*   *   *   *   *

To the best of my knowledge at the time of writing there did not exist a comparable strategy as detailed as this throughout the entire extensive RET literature. We actually have about 90 such iB-rB examples plus several other strategies. One of them is related to anxiety production:

The "What Ifs"

Very often, anxiety is produced by our focusing on some future possibility, evaluating it as a disaster or catastrophe, and telling ourselves that we would be helpless to deal with it if it occurred. Thoughts such as these are implied in the question, "What if . . . ?" Some examples of these "what ifs" are:

WHAT IF

_____ I can't find a job
_____ I panic
_____ I lose my job
_____ I get criticized
_____ I fail
_____ I do something foolish
_____ I make a mistake
_____ I can't pay my bills
_____ I die

Many clients accept the reality of such questions and admit their involvement in anxiety production. Yet it is rare to find anyone who has actually *answered* his or her "what if" questions. People merely assume that the consequences will be "awful" and very rarely "deawfulize" by answering their questions: "So what if such and such *does* happen? What could you possibly do to handle, cope, or deal with it?" Thus the approach is to focus on the formulation of some answers. Take as an example, "What if I lose my job?" Here is a model for a response:

1. First of all, I can resist the temptation to focus exclusively on all the problems and hassles that getting fired or laid off might create.

There is actually no guarantee that losing my job will even be bad. It may turn out that it might be one of the better things to happen to me. I might find a better job, with higher pay, greater personal satisfaction, or much improved working conditions.

2. While resisting the temptation to focus on the problems created by my loss of the job, I can look for and write down all of the things I can think of that I could possibly do if I did lose my job.

For example, I could

- Register with the state employment agency.
- Register with private employment agencies.
- Check the want ads daily and follow up on any that sound appropriate.
- Call people I know in other businesses or companies.
- Contact those who have offered me jobs before.
- Prepare a résumé and circulate it with an appropriate covering letter.
- Put an ad in the newspaper.
- Get a book on job-hunting strategies and look for other ideas.
- Consider retraining in another field, with the help of government loans.

When the client realizes that there are many things that can be done, the net effect is "deawfulizing" the previous assumed catastrophe and, hence, markedly reducing anxiety over the "what if" question.

BUILDING POSITIVE SELF-REGARD: AN INELEGANT STEP ALONG THE WAY TO UNCONDITIONAL SELF-ACCEPTANCE

Building self-esteem is not a therapeutic strategy recommended by RET because, although temporarily helpful, it nevertheless involves self-rating rather than the more elegant self-acceptance. Occasionally, however, I find a strategy requiring the client to make a series of positive statements about himself or herself to be dramatically useful as a step toward the elegant solution. Some people have been selectively attending to and emphasizing their faults, weaknesses, mistakes, and failures to such an extent that they have great difficulty in comprehending a nonjudgmental, self-accepting view.

I have selected a large number of traits, qualities, and characteristics from a compulsively thorough search of the English language conducted many years ago by Allport and Odbert (1936). They found 17,953 terms used to describe traits, moods, personal conduct, and so on, and I have selected a large number of these to constitute a stimulus pool that contains a wide variety of suggestions for the client.

I once introduced this strategy to a client by saying, "You've been telling me a lot of your faults, mistakes, and weaknesses. How about making a list of some of your good qualities?" Her response was "Dr. Woods, that's a list that will never begin." Over the next 20–30 minutes, she then created, in response to my suggestions of individual traits, qualities, and characteristics, 10 or 12 positively-stated short paragraphs about herself. Each paragraph elaborated on a single stimulus term and was an unexaggerated, realistic statement that she felt was honest and true. After we finished with just these 10 or 12, I had her read them over and asked how she then felt about herself. She grudgingly admitted that she did, indeed, feel better. Her mood improved even more when it was pointed out that all of the characteristics we had thus far explored began with the letter *a*. We had the entire remaining alphabet to continue with! The "shock value" of such a realization then made it unnecessary to continue.

You can have people write these sorts of positive descriptions on 3 × 5 cards to be posted in private places, carried around, and reviewed. It is a worthwhile strategy to consider with those who are depressed and/or self-downing.

One Strategy for Coping with Depression

These are personal characteristics that many people have but don't take much notice of. When feeling "down" or depressed, it is worthwhile to "look at the other side" and remind oneself that there are good things, too. Look at this list and write a sentence or two about yourself using as many of these as apply to you. Don't be overly modest! Be truthful and honest with yourself. You are the only one who is going to look at this.

Example with a positive "trait":
     Considerate. "I would say that I am generally a very considerate person. I care about others and their feelings. Considering that there are many who are not considerate, I am pleased and proud of this trait in me."

Example with a negative "trait":
     Hostile. "I am definitely not a hostile person. I am generally quite friendly and positive towards others."

Argumentative	Decent	Musical
Artistic	Devoted	Mature
Angry	Dishonest	Mean
Attentive	Enthusiastic	Neat
Agreeable	Flexible	Neighborly
Approachable	Forgiving	Nagging
Brutal	Friendly	Normal
Busy-body	Fortunate	Optimistic
Beloved	Generous	Orderly
Calm	Gentle	Passionate
Careful	Good-natured	Patient
Cheerful	Grateful	Peaceful
Caring	Genuine	Pretty
Concerned	Healthy	Pleasant
Capable	Helpful	Polite
Clean living	Honest	Proud
Clean	Hostile	Reasonable
Compassionate	Irrational	Responsible
Confidant	Interesting	Reverent
Considerate	Jealous	Respectable
Cooperative	Kind	Sensitive
Cruel	Level-headed	Sexy
Deceitful	Loving	Tender
Dependable	Loyal	Warm

For some of these, it is more appropriate to make a list, e.g., a list of things you are capable of doing, a list of things you are grateful for, etc.

Keep what you have written available. Study these statements so that you remember them, especially look at them whenever you begin to feel depressed.

FIG. 13. Selected items from a stimulus pool of traits, qualities, and characteristics with instructions for use in coping with depression.

An abbreviated version of the list with instructions that I have prepared as a hand-out appears in Figure 13.

EVIDENCE OF THE EFFECTIVENESS OF THE ABOVE STRATEGIES

The procedures for applying RET described in this chapter have been developed over a period of time, and they will continue to evolve and change with experience and critical feedback from colleagues and clients. The homework forms, for example, were improved after several years of experience and valuable suggestions from a number of colleagues with whom they were shared.

Also, the therapeutic approach varies with the needs of the client, and each series of individual therapy sessions is unique. Yet, in recent years, the general plan and sequence have been reasonably consistent with the outline of this chapter for almost all clients seen for emotional-behavioral problems.

Motivated by the preparation of this chapter, I searched all my client files for a five-year period (1984–1988) seeking data relevant to the effectiveness of the general RET approach described. Because I have full-time obligations as a professor of psychology, my private practice is of necessity a part-time venture. And because we are interested only in data relevant to client work dominated by my application of RET, my search excluded from consideration all persons seen for injury-related pain problems, weight control and smoking control, and any parents advised on child management problems. RET is, of course, appropriate in these areas, and it was applied, but not in the same consistent manner as is outlined in this chapter. To describe the file search in another way, I selected only those people who had sought my services exclusively for psychoneurotic problems (i.e., severe inappropriate emotional reactions). As a final restriction, I excluded anyone seen in therapy for less than four hours. All of these restrictions produced a final sample of 176 clients for study.

Everyone initially responded to a battery of diagnostic tests; many were then retested on selected instruments relevant to their problems, following a sequence of therapy sessions. The instrument I have most commonly used on these limited retests has been the Trait Scale of the State-Trait Anxiety Inventory (STAI; Spielberger, Gorsuch, & Lushene, 1970). This instrument was chosen because high levels of anxiety are among the most common presenting problems in the clients I see (as will be documented below). Anxiety is also defensible as a choice for study because of the role it plays in human misery and physical suffering (see, for example, Woods & Lyons, 1990). The client files that contained retests on the STAI numbered 109, representing 61.9% of those seen in therapy for psychoneurotic problems over the five-year period under study.

Data pulled on these 109 retested clients included their retest STAI scores and the number of therapy sessions before the retest. The data pulled on all 176 clients included the initial STAI score, age, sex, and total number of sessions up to termination of therapy.

The distributions for the retested group of initial STAI scores and retest scores are shown in Figure 14. Large dramatic reductions in anxiety are clearly apparent in this figure. On the initial testing, the median score was 55, which is approximately the 95th percentile. By retest, the median

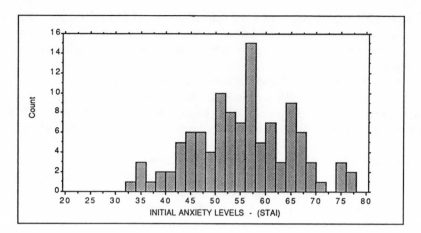

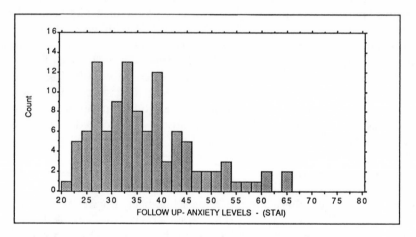

FIG. 14. Initial and follow-up tests on anxiety (STAI).

had dropped to 34, which is about the 50th percentile. At retest, 93.6% of the clients scored below the median of the initial test. Inferential statistics are hardly necessary, as the means of these two distributions are almost two standard deviations apart! (Initial test: $M = 54.8$; $SD = 9.7$. Retest: $M = 35.8$; $SD = 9.8$. $t(108) = 18.93$, $p < .0001$.)

How long did it take clients to achieve such an effect with RET? The mean number of sessions before retest was 8.5, and the median was 7. Note that it took *at most* this number of sessions to produce this lowering in anxiety scores. Some may have achieved lower anxiety in fewer sessions; it was just not measured until a "convenient" time. Clients, after all, are not research subjects to be tested at predetermined intervals. What happened was more like "Well, you appear to be doing much better. Let's recheck a few of the scales we initially used to see how much progress you have really made." Because this rechecking did not occur in 67 cases, it is not known whether nonretested clients were different in any important ways from the retested group. Differences would clearly limit the generality of the reported results.

Table 1 summarizes the results of the data that were obtained. There were no significant differences in age or sex composition between the retested and the nonretested groups, but the nonretested group was slightly, but significantly, less anxious initially and had been seen for a smaller total number of therapy sessions at termination. The nonretested group terminated, on the average, at about the time that the remaining clients were retested. Thus, some of them would have been retested soon had they not finished therapy. The reason that some of the remaining clients were not retested with the STAI was that they had scored lower on anxiety initially. (Eleven people, or 16.4% of this group were at or below the 50th percentile initially, compared to only one person in the retested group.)

In any case, the retested group was slightly more anxious initially and was seen for a longer time. These differences make even more impressive the finding that, typically, 7–8.5 hours of rational-emotive therapy, applied as described, was successful in reducing anxiety from the 95th to the 50th percentile.

One could, of course, argue that these results were achieved not because of RET, but because of something like the "unique persuasive power over clients" possessed by the author, that is, idiosyncratic characteristics of the therapist rather than the therapeutic strategy itself. The continued

TABLE 1. A Comparison of Retested and Nonretested Groups

		Retested group ($n = 109$)	Nonretested group ($n = 67$)	Statistic
Initial anxiety level (STAI)				
	M	54.8	51.3	$t(174) = 2.00$
	SD	9.7	13.3	$p < .05$
Age				
	M	35.3	37.3	$t(174) = 1.14$
	SD	11.5	11.0	ns
Sex composition				
	Male	41.3%	47.8%	$X^2(1) = 0.71$
	Female	58.7%	52.2%	ns
Number of therapy sessions at termination				
	M	12.4	7.5	$t(174) = 4.54$
	SD	8.3	4.2	$p < .001$

accumulation of evidence can answer this argument, and much has already appeared in the literature (DiGiuseppe & Miller, 1977; Lyons & Woods, in press; McGovern & Silverman, 1984). It is to be hoped that, as strategies for increasing the effectiveness of RET are applied by therapists motivated to collect, analyze, and report additional relevant data, we will be able to present increasingly definitive results showing that it is the reasonableness and validity of the theory and therapy of RET that are working rather than some unique characteristics of individual therapists.

REFERENCES

Allport, G. W., & Odbert, H. S. (1936). Trait-names. A psycho-lexical study. *Psychological Monographs, 47*(211).

Bredekin, T. (1988). *Irrationality profiles for inward and outward expression of anger.* Unpublished master's thesis, Hollins College, Roanoke, VA.

DiGiuseppe, R. A., & Miller, N. J. (1977). A review of outcome studies on rational-emotive therapy. In A. Ellis & R. Grieger (Eds.), *Handbook of rational-emotive therapy.* New York: Springer.

Ellis, A., & Dryden, W. (1987). *The practice of rational-emotive therapy.* New York: Springer.

Gentilini, J. M. (1988). *Suicide ideation and irrational beliefs in a college population.* Unpublished honors thesis, Hollins College, Roanoke, VA.

Grieger, R., & Boyd, J. (1980). *Rational-emotive therapy: A skills based approach.* New York: Van Nostrand Reinhold.

Luttrell, V. R. (1987). *Irrational beliefs, stressful thoughts, anger expression, and anxiety and their relationship to premenstrual syndrome.* Unpublished master's thesis, Hollins College, VA.

Lyons, L. C., & Woods, P. J. (in press). The efficacy of rational-emotive therapy: A quantitative review of the outcome research. *Clinical Psychology Review.*

McGovern, T. E., & Silverman, M. S. (1984). A review of outcome studies of rational-emotive therapy from 1977 to 1982. *Journal of Rational-Emotive Therapy, 2,* 7–18.

Oesterle, S. (1984). *Anxiety, anger, and anger expression and their relationship to physical illness.* Unpublished master's thesis, Hollins College, Roanoke, VA.

Secrist, L. K. (1986). *A split-half test of reliability on the Jones Irrational Beliefs Test and irrationality profiles for inward and outward expression of anger.* Unpublished master's thesis, Hollins College, Roanoke, VA.

Spielberger, C. D., Gorsuch, R. L., & Lushene, R. E. (1970). *The State-Trait Anxiety Inventory.* Palo Alto, CA: Consulting Psychologists Press.

Woods, P. J. (1983). On the relative independence of irrational beliefs. *Rational Living, 18,* 23–24.

Woods, P. J. (1984). Further indications on the validity and usefulness of the Jones Irrational Beliefs Test. *Journal of Rational-Emotive Therapy, 2,* 3–6.

Woods, P. J. (1987a). Do you really want to maintain that a flat tire can upset your stomach? Using the findings of the psychophysiology of stress to bolster the argument that people are not directly disturbed by events. *Journal of Rational-Emotive Therapy, 5,* 149–161.

Woods, P. J. (1987b). Reductions in Type A behavior, anxiety, anger, and physical illness as related to changes in irrational beliefs: Results of a demonstration project in industry. *Journal of Rational-Emotive Therapy, 5,* 213–237.

Woods, P. J., & Coggin, S. (1985). Irrationality profiles for anger and anxiety. *Journal of Rational-Emotive Therapy, 3,* 124–129.

Woods, P. J., & Lyons, L. C. (1990). Irrational beliefs and psychosomatic disorders. *Journal of Rational-Emotive & Cognitive-Behavior Therapy, 8,* 3–20.

Woods, P. J., & Muller, G. E. (1988). The contemplation of suicide: Its relationship to irrational beliefs in a client sample and the implications for long range suicide prevention. *Journal of Rational-Emotive & Cognitive-Behavior Therapy, 6,* 236–258.

REGIME

A Counseling and Educational Model for Using RET Effectively

ROBERT W. DAWSON

Cognitive-behavioral approaches, in general, and RET, in particular, have been criticized for overfocusing on cognitive dimensions and cognitive techniques while inadequately dealing with the affective dimensions of patients' problems (e.g., Corey, 1982). The six-stage model outlined in this chapter under the acronym of *REGIME* emphasizes the affective, cognitive, and action dimensions of behavior. By highlighting microcounseling skills, the cognitive BC link, goal setting, and a multimodal approach to both assessment and intervention, it also sequences the therapeutic processes that are necessary for positive outcomes.

REGIME was developed as a result of my experience as a practitioner and teacher of rational-emotive therapy. In my first psychology position after completing graduate school, I was for some time what I now call a "mad-dog disputer." I was so well trained to "look for the should's, look for the must's" that I tended to attack them as soon as they reared their irrational heads. I tended to neglect completely the importance of first establishing with the client an understanding of the link between irrational thinking and disturbing emotions and self-defeating behaviors.

I am sure that I confused the hell out of a number of clients, turning at the drop of a *should* from an active listener to an active, argumentative disputer. In retrospect, I now realize that not only did this seem out of character for me in terms of my client's expectations of my active, empathic listening, but my clients also failed to understand why I suddenly ques-

ROBERT W. DAWSON • Australian Institute for Rational-Emotive Therapy, P.O. Box 1160, Carlton, Victoria, Australia 3053, and Community Training Systems, 459 Swanston Street, Melbourne, Australia 3000.

tioned their sensibilities. Giving the spiel of "It's as simple as ABC" too early in the counseling process often failed to result in the client's comprehension of the BC link, for this explanation seemed to be met with only limited enthusiasm and understanding from average clients, who wanted to do the talking and who were strongly distracted from listening and comprehending by the intensity of their emotionality. I now clearly see that there is little point in disputing the client's thinking if the client isn't ready to listen and, even if listening, doesn't understand or believe in the link between such thoughts and problem emotions and behaviors.

In my early days, I overlooked the importance of microcounseling skills (e.g., Egan, 1986) and of establishing good rapport with my clients. In view of the vigor with which Albert Ellis (1977) stresses the basics of RET, to look for "shoulds" and "musts" and to determinedly dispute them, it is easy to understand how students of RET might overlook the importance of giving clients an opportunity to express their feelings and might overlook the power of empathy in allowing the client to feel she or he is understood and, as a result, to be willing to listen, to understand, and to effectively use the ABC model of RET.

Some 10 years after my first psychology job, I was reminded of my mad-dog disputing behavior by the enthusiasm for disputation shown by the graduate students whom I was training in RET. However, I discovered through a considerable amount of trial and error that this enthusiasm could be channeled effectively through following a framework that highlighted and ordered the application of strategies in the counseling process.

REGIME offers both the neophyte and the experienced RET practitioner a convenient method of teaching and remembering the framework of processes, steps, and strategies that order and assimilate microcounseling skills within the broad spectrum of RET. Moreover, REGIME promotes the sequencing of the initial stages of RET in order to produce the most efficacious results (e.g., it stresses the importance of teaching emotional responsibility and of setting emotional and behavioral goals before launching into disputational interventions).

REGIME: Objectives, Therapist Strategies, and Client Behaviors

The six stages of the model emphasize the importance of:

R: The therapeutic relationship
E: Emotional responsibility
G: Goal setting
I: Interventions that are specifically goal-directed
M: Monitoring homework
E: Evaluating change, and eventually exit

Table 1 gives an overview of objectives, illustrative therapist strategies, and desired client behaviors during sessions for each stage of the model. Examples of therapist strategies are meant to be illustrative rather than prescriptive. It is assumed that therapists will use their own mix of RET techniques to achieve the goals and desired client behavior at each stage.

REGIME: STAGES OF THERAPEUTIC PROCESS

Stage 1: The Relationship between Client and Therapist

An effective therapy outcome depends on the establishment of a "special" relationship between therapist and client (e.g., Garfield, 1989), and RET is no exception. This relationship is made qualitatively different from the many existing relationships between the client and other individuals by the willingness of the therapist to listen accurately to, to reflect back, and to talk about the client's emotions without offering opinions or judgments in return. The importance of the relationship stage of REGIME is to help clients recognize and clarify both their practical and their emotional problems while building rapport with their therapist.

Rapport is often regarded as a basic ingredient serving as a prerequisite for the establishment of such a relationship. Suggestions of maintaining unconditional positive regard and staying in the frame of reference of the client are good advice for the RET therapist on how to achieve rapport.

However, it is necessary to go beyond rapport to establish the special nature of the relationship required for effective outcomes. This relationship within the REGIME model is created through the therapist's making reflections of the type: "You feel (some range of emotional experiences), when (some set of circumstances or events)," or "When (circumstances), you feel (emotions)."

A common mistake made by therapists during this stage is to make reflections preceded by "You feel" or "You feel that," which are really reflections of the client's opinions, judgments, or viewpoints, for example, "When your boyfriend flirts with other women at parties, you feel betrayed. You feel that he doesn't care enough for you."

Such reflections can lead the therapist to think that he or she is coming to grips with the emotional disturbance of the client, when in fact he or she is reflecting the client's cognitions, not experienced emotions. With the above example, reflections of emotions could be "When your boyfriend flirts with other women at parties you feel angry" or "You feel hurt and anxious."

The relationship stage is finished when the therapist accurately hears, understands, clarifies, and reflects back to clients their practical and emotional disturbances.

In practice over the years, I have come to appreciate the thoroughness

TABLE 1. REGIME: A Six-Stage Model for Teaching and Using Rational-Emotive Therapy

Objectives	Therapist strategies	Client behaviors
Stage 1. Relationship Develop rapport with the client through a trusting and accepting relationship. Increase client awareness of the A,B,C's.	Emphatic reflective listening, unconditional positive regard, helpful questioning, summarizing.	Identify the variety of different problem circumstances and associated reactions (emotions, actions, sensations). Assess intensity of emotions.
Stage 2. Emotional responsibility Break the direct link between circumstances and feelings. Highlight B's both specific irrational beliefs in specific situations and the overall irrational belief system. Have the client take responsibility for problem emotions and behavior.	Sentence completion questioning, reframing and developing different viewpoints, outlining, summarizing.	Demonstrate understanding of the "When . . . .(A) . . . " "You feel . . . .(C) . . . " "Because you think. . . . .(B). . . " link
Stage 3. Goal setting Work on one problem at a time from the initial set of problem circumstances; establish emotional and behavioral change goals. Achievement of these goals requires the identification of problem BC links, as well as the practical problems faced by the client. Ongoing work will return to this stage to address new goals as appropriate.	Questioning; clarifying; facilitating a consideration of consequences.	Involvement in prioritizing of problems and associated goal setting. Demonstration of consequential thinking. Accepting responsibility for change.

Stage 4. Intervention Dispute and restructure cognitions acting as obstacles to goals. Generate goal-facilitating cognitions. Remedy behavioral skills deficits (physiological, emotional, and behavioral).	Full range of cognitive, emotional, behavioral, and physiological techniques. Establishing session agendas, negotiating homework. Returning to earlier stages of the model as necessary.	Work on the disputation of irrational and antiempirical cognitions; acquire behavioral skill resources.
Stage 5. Monitoring homework Enable clients to apply skills acquired in therapy in their natural environment; generalize and maintain RET self-management skills. Help clients overcome low frustration tolerance.	Set and review homework; monitor and contrast progress against goals; encourage generalization of skills; recycle to Stage 3 to deal with different problems.	Discuss difficulties and successes in homework. Fine-tune the implementation and generalization of skills. Help evaluate the therapeutic process.
Stage 6. Evaluation and exit Assess outcomes. Initiate client evaluation and closure of therapy.	Reassess client, e.g., using the BASIC ID evaluation of goal attainment, encourage continued personal responsibility, self-generated homework, and self-rewards. Set date for follow-up session.	Show readiness for therapy termination, become involved in review process, outline planned program to consolidate self-help skills, and agree to attend follow-up session.

provided by the BASIC ID and Multi-Modal Therapy (Kwee & Lazarus, 1986; Lazarus, 1981) in the initial assessment of my clients. I rely on the dynamics outlined in the above relationship phase to ensure the development of a therapeutic relationship with my clients. However, I use the seven dimensions of Lazarus's approach to guide my assessment of the totality of my client's presenting problems.

I do not use these dimensions as a shopping list in asking clients about their life. At the end of the initial session, I review the notes that I have taken (I was trained under the premise that, if I am comfortable in taking notes, my clients will also be, and that has been my experience) and re-write them across the seven dimensions of behavior, affect, sensations, imagery, cognitions, interpersonal relationships, and, finally, diet, drugs, and lifestyle. It frequently occurs that I have insufficient or no detail on one or more dimensions.

At the beginning of the second session, I ask specific questions of my client regarding the dimensions in question. When I have adequate detail on all seven dimensions, I summarize my assessment to the client. The BASIC ID framework lends a thoroughness and understanding to a summary that rarely fails to impress. Impressing clients at this stage of counseling significantly enhances the likelihood of their cooperation, their motivation, and their acceptance of responsibility for their emotional disturbance.

Stage 2: Emotional Responsibility

In the second stage of the REGIME model, the therapist helps clients recognize their own contributory role in their emotional reactions to themselves, others, and environmental circumstances. The therapist does this by didactically teaching the relationship between the As, the Bs and the Cs.

The message being communicated in this stage is that different people react differently in the same circumstances—even if the difference is one of intensity rather than necessarily of kind—because each person is contributing differently to her or his own reactions. For example, under the same conditions someone else may be angry like the client but, unlike the client, may be much more angry.

There are a number of different ways in which a therapist can assist the client to reach this insight. The method that I have developed is to use a sentence completion task couched in the context of concomitant As and Cs. We know that correlation does not necessarily imply causation. By asking a question that implies that some information is missing, we can facilitate our clients' discovering this wisdom for themselves. For example, "When (circumstances) happen, you feel . . . "(N.B.: The feelings reflected here are the client's emotions and sensations, not their cognitive feelings, i.e., opinions, guesses, forecasts, etc.). Then I add the question, "Because?" This powerful one-word extractor of the cognitive causal links between As and Cs works best when it is stated in a clearly questioning tone. For example, "When you were about to give your talk, you felt anxious, tense, and sweaty—because . . . ?"

Many clients respond to this question by repeating the circumstance (the when), for example, "Because I was about to stand up and give my talk!" When this occurs, the therapist wants to persevere with the question: "Yes, when you stood up and were about to talk you felt anxious and sweaty—because?" The message that there is something clearly missing in the client's explanation can be most clearly given by therapists' raising their tone of voice on the second syllable of *because* and at the same time drawing it out somewhat.

Through this line of questioning, the therapist seeks to draw attention to and then to identify and clarify the cognitive (perceiving and evaluating) link or connection that the client is making between the circumstance and the experienced emotions.

On occasion, this approach will not work. Clients sometimes persist in answering the "because" question with restatements of the circumstances without any detail of associated cognitions. When this occurs, a fall-back position is to ask the client to imagine the hypothetical situation of 10 or even 100 other people in the same circumstance and to guess at what they would be feeling. Would they all be feeling the same things? If the client believes that all others would feel the same, the therapist asks whether the client can imagine someone else having the same feelings but feeling it more intensely than the client, in other words, feeling worse than the client. Most clients answer "Yes" to this question.

From here, the therapist capitalizes on the report by the client that someone else could feel differently with a question like "What would be responsible for this other person's being even more angry (anxious, guilty, depressed, etc.) than you?" Once answers to this question have been obtained, the therapist goes on to ask the client to consider the possibility and reasons for others' being less emotionally disturbed. The reasons being looked for relate to the way the hypothetical clients perceive and evaluate the situation.

As these reasons are uncovered, the therapist responds to each with something like "Ah, so you felt . . . because you thought . . ." or "Because you thought . . . , you felt . . ."

After a number of these reflections (repetition is important at this stage), the therapist again summarizes the situation with reflections like "Oh, so when . . . ," "You feel . . . ," "Because you think (perceive, judge) . . . ," "Is that the way it seems?" or "Does this seem right to you?" or "How am I doing?"

Repeating a number of summary statements like these ensures that the client will begin to think in ways that will foster emotional responsibility. However, one can be sure that a client is accepting emotional responsibility only when the client can satisfactorily answer the following question: "Just so I know that I am understanding this correctly, can you tell me why you were so upset (specifically, angry, depressed, frustrated, anxious, guilty) when this circumstance (describe in detail) occurred?" The answer sought is "Because I was thinking . . ."

Stage 3: Goal Setting

Goal setting is a step that is often overlooked by enthusiastic new therapists who are rightly focusing on the application of core skills (e.g., disputation) and on formulating hypotheses of problem etiology and maintenance. Once having identified emotional and practical problems, the most common mistake made by the therapist at this point is to leap into the use of intervention techniques motivated by nothing other than the knowledge that such techniques work for the presenting problems. While working problems one at a time, it is important for the therapist to establish goals for each one. This requires the therapist to take enough time to ascertain how the client would like to feel and act in each stated circumstance. The client is asked questions like "If we assume that, initially at least, you cannot change the circumstances, how would you like to feel and how would you like to be able to act if the same thing happened again?" Having achieved a list of different emotional and behavioral goals in the given circumstances, the therapist involves and may influence the client in setting priorities for intervention.

Setting priorities depends on the wants of the client, the likelihood that positive change will facilitate early success experiences, and the assessment of core irrational beliefs identified by the therapist. A common practice of RET is to target secondary self-acceptance emotional stress as an initial goal for change. However, this is not by any means a rule of thumb. Where a primary emotion (e.g., anger) is particularly intense, it may well pay to work first on the anger and to deal with the guilt second. By first seeking what personal change clients can make in the given circumstances, clients are reminded of the importance of gaining emotional and behavioral control over themselves before attempting to change others' behavior or to change the environment. Also, this involvement emphasizes the emotional-and-personal-responsibility theme of REGIME and maximizes client cooperation in the subsequent intervention process.

While hypothesizing about the range of the irrational beliefs contributing to problem etiology and maintenance, intervention should target specific areas and behaviors for change. A thorough understanding of RET will guide considerations of which irrational beliefs, when effectively disputed and replaced, will have the greater ripple effect on the disputation and replacement of other irrational beliefs, and/or which emotional disturbance(s) is acting as the greatest obstacle to achieving behavioral goals.

Sometimes, clients persist in working on goals that are unrealistic or that may not be seen by the therapist as optimum. Unrealistic goals include not only the unattainable but also the inappropriate. For example, instead of feeling down, angry, or very frustrated, the client may want to feel unconcerned or, perhaps, even happy in circumstances that, indeed, may be objectively bad. The realistic goals in such circumstances are to moderate extreme, destructive emotions into more manageable emotions even if these are still negative to the client. Realistic goals in such circumstances would not include obliterating negative feelings or attempting to replace them with positive feelings.

Nevertheless, in order to maximize client cooperation, the therapist stays with the client's initial choices of change. There will always be time to work on more optimum goals, and in the case of unrealistic goals, the client may be helped to see this reality at the stage of planning and implementing change interventions.

Stage 4: Intervention

Although RET is recognized by its use of cognitive disputational strategies, it is important for the RET therapist to become competent with a full range of RET behavioral, emotional, and cognitive change techniques. Any technique is appropriate provided it is aimed at an eventual change in clients' beliefs that will encourage, generalize, and/or maintain goal-appropriate emotions and behaviors.

Such "multimodal" techniques (e.g., Lazarus, 1981) may be borrowed from various therapeutic schools and should be chosen on the basis of whether they suit the trainee therapist's interactional style; whether they suit the client's style and particular problem; and, especially, whether the problem is proving to be intractable with the use of "orthodox" RET methods.

In my experience in using RET over the last 15 years, clients show very real differences in the ways that they react to the disputational methods used in RET. Watching Albert Ellis dispute the irrational beliefs of his clients we see a forceful and didactic approach working very effectively. Although this style has worked with some of my clients over the years, it has certainly not worked for all of them. A significant number of my clients resist being given insights. They resist being told what is wrong with their thinking and what they can do about it when they are still in the grip of their irrational demandingness, unscientific reasoning, and associated intense emotional disturbance. As a result of this experience, the approach that I now generally lean toward is interaction of a Socratic dialogue type with my clients. Through the asking of questions, Socratic dialogue seeks to direct listeners to their own insights into the irrationality of their thinking and its aversive and goal-defeating emotional and behavioral concomitants. Skill in using Socratic dialogue is based, first, on knowing what the answers are and, then, on being able to ask a series of questions that draw the respondent inexorably to giving these and only these answers.

Like any skill, this technique takes some practice to master. However, if one knows what the answers are, it takes practice only in thinking of the right questions. The theory of RET gives powerful answers to the question of why and how people disturb themselves. With a good theory (i.e., giving clear and valid answers), Socratic RET is not only possible, it is profound in facilitating insight that promotes lasting therapeutic change. However Socratic RET does take a little more time than the active didactic approach often modeled by Albert Ellis.

A modern-day proponent of this age-old technique is the apparently bumbling and disheveled detective played by Peter Falk in the television series "Columbo." The Columbo technique has the therapist looking and sounding somewhat uncertain or even confused (and sometimes saying so) when faced with the irrational thinking and behaving of the client: "You say you want to improve your job performance, but at the same time, you won't do paperwork. Can you explain that to me?"

I now have a client who is dissatisfied with her current relationship because of the restrictions that her partner puts on her time with other people. He dislikes her going out anywhere without him and states that, as she provides sufficient companionship and stimulation for his needs, he in turn should be adequate for her needs. Although Mary's dissatisfaction (and increasing frustration) has prompted her to discuss this problem with her partner, she reports always bending to his will (and as a result getting angry at herself and at him) because she is afraid of her relationship's ending and, as a result, of feeling alone and desperate. Her failure to be assertive leads to increasing dissatisfaction with herself and her relationship, and to dissatisfaction with and resentment of her partner. If this situation continues, it is likely that her relationship will come to an end. On the other hand, fearing that it may end if she asserts herself prevents her from taking constructive action. Either way, she is on course to an ending of the relationship. Mary sees this but still doesn't change her behavior. RET theory suggests that the causes of her destructive nonaction are, in combination, her need to be approved of and her need for comfort at all costs; her awfulizing about how bad it would be to confront her partner about his "one-eyed" view and his subsequently leaving her; and low frustration tolerance and global putdowns of herself and her rights.

The usual didactic method of disputing absolutistic expectations or demands is to ask the question "Why should it be the way that you want?" Most clients answer this question with justifications of their wants and are confused by the RET therapist's disagreeableness because they believe that their wants are reasonable—as, indeed, in most cases they are. The RET therapist usually clears up this confusion by telling a story to illustrate the difference between wants and needs and concludes by telling clients that they have been irrationally "needing what they want" instead of rationally "desiring or preferring what they want." Didactic RET usually continues at this point by explaining that emotional reactions to not getting what one believes one "absolutely needs" are more extreme than emotional reactions to not getting what one "merely wants," because of catastrophizing, the accompanying low frustration tolerance, and global ratings of self, others, and the world. This process can be didactic RET at its best.

Like didactic RET, Socratic RET has the same insight as its goal but assumes that a client's self-discovery of the difference between wanting and demanding will have a greater influence on reducing future demanding behavior. For example a Socratic method of leading clients to the discovery of their own demandingness and its negative consequences is a technique I call "validating wants." Validating wants is a technique that reality tests and then supports what the client wants as being rational (scientific, logical, goal-directed) and reasonable and then disputes clients' expectation or demand that they get what they "reasonably want." By validating and supporting the client's wants, the therapist clears the way for a focus on the getting (demandingness) of the wants rather than on the wants themselves (their reasonableness). In the case of Mary and her fear of losing her intolerant partner, this technique might begin with the question "Mary, why do you want to be in a close, intimate relationship with someone?" By tacking onto the end of each elicited answer the question "Because?" the therapist uncovers the range of Mary's wants and their reasons. These reasons are then checked in terms of their rationality (e.g., vis-à-vis Mary's higher order goals of happiness and long life) and Mary's assessment of their reasonableness. As I stated earlier, most of these reasons will be rational and reasonable. Humans are innately both rational and irrational. We have a clear capacity to be logical, scientific, reasonable, and fair, but then, we irrationally demand that, because we are, we need and should get what we want.

The dialogue might continue as follows:

T: Mary, it seems that the reasons you have for wanting to be in a close, intimate relationship with someone are quite important and reasonable.

C: I think so.

T: Is "important" reason enough for you to insist on getting what you want?

C: What do you mean?

T: Do you feel as if you need this sort of relationship?

C: Yes.

T: So you feel that you need it, you must have it, and you should have it because it is very important to you and because it is quite a reasonable thing to want. Is that it?

C: Well, yes, I suppose so.

T: That seems right to you?

C: Yes.

T: I agree, Mary, that seems to be what I am hearing, but I am not sure I properly understand. Can you help me with this?

C: If I can.

T: OK. You seem to be saying that, if a person wants something that is very important to them and it is reasonable and fair to want whatever it is, then the want becomes a "must-want."

C: What is a "must-want?"

T: Oh, I'm sorry. A must-want is a want you must have, a want that becomes a need. A need is a must-want.

C: Oh.

T: Do you understand what I mean by a must-want?

C: Yes, I think so. A must-want is something that you must have, something that you need.

T: Right! And if that is a must-want, what is a maybe-want?

C: A what?

T: A maybe-want. If a must-want is something that you must have, then a maybe-want is something that . . . ?

C: Is it something that you want but don't have to have?

T: Right on! So what is the difference between a maybe-want and a must-want?

C: A maybe-want is something that you want, but that you could do without; a must-want is something that you want that you must have, something that you need.

T: Good, you understand me, but I am still confused about something you said before. Will you help me sort this out?

C: Yes.

T: Is wanting an intimate relationship with someone a must-want or a maybe-want? Do you feel you need it?

C: Yes, it feels like a need to me.

T: Then it's a must-want?

C: Yes.

T: And it's a must-want because it's very important to you and it's a reasonable thing to be wanting?

C: Right!

T: Are "very important" and "reasonable" good enough reasons to feel something is a must-want, a need?

C: Yes they are. They are to me!

T: Mary, is it reasonable and very important that all adults who want to work are able to?

C: Well, yes it is.

T: Are all adults who want to work able to find jobs?

C: No, I suppose not.

T: Well then, are "reasonable" and "very important" good enough to guarantee all people jobs?

C: No, it isn't.

T: Do you think that those people who want to work see work as must-wants?

C: Yes, I do.

T: Because they feel that working is very important and only fair in our modern society, they feel that working should be and is a must-want.

C: Yes.

T: Is feeling something is a must-want good enough to guarantee that it will happen?

C: No, I guess it isn't.

T: And do people manage when they don't get their must-want job?

C: Well, I suppose they do, but not very well.

T: But do they manage in some way?

C: I suppose that most people do.

T: OK, here is where I get confused. If a maybe-want is something that you want but don't absolutely need—you can manage without it—it seems to me that a job is a maybe-want because people can manage, even if somewhat badly, without it. If you can manage without the job that you want, then the job is a maybe-want.

C: Yes, if you can manage without it, then it is a maybe-want.

T: But you agreed earlier that most of these people would feel that a job is a must-want.

C: Yes.

T: Well, then, can thinking or feeling change reality?

C: What do you mean?

T: Take a maybe-want, add heaps and heaps of worry, and start thinking that it is a must-want. Will the worried-about maybe-want become in reality a must-want?

C: Not in reality.

T: Can thinking alone turn a real maybe-want into a real must-want?

C: No. It could make you feel that something is a must-want when it isn't.

T: Exactly! Can you remember the difference between a must-want and a maybe-want?

C: Yes. A maybe-want is something that you want but that you can, in reality, manage without. A must-want is something that you want that you can, in reality, not manage without.

T: Excellent! Now let's look once again at your want for a close, intimate relationship with someone. You feel that you need such a relationship, but what sort of want is this, a must-want or a maybe-want?

C: I want to say it is a must-want.

T: Can you manage without this want being satisfied?

C: Well, I suppose I have.

T: So what sort of want is it?

C: A maybe-want.

T: What would be worse, not getting a maybe-want or not getting a must-want?

C: Not getting a must-want.

T: What feels worse, worrying about not getting a maybe-want or worrying about not getting a must-want?

C: Worrying about not getting a must-want.

T: Exactly! So what can you do about the wants that you regularly don't get in order to feel a minimum of distress?

C: Decide which are maybe-wants and which are must-wants.

T: And?

C: If I correctly recognize which wants are maybe-wants, then I will be less upset about not getting them.

T: OK. Now, what can you do about your worries about not getting what you want in order to feel a minimum of distress?

C: The same. If I am worrying about a maybe-want, then I will be less upset than if I am worrying about a must-want.

T: You have been worrying about losing your close relationship with your partner, right?

C: Yes. And I can see where you are heading. This relationship is really a maybe-want. I have been thinking that it is a must-want, and as a result, worrying about it has been upsetting me more than it needs to.

T: Could you manage if indeed you lost this maybe-want?

C: It would be awful, but I suppose I could.

T: Do you really mean awful, really mean 100% bad? That's what awful means. Is not getting a maybe-want 100% bad?

C: No, it would be bad, but not 100% bad.

T: Not awful?

C: No, not awful.

T: So if the worst happened in regard to this relationship and it ended suddenly because your partner would not tolerate your friendships outside it, could you manage?

C: Yes.

T: Would you manage?

C: Yes.

T: Will you manage?

C: Yes.

Irrespective of the disputational style chosen, RET works on identifying and replacing irrational beliefs with rational beliefs along a continuum from the specific to the general. Specific irrational beliefs relevant to specific As are disputed and replaced with specific rational beliefs. As a series of specific As and Bs are dealt with, clients are encouraged to achieve the insight that they not only are able to handle specific situations should they happen again (inelegant disputation) but also would be able to handle the worst possible situations in the present and the future (elegant disputation).

In seeking to give clients the benefit of the power of elegant disputation, RET therapists can be overzealous in jumping too quickly to the "What's the worst thing that could happen, and where is the evidence that you can't stand that?" question. This is another example of the mad-dog disputing style mentioned earlier that is caused by a mistaken belief that the necessary and sufficient requirement for the effectiveness of RET is to dispute the should's inelegantly and elegantly.

There are two general negative consequences of mad-dog disputing.
The first consequence is that, if one disputes should's as soon as they
are heard, it becomes very difficult to stick to one should long enough to
achieve an adequate and meaningful disputation. Demanding clients (the
average client) are full of should's. Unless we deal with should's one at a
time, the complexity of the disputational task quickly increases and prevents effective outcomes.

The second consequence comes from overzealously pushing elegant
disputation onto a client too soon and too fast. It makes sense that if clients
can believe that they can deal with the worst that can happen, then they
can certainly deal with what has already happened. However, it also
makes sense that, if clients are suffering significant low frustration tolerance over what has already happened, then they are certainly not ready to
consider the worst possible consequences.

Where low frustration tolerance is a significant variable in the presentation of a client's problems (as it often is), it needs to be addressed before
the process of elegant disputation is introduced.

Effective disputation of irrational beliefs is a necessary step before the
development of a new, more rational belief system. However, it is not
sufficient for lasting therapeutic change. Unless the client is set homework
tasks of acting consistently with the new rational thoughts, these will not
become beliefs.

Stage 5: Monitoring Homework

This stage recognizes that the application by a client of skills learned in
therapy requires therapeutic planning. Clients had better be set homework
that regularly requires the rehearsal, practice, and implementation of new
skills. Homework exercises should be designed along a hierarchy of difficulty in order to promote the client's acquiring "high frustration tolerance."
That is, when the client is confronted with applying new skills outside the
security of your office, he or she will find it "hard work" and will frequently fail to comply with homework assignments because of his or her
"low frustration tolerance" (LFT).

Each therapy session should begin with a review period that monitors
the client's application of new skills. It is important to give this time to
reinforce and reward clients for their effort and to identify and resolve
"plateaus" in client progress.

Even if care is taken to establish client cooperation by following the
steps earlier outlined in this chapter, client resistance will still be a function
of both the nature of the problem and the client's LFT (e.g., Ellis, 1985).
Resistance can also occur as a result of the therapist's not being specific
enough in setting homework or, alternatively, attempting to push the client

too fast. Careful examination of homework not achieved is important in order to clarify understanding or to modify the rate of the desired progress.

Progress plateaus can also occur as a result of clients' discouragement caused by applying their own standards of success, standards that they keep raising as they make progress. This process can be illustrated by the following lines of thought: "I was doing really well, so I should be able to continually improve!" or "Given that I am now more in control of my disturbance, I should be able to do this task more easily than I can. But I can't and I should be able to. I'll always be worse off than others!" or "I could do it yesterday, so I should be able to do it today. What's wrong with me?"

Associated with this self-talk is the tendency for clients to down themselves globally whenever they see themselves failing on specific tasks. Plateauing is often seen by clients failing their own expectation that, once on the road to recovery, they "must" continue to improve consistently. If this rating is allowed to become entrenched, this perceived global "failure" will almost inevitably lead to a general "backslide" or relapse as a result of the general "giving up" that such damning self-downing leads to. When clients do plateau, they may be helped if they are informed that (1) gradients of improvement marked by plateaus are the norm and smooth progress curves just do not occur; (2) they had better be aware of their tendency to be continually raising the standards by which they judge themselves and that this can be a destructive process; (3) they had better allow themselves to have off days just like everyone else; and (4) they had better not expect perfection unless they plan to be saintlike, and that to achieve this they have to die first!

The expectation that plateaus in progress will occur makes the experience of a plateau easier to cope with, and thus, backslides are less likely.

Stage 6: Evaluation and Exit

Progress in therapy is measurable by a number of factors, most commonly by those that are overtly discernible, for example, by behavioral change and by self-reports of cognitive change. However, evaluation within the REGIME model specifies that the therapist would also do well to evaluate progress by assessing the ongoing changes and associated intensities of the client's emotional behavior.

Progress occurs when the client's emotional intensity moves from disturbance to dissatisfaction. Examples of this movement show up when fear and extreme incapacitating anxiety change to moderate to mild anxiety; when extreme frustration associated with anger and destructive behavior changes to the moderate to mild frustration associated with constructive behavior; when guilt changes to regret; and when depression changes to sadness.

The evaluation stage of REGIME requires the RET therapist to be aware that the rate of change across the behavioral, emotive, and cognitive dimensions is not always constant or in synchrony (Barlow & Mavissakalian, 1981). However, synchrony must occur if changes are going to be long-lasting. Desynchrony across cognitive, behavioral, and emotional dimensions is an indication of work remaining for both client and therapist. For example, if the client's goal is to accept her or his spouse's behavior, but the client continues to experience ongoing anxiety and resentment in the attempt, then this is clear evidence that irrational beliefs regarding self-acceptance and fairness have yet to be addressed.

When changes in problem-focused emotionality are consistent with changes in cognition and overt behavior, the exit stage of REGIME has been reached. Most clients are aware that they are reaching or have reached this stage; some have to be encouraged to recognize their achievement. When encouragement is required, the best way to approach it is to summarize the therapy process to date, identifying the initial and changed goals (both practical and emotional) and their successive achievements. Encouragement is usually all that is required at this point if emotional and personal responsibility has been consistently emphasized throughout the therapy process.

REGIME Intervention Matrix

The entire REGIME model can be represented in a two-level matrix (see Table 2) that helps the therapist keep in mind the appropriate steps of the model and the order of progression through the model. By visualizing this matrix at any time, the RET therapist will never be in doubt about where he or she is in the therapeutic process and consequently where he or she is going next—a confusion often expressed by trainee RET therapists.

This intervention matrix can also be usefully taught to clients as a way of operationalizing their awareness of emotional responsibility into steps to change their emotional and behavioral distress. The matrix becomes useful for this purpose only after the therapist has guided the client to a full understanding and acceptance of emotional responsibility.

Transcript

The following excerpts from a therapy transcript illustrate the first three stages of REGIME. Sufficient guidelines for the last three stages are shown in Table 1, and many examples of specific intervention strategies are detailed elsewhere (e.g., Ellis & Dryden, 1987; Walen, Wessler, & DiGiuseppe, 1980).

TABLE 2. Intervention Matrix

	Circumstances	Feelings/actions	Thoughts
Insight level	(1) Identify the circumstances. When . . .''	(2) Identify the *associated* feelings and actions. You felt . . .'' You did . . .''	(3) Identify the *causal* cognitions. "Because you thought . . .''
Change level	(4) Assume the *same* circumstances.[a]	(5) Identify how the client would like to feel (or behave) given the same circumstances; i.e., establish goals.	(6) Modify cognitions to achieve these goals and then address skill deficits in order to modify circumstances.[b]

[a]Only after the client can appropriately deal with the circumstances as they are is the issue of changing the activating events addressed.
[b]Obstacles and skill deficits occur in the cognitive, physiological, and behavioral (action) domains. The therapist normally begins with disputing and changing the contents of Item 3.

STAGE 1: RELATIONSHIP

THERAPIST: What would you like some help with?
CLIENT: I have this problem with my face.
T: What do you mean?
C: Well, it's happened a lot recently. People seem to be startled by the look I get on my face.
T: Can you tell me about a recent example of when this happened?
C: I was with two friends waiting to get served in a shop when Brian said something to Rachel. I didn't quite hear what he said at that time—I guess it was that he was leaving—but anyway, I looked around when I became aware of his walking away. I don't know how I looked, but whatever it was, Rachel said, "Don't look at me like that!" in an aggressive manner.
T: When she responded in that manner, how did you feel?
C: I wondered what made her say that. I wasn't aware of looking any particular way, and I don't want to make other people respond that way to me.
T: When she did respond aggressively and you were wondering what made her say that, what were you feeling inside?
C: Well, I suppose I felt a little bit uptight.
T: When you are uptight, what does that feel like?
C: I guess I get tense across here (*indicating his stomach*).
T: Anything else? (*T runs through a range of anxiety symptoms.*)
C: My heart seems to pound a bit.
T: How tense did you become on that occasion? On a scale of 1 to 10, where 10 is very, very tense and your heart is really pounding, how tense do you think you were?

C: I suppose about 6.

T: After Rachel spoke to you aggressively and you felt that way, what did you do?

C: I felt surprised and just kept looking at her.

T: For how long?

C: Not for long. I felt embarrassed and red in the face, and I looked away quickly.

T: So after she spoke to you aggressively, you felt embarrassed and in shock sort of . . . and you looked away quickly.

C: Yeah.

T: Then what did you do?

C: I ordered my lunch and worried about what I was doing, what was wrong with my face.

T: Did you say anything further to Rachel?

C: No.

Stage 2: Emotional Responsibility

T: So when you looked suddenly around at your friends and Rachel said, "Don't look at me like that!" you felt tense in the stomach and you were aware of your heart pounding quite a bit. You felt this tension because?

C: Because Rachel said, "Don't look at me like that!"

T: Right, when Rachel said, "Don't look at me like that!" you felt 6 out of 10 tense, because?

C: Well, because of what Rachel said, the way she reacted to the way that I looked.

At this point the client's understanding of his emotional reaction puts the causal explanation on the circumstances: Rachel's behavior has made him feel tense, concerned, and anxious. Establishing emotional responsibility requires the breaking of this bond and the establishment of a new causal one, a bond between what the client thinks and what the client feels:

T: Can you imagine someone else being in this same situation, being confronted with Rachel's words and feeling even more tense, more concerned, more anxious than you felt, say, 9 or 10 of 10 on our 10-point scale?

C: Well, I suppose so.

T: Another person who in the same situation would feel worse than the way you felt?

C: Yes.

T: How could that be? What would make this other person feel even more tense than you?

It can happen that the client is not able to answer this question, especially if the client has never thought that what goes on inside her or his head could contribute to feelings like tension or anger. In such a case, the therapist might have to prompt with something like "Here is this other person, in the same situation as you, feeling more tense than you. We know it's not the situation because you are in the same situation and you are not as tense. If it's not the situation and it's not Scottie beaming down tension from the *USS Enterprise,* what could it be, what could this more tense person be doing that would make her or him more tense than you?" If no answer is forthcoming or the answer does not include "what the person thinks," the therapist should try "Is there something that this other person could think that would make him more tense?"

C: He could be thinking that Rachel was thinking bad things about him.

T: Like what?

C: That he was a terrible person, that she didn't like him.

T: And if he thought that, if he thought that Rachel was thinking that he was a really terrible person and that she didn't like him, that would make him feel even more tense and uptight than the way you felt when Rachel said, "Don't look at me like that!"?

C: Yeah, I suppose it would.

T: Now, can you imagine a person in the same situation—being spoken to aggressively by Rachel—who would feel less tense, less anxious than the way you felt, say, 2 or 3 out of 10 on out 10-point scale?

C: Yeeeaah *(client obviously thinking).*

T: How could this person be like this? How could he feel less uptight in the same situation?

C: He could be saying to himself that it doesn't matter what Rachel says or what Rachel thinks about him.

T: Are you saying that if he doesn't care what Rachel thinks about him, he wouldn't feel as tense as you did when Rachel said, "Don't look at me like that!"?

C: Yes.

T: So we have three people who were in the same situation when Rachel said, "Don't look at me like that!" and who each felt differently because each thought differently. One thought, "She thinks I'm really terrible and she doesn't like me," and that made him feel 9 or 10 out of 10; one thought, "I don't really care what Rachel thinks about me," and this thought made him feel 2 or 3 out of 10; and you felt 6 out of 10. What did you think that made you feel this way?

C: Well, that she might think I am terrible, that I am a terrible person, and that she might not like me.

T: So three people in the same circumstances felt differently. What made them feel differently?

C: What they were thinking about.

T: And what made you feel 6-out-of-10 tense and anxious when Rachel said, "Don't look at me like that!"? Was it what she said?

C: It was what I was thinking, that she might think I was terrible and that I might be a terrible person.

T: Right. So when Rachel said, "Don't look at me like that!" your heart was pounding, and you felt tension, anxiety, and concern because?

C: Because of what I was thinking.

T: So what made you feel bad?

C: What I was thinking. (*If the client answers this question with "Rachel yelled at me," the therapist starts Stage 2 all over.*)

Breaking the causal links that clients make between circumstances and their problem emotions and actions is a difficult but not impossible exercise if the therapist is prepared for repetition. Repetition is necessary to overcome years of social conditioning and humans' tendency to base their worth on the approval of others. Of course, therapy doesn't always run as smoothly as the transcripts that one reads. However, the above demonstrates the steps necessary for establishing emotional responsibility.

STAGE 3: GOAL SETTING

T: Let us assume, for the moment at least, that circumstances like the one you describe will continue to happen at the same frequency that you have recently experienced. Could you do that?

C: Yes.

T: If it continues to happen every now and again, how would you prefer to feel when it happens?

C: I would like it to stop happening at all.

T: Right. You may be able to make it stop happening sometime in the future, but for now, suppose that it still happens every now and again. How would you prefer to feel, instead of feeling 6-out-of-10 tense, instead of your heart pounding, instead of feeling anxious and very concerned. How would you like to feel when someone unexpectedly says, "Don't look at me like that!"?

C: Well, I suppose I would like to feel less tense or anxious or less concerned, or maybe not concerned at all.

T: OK. Now we have recognized that what you think determines how tense you feel. If you continue to think what you have been thinking, will this help you feel less tense or anxious?

C: No.

T: If you keep thinking the way that you have been about this situation, how will you be feeling?

C: The same as I was before.

T: Right, so in order to achieve your goals, to feel less tense and anxious and maybe not concerned at all, what will you have to do first?

C: Stop thinking what I have been thinking whenever this happens.

CONCLUSION

REGIME is presented as a six-step framework for teaching and using RET. Its importance lies in its emphasis on setting the stage for the power of RET theory and process to achieve optimum results.

There is a tendency for trainee RET therapists to become overfocused on the uniqueness of RET—the elegant disputation of irrational beliefs—and to become mad-dog disputers every time they hear the word *should*, spurred on by Ellis's words of "look for the shoulds, look for the musts."

RET is a powerful therapeutic approach that can be suited to most clients, providing the therapist is willing to develop rapport, establish emotional responsibility, set emotional and behavioral outcome goals before intervention, monitor homework, and evaluate outcome.

REGIME provides an effective framework for teaching RET, makes it palatable to a broader range of therapists, and makes it effective on a broader range of clients.

REFERENCES

Barlow, D. H., & Mavissakalian, M. (1981). Directions in the assessment and treatment of phobia: The next decade. In M. Mavissakalian & D. H. Barlow (Eds.), *Phobia: Psychological and Pharmacological Treatment* (pp. 199–245). New York: Guilford Press.

Corey, G. C. (1982). *Theory and practice of counseling and psychotherapy*. Monterey, CA: Brooks/Cole.

Egan, G. (1986). *The skilled helper: A systematic approach to effective helping*. Monterey, CA: Brooks/Cole.

Ellis, A. (1985). *Overcoming resistance*. New York: Springer.

Ellis, A., & Dryden, W. (1987). *The practice of rational-emotive therapy*. New York: Springer.

Ellis, A., & Grieger, R. (1977). *Handbook of rational-emotive therapy*. New York: Springer.

Garfield, S. L. (1989). The client-therapist relationship in rational-emotive therapy. In M. E. Bernard & R. D. DiGiuseppe (Eds.), *Inside rational-emotive therapy: A critical analysis of the theory and practice of Albert Ellis*. New York: Academic Press.

Kwee, M. G. T., & Lazarus, A. A. (1986). Multimodal therapy: The cognitive-behavioural tradition and beyond. In W. Dryden & W. Golden (Eds.), *Cognitive-behavioural approaches to psychotherapy*. London: Harper & Row.

Lazarus, A. A. (1981). *The practice of multi-modal therapy*. New York: McGraw-Hill.

Walen, S., Wessler, R., & DiGiuseppe, R. (1980). *The practitioner's guide to rational-emotive therapy*. New York: Oxford University Press.

5

Flexibility in RET
Forming Alliances and Making Compromises

WINDY DRYDEN

In this chapter, I discuss two concepts that I have found useful in my clinical practice of RET. The first concerns Bordin's (1979) reformulation of the psychoanalytic concept of the therapeutic alliance, an idea I have found helpful in my struggles to develop a general framework for the conduct of RET. The second addresses the clinical reality that sometimes one is called on to make compromises with "elegant" RET while attempting to help clients achieve a "good enough" therapeutic outcome but not necessarily an "elegant" one. These two concepts have encouraged me to be flexible in my practice of RET—an important ingredient in making RET more effective.

THE THERAPEUTIC ALLIANCE

Bordin (1979) argued that the term *therapeutic alliance* refers to the complex of attachments and shared understandings formed and activities undertaken by therapists and clients as the former attempt to help the latter with their psychological problems.

Bordin stressed that there are three major components of the therapeutic alliance: (1) *bonds*, which refer to the interpersonal connectedness between therapist and client; (2) *goals*, which refer to the aims of both therapist and client; and (3) *tasks*, which are activities carried out by both therapist and client in the service of the latter's goals.

This chapter has been adapted from material previously published in W. Dryden (1987). *Current Issues in Rational-Emotive Therapy.* London: Croom-Helm.

WINDY DRYDEN • Department of Psychology, Goldsmiths' College, University of London, New Cross, London, England SE14 6NW.

133

I consider each of these components separately and show that rational-emotive therapists have important clinical decisions to make in each of the three alliance domains if they are to individualize therapy for each client and thus maximize therapeutic benefit.

At the outset, it should be noted that Bordin (1979) speculated that effective therapy occurs when therapist and client (1) have an appropriately bonded working relationship; (2) mutually agree on the goals of the therapeutic enterprise; and (3) understand their own and the other person's therapeutic tasks and agree to carry out these in order to implement the client's goals.

Bonds

The major concern of rational-emotive therapists in the bond domain should be to establish and maintain an appropriately bonded relationship that will encourage *each* individual client to implement his or her goal-directed therapeutic tasks. It should be underscored that there is no *single* effective bond that can be formed with clients in RET; different clients require different bonds.

This fact became clear to me when I was on a six months' sabbatical at the Center for Cognitive Therapy in Philadelphia in 1981. As reported elsewhere (Dryden, 1984), I saw two clients on the same afternoon who benefited from a different bonded relationship with me. At 4 P.M. I saw Mrs. G., a 50-year-old married businesswoman who was impressed with my British professional qualifications, and whose responses to my initial questions indicated that she anticipated and preferred a very formal relationship with her therapist. I provided such a relationship by using formal language; citing the research literature whenever appropriate; wearing a suit, shirt, and tie; and referring to myself as "Dr. Dryden" and to the client as "Mrs. G." On one occasion, I inadvertently used her first name and was put firmly in my place concerning the protocol of professional relationships. On another occasion, I disclosed a piece of personal information in order to make a therapeutic point and was told in no uncertain terms, "Young man, I am not paying you good money to hear about your problems." Here, a therapist is faced with the choice of respecting and meeting a client's bond anticipations and preferences or examining the reasons why, for example, this client was so adamantly against informality in her therapist. In my experience, the latter strategy is rarely productive, and rational-emotive therapists are recommended to meet their clients' preferences for therapeutic style as long as doing so does not reinforce the client's psychological problems.

At 5 P.M. on the same afternoon, I regularly saw Mr. B., a 42-year-old male nurse who indicated that he had not responded well to his previous therapist's neutrality and formality. Our therapy sessions were thus characterized by an informal bond. Before seeing him, I would remove the jacket and tie that I wore for Mrs. G.; in sessions, we used each other's first names and both had our feet up on my desk. We also developed the habit of taking turns in bringing in cans of soda and my client referred to our meetings as "rap sessions," whereas I conceptualized my work as therapy within an informal context.

I maintain that Mrs. G. would not have responded well to an informal therapeutic relationship, nor would Mr. B. have done as well with a highly formal mode of therapy. Thus, I argue that it is important that rational-emotive therapists pay attention to the question: "Which bond is likely to be most effective with a particular patient at a given time in the therapeutic process?" Drawing on social-psychological principles, certain writers have argued that some clients show more progress when the therapeutic bond is based on liking and trust, whereas others flourish more when the bond emphasizes therapist credibility and expertness (Beutler, 1983; Dorn, 1984; Strong & Claiborn, 1982). Future research in RET could fruitfully address the issue of which bond is effective with which clients. However, until we have such data, therapists can make decisions about which type of bond to foster on the basis of an early assessment of the client's anticipations and preferences in the bond domain and can try to meet such expectations, at least initially. This is one reason why I would caution novice therapists against emulating the therapeutic style of leading RET practitioners, whose bond with clients may be based mainly on prestige and expertness. Rational-emotive therapists should thus be prepared to emphasize different aspects of themselves with different clients in the bond domain without adopting an inauthentic facade, and to monitor transactions in this domain throughout therapy.

How can this best be done? One way would be to administer a portion of Lazarus's Life History Questionnaire (1981), which focuses on clients' expectations regarding therapy. The items "How do you think a therapist should interact with his or her clients?" and "What personal qualities do you think the ideal therapist should possess?" are particularly relevant and can provide an impetus for further exploration of this issue at the outset of therapy. If the client has had therapy previously, the current therapist can explore which aspects of the previous therapist's interactive style and behavior were deemed by the client to be both helpful and unhelpful. Particular emphasis should be placed on the exploration of the instrumental nature of previous therapeutic bonds, as statements such as "he was warm and caring" are of little use unless the client values these qualities and attributes therapeutic potency to them.

Furthermore, and for similar reasons, I have found it helpful to explore clients' accounts of people in their lives who have had both positive and negative influences on their personal development. Such an exploration may provide the therapist with important clues to which types of therapeutic bonds to promote actively with certain clients and which bonds to avoid developing with others.

Therapeutic style is another aspect of the bond domain that requires attention. Interpersonally oriented psychotherapists (e.g., Anchin & Kiesler, 1982) have argued that clinicians need to be aware that therapeutic styles have a "for better or worse" impact on different clients. Rational-emotive therapists tend to be active and directive in their style of conducting therapy. This therapeutic style may not be entirely productive with passive clients and, as Beutler (1983) argued, with clients who are highly reactive to interpersonal influence. Clients who tend to be passive in their interpersonal style of relating may "pull" an increasingly active style from their therapists, who may in turn reinforce these clients' passivity with their increased activity. Clients whose psychological problems are intrinsically bound up with a passive style of relating are particularly vulnerable in this regard. It is important that rational-emotive therapists be aware of the danger of becoming enmeshed in such unproductive vicious circles, which have unfortunate self-fulfilling prophecy implications for their passive clients. The therapist needs to engage clients productively at a level that constructively encourages increased activity on their part, but without threatening them through the use of an *overly* passive style of practicing RET.

Beutler (1983) argued that all approaches to psychotherapy can be viewed as a process of persuasion; this is particularly true of RET practitioners, who aim to "persuade" clients to reevaluate and change their irrational beliefs. Thus, rational-emotive therapists need to be especially careful in working with clients for whom such persuasive attempts may be perceived as especially threatening (i.e., highly reactant clients). Here, it is important that therapists execute their strategies with due regard to helping such clients to preserve their sense of autonomy, emphasizing throughout that these clients are in control of both their own thought processes and their own decisions concerning whether or not to change their beliefs. At present, the above suggestions are speculative and await full empirical inquiry, but my clinical work has led me to question the desirability of establishing the same therapeutic bond with all clients and of practicing rational-emotive therapy in an unchanging therapeutic style.

Goals

The major concern of rational-emotive therapists in the goal domain of the alliance is to ensure that there will be agreement between therapist and client on the client's outcome goals for change. A prerequisite of such agreement concerns clients' and therapists' arriving at a shared understanding of the clients' most relevant problems as defined by the clients (Meichenbaum & Gilmore, 1982). Difficulties may occur here when the therapist uncritically accepts the client's initial account of his or her problem, as such accounts may well be biased by the client's internalized values, for example, the view of significant others in the client's life.

In addition, although most rational-emotive therapists believe that early goal setting with the client is important, clients' initial statements about their goals for change may well be colored by their psychological disturbances as well as by their internalized values concerning what these goals *should* be. Rational-emotive therapists need to walk a fine line between uncritically accepting clients' initial goals for change and disregarding them altogether. A helpful solution here involves the establishment and maintenance of a channel of communication between client and therapist that deals with metatherapy issues (i.e., issues concerning matters relating to the therapy itself). Dryden and Hunt (1985) referred to the activities that occur within this channel as involving negotiations and renegotiations about therapeutic issues. Rational-emotive therapists need to take a major responsibility for keeping this communication channel open in order to monitor clients' goals over time and to determine the reasons for shifts in these goals.

Pinsof and Catherall (1986) have made the important points that clients' goals occur (implicitly or explicitly) in reference to their most important relationships and that their therapists need to be mindful of the impact that these systems are likely to have on both the selection of such goals and the clients' degree of progress toward goal attainment. Adopting this focus may well mean involving parts of the client's interpersonal system in therapy itself. It also suggests that future theorizing in RET can profitably assign a more central role to interpersonal issues (cf. Safran, 1984).

Tasks

Rational-emotive practitioners tend to subscribe to the following therapeutic process. Initially, having agreed to offer help to the client, the therapist (1) attempts to structure the therapeutic process for the client and (2) begins both to assess his or her problems in rational-emotive terms and to help the client to view his or her problems within this framework. Goals are elicited based on a rational-emotive assessment, and therapeutic strategies and techniques are implemented to effect the desired changes. Finally, obstacles to client change are analyzed and, it is hoped, overcome, and therapeutic gains are stabilized and maintained.

Therapists have tasks to execute at each stage in the rational-emotive therapeutic process; these are now outlined.

Structuring

Effective RET depends in part on both participants' clearly understanding their respective responsibilities in the therapeutic endeavor and on both participants' agreeing to discharge these responsibilities in the form of carrying out therapeutic tasks. It is the therapist's major responsibility to help the client to make sense of this process by providing an overall structure of mutual responsibilities and tasks. It is important to stress that structuring occurs throughout therapy and not just at the outset of the process. Sensitive clinicians who pay attention to alliance issues structure the process using language that the client can understand and analogies that make sense to the individual client. Thus, it is often helpful to discover clients' hobbies and interests so that apt and personally meaningful structuring statements can be made. Thus, if a client is interested in golf, ascertaining how that person learned the game may be valuable in drawing parallels between the processes of learning coping skills and learning golfing skills. Both involve practice, and failures can be realistically anticipated in each activity.

Assessment and Conceptualization of Clients' Problems

During the assessment process, rational-emotive therapists traditionally attempt to gain a full understanding of the cognitive and behavioral variables that are maintaining their clients' problems. During this stage, two issues become salient from an alliance theory perspective. First, it is important for therapist and client to arrive at a shared *definition* of the client's problems (i.e., what these problems are). Second, as Meichenbaum and Gilmore (1982) noted, it is important for them to negotiate a shared *conceptualization* of the client's problems (i.e., an explanation of what accounts for the existence of these problems), so that they can work productively together in the intervention stage of therapy.

When working toward shared problem conceptualization, I argue that it is important for RET therapists to use, wherever possible, clients' language and concepts, particularly when providing alternative explanations of their problems. This approach helps therapists to work within the range of what clients will accept as plausible conceptualizations of their problems. If clients' own ideas about the origins of their problems and, more particularly, about what maintains them are ignored, then they may well resist accepting their therapists' conceptualizations. As Golden (1985) noted, sometimes therapists have to accept initially, for pragmatic purposes, a client's different (i.e., from the therapist's) conceptualization of his or her problems in order to arrive later at a shared one. In addition, rational-emotive therapists may well privately (i.e., for themselves) conceptualize a client's problems in rational-emotive terms (irrational beliefs) while publicly (for the client) using the client's conceptualization (e.g., negative self-hypnosis). To what extent the effectiveness of RET is based on negotiation or on the unilateral persuasion attempts of the therapist is a matter for future empirical enquiry.

Change Tactics

Once the therapist and the client have come to a mutually agreed-on understanding of the client's problems, the therapist discusses with the client a variety of techniques that the client can use to reach his or her goals. Here, it is important to realize that both client and therapist have tasks to execute.

Effective RET in the task domain tends to occur when:

1. Clients understand what their tasks are.
2. Clients understand how executing their tasks will help them achieve their goals.
3. Clients are, in fact, capable of executing their tasks and believe that they have this capability.
4. Clients understand that change comes about through repeated execution of their tasks.
5. Clients understand the tasks of their therapists and can see the link between their therapists' tasks, their own tasks, and their own goals.
6. Therapists adequately prepare their clients to understand and execute the latter's tasks.
7. Therapists effectively execute their tasks (i.e., they are skilled in the techniques of RET) and use a wide range of techniques appropriately.
8. Therapists use techniques that are congruent with their clients' learning styles. Whereas some clients learn best through action, others learn best through reading bibliotherapy texts and so on.
9. Therapists use techniques that clients have selected (from a range of possible procedures) rather than unilaterally selecting techniques without client participation.
10. Therapists pace their interventions appropriately.
11. Therapists use techniques that are potent enough to help clients achieve their goals (e.g., using exposure methods with clients with agoraphobic problems; Emmelkamp, Kuipers, & Eggeraat, 1978).

In conclusion, it is my contention that it is *insufficient* for therapists to practice RET in a way that is theoretically correct for effective therapy to occur. Rather, RET is made more effective, I hypothesize, when therapists also attend to the components of the therapeutic alliance outlined above and are prepared to intervene flexibly based on their understanding of these components.

COMPROMISES IN RET

In this part of the chapter, I discuss the notion that, although RET therapists prefer to encourage their clients to achieve a profound philosophical change by replacing their irrational beliefs with rational beliefs, this is not always possible. In such cases, RET therapists are advised to make various compromises in helping clients deal with their problems in ways that do not involve philosophical change. These alternative strategies are termed *compromises* in that, although not ideal, they often bear more fruit than the preferred strategies of RET.

When it is clear that the client is not able to achieve philosophical change, whether on a particular issue or in general, the therapist often uses other cognitive-behavioral therapeutic methods to effect less "profound" change. Because, in such cases, these methods yield better results for the client than can be achieved by standard rational-emotive methods, they are regarded as compromises yielding an outcome between no change, on the one hand, and profound philosophical change, on the other.

Inferentially Based Change

Inferentially based change occurs when clients do not change irrational beliefs but do succeed in correcting distorted inferences, such as negative predictions, and overly negative interpretations of events and of the behavior of others.

A good example of such a change was reported by a therapist of my acquaintance. He was working with a middle-aged woman who reported feeling furious every time her aging father would telephone her and inquire, "Noo, what's doing?" She inferred that this was a gross invasion of her privacy and absolutistically insisted that he had no right to act in this way. The therapist initially intervened with the usual rational-emotive strategy by attempting to dispute this client's dogmatic belief and tried to help her see that there was no law in the universe that stated he must not invade her privacy. Meeting initial resistance, the therapist persisted with different variations of this theme—all to no avail. Changing tack, he began to implement a different strategy designed to help the client question her inference that her father was actually invading her privacy. Given her father's age, the therapist inquired, was it not more likely that his question represented his usual manner of beginning telephone conversations rather than an intense desire to pry into her affairs? This inquiry proved successful in that the client's rage subsided because she began to reinterpret her father's motives.

Another example of inferentially based change occurred with one of my clients, Robert, who was anxious because people might stare at him for spilling his drink. His hands would shake whenever he attempted to drink in public. I first used the customary philosophically based RET strategy, encouraging him to assume the worst and imagine that people would actually stare at him when he spilled his drink. This approach yielded his irrational belief: "If they stare at me, it would prove I am a worthless freak." However, I could not encourage him to dispute this belief successfully, and he still adhered strongly to it after my varied disputing efforts. Changing tack, I took him to several pubs and asked him to observe other people's reactions as I deliberately spilled drinks in public. He came to realize that other people, in general, did not stare at me when I spilled my drink, and this observation helped him to change his own inference to "It is unlikely that most people will stare at me when I spill my drink." This inferentially based change enabled him to order and consume drinks in public and reduced his social anxiety, although he never did change his aforementioned irrational belief.

Interestingly, in both examples, although my fellow therapist and I returned to disputing our clients' irrational beliefs *after* helping them to modify their distorted inferences, we never succeeded in helping them to change these beliefs. However, some clients are more willing to reevaluate their irrational beliefs after they have been helped to correct distorted inferences. Rational-emotive theory holds that irrational beliefs are the breeding ground for the development of negative inferences and that, thus, when clients succeed in changing their irrational beliefs, spontaneous reduction in the negativity of inferences will follow. However, these two examples show that inferentially based change can occur in the absence of philosophically based change.

Behaviorally Based Change

Behaviorally based change occurs when clients do not change irrational beliefs but improve by effecting constructive changes in behavior. Such behavior changes, in my experience, occur when clients (1) replace dysfunctional behavior with constructive behavior and (2) acquire constructive patterns of behavior that have previously been absent from their skill repertoire. An example of each follows.

Replacing Dysfunctional Behavior with Constructive Behavior

Sylvia, a first-year university student, sought therapy for extreme examination anxiety. She predicted that she would fail her first-year exams, demanded that she must pass them, and concluded that, should she fail, this failure would be the "end of the world." No amount of disputing her irrational beliefs yielded any therapeutic gain, so I shifted attention to her test-taking behavior. I discovered that Sylvia approached an examination in the following way: She would choose to answer the first question that she knew anything about; she would write everything she knew about that question without first making an answer plan and would often answer only two out of four questions in the entire examination. It thus transpired that her inferences concerning failure were accurate rather than negatively distorted.

My subsequent therapeutic approach focused on teaching Sylvia the following examination techniques: allocating sufficient time to answer all questions; analyzing the wording of the examination questions; making answer plans; answering all parts of a given question; and dealing with "mind-blank" experiences through cognitive distraction. With the help of her department, I arranged for Sylvia to take several practice examinations so that she could develop her newly acquired skills; the result was that she performed very well on these examinations. These experiences helped Sylvia to predict success, rather than failure in her end-of-year examinations. This prediction led to a significant decrease in her examination anxiety. However, although Sylvia did in fact do very well on her exams, she still held the same irrational beliefs about failure as she did at the outset and did not want to focus on these later, as she thought failure to be "so unlikely that it's not worth considering."

This example clearly shows that behavior change often leads to inferentially based change but not necessarily to philosophically based change.

Acquiring New Skills

Mrs. Anderson was referred to me with problems of anger and depression. Her husband and two teenaged children expected her to go out to work, do all the housework without help, and cater to their every whim. She had done this for several years but had become increasingly angry and depressed. Her anger was based on the irrational belief that they must not treat her this way, and her depression stemmed from the belief that she was no good for failing to please her family. Traditional rational-emotive disputing methods failed to yield any therapeutic gains, so I shifted the focus of therapy to a discussion of assertion and the value of politely declining to do the bidding of her family. Through role-playing methods, it transpired that Mrs. Anderson did not have assertive skills in her repertoire, as she could communicate only in an aggressive and demanding manner. I thus trained her intensively in polite, negative assertive skills, which she was able to put into practice with her family. Surprisingly, her family responded quite well to her behavior, began to share household tasks, and made fewer demands on her. The result was that Mrs. Anderson's depressed mood lifted appreciably and she became far less angry. As in the other examples in this chapter, I returned to disputing her irrational beliefs as outlined above, but again without success.

This example shows that a client's behavioral changes can sometimes elicit constructive behavior from others, leading to healthy changes in the interpersonal system of which the client is a part.

Changing Activating Events

I concluded the above example with the observation that a client's change in behavior can promote healthy system-based change. However, this does not always occur. In a case similar to the one described above, I had to involve the client's husband and children in therapy and encourage them to change their behavior toward the depressed client, Mrs. Curran, as her own assertive efforts did not on this occasion elicit constructive responses from her family. Once they changed their behavior toward Mrs. Curran for the better, her mood lifted. Again, disputing efforts aimed at helping Mrs. Curran to reevaluate her irrational beliefs, pre- and postimprovement, did not lead to philosophically based change.

In another example of helping clients by promoting changes in activating events, I helped Mr. Brown to overcome his depression by encouraging him to change his vocation from accountancy to law. He was depressed because he believed, "I have to enjoy my job in order to be happy." No amount of disputing this belief yielded any therapeutic gain, so I switched the focus of the sessions to exploring his vocational interests and aptitudes. This change led Mr. Brown to conclude that he would be happier as a lawyer than as an accountant. Accordingly, he decided to go to law school. Years later, after he had qualified as a lawyer, I met Mr. Brown, who had effected a successful career change. He still believed that he had to be vocationally satisfied in order to be happy, but as he was happy working in the law, he had concluded that there was no need to reevaluate this irrational belief.

Challenging but Not Overwhelming: A Compromise in Negotiating Homework Assignments

Ellis (1983) has criticized the use of gradual approaches to helping clients overcome their emotional and behavioral problems. His argument was that the use of gradual methods in psychotherapy and behavior therapy reinforce

> a philosophy that states or implies that (1) emotional change has to be brought about slowly and cannot possibly occur quickly or suddenly; (2) that it must be practically painless as it is occurring; and (3) that it cannot occur with the use of jarring, painful, flooding methods of therapy. (p. 142)

Thus, psychotherapeutic gradualism is seen by Ellis as countertherapeutic in that it basically reinforces clients' discomfort anxiety or philosophy of low frustration tolerance (LFT), which serves to perpetuate rather than ameliorate their problems. He thus prefers, wherever possible, the use of flooding or "full-exposure" methods and homework assignments in RET, primarily because they help clients to overcome their discomfort anxiety and to raise their tolerance level for frustration.

However, "wherever possible" is the important phrase to note here, as not all clients will agree to execute flooding or "full-exposure" homework assignments. That this should be rational-emotive therapists' initial approach to negotiating homework assignments is not questioned here. In taking this stance, therapists should explain the rationale for this type of homework assignment, should emphasize the benefits of such an approach, and should encourage clients to implement these assignments after thoroughly disputing clients' LFT ideas. What therapists are in fact saying is "Such methods are the most efficient means of helping you achieve your therapeutic goals." It is not surprising that Ellis should recommend such assignments, given his belief in the value of efficiency in psychotherapy (Ellis, 1980b).

However, no matter how therapists try to encourage (or persuade) some clients to execute full-exposure homework assignments, clients may steadfastly refuse to do so. In the face of such opposition, if therapists persist in their persuasive tactics, they commit two therapeutic errors. First, they threaten the therapeutic alliance between themselves and their "resistant" clients. In such instances, the therapeutic alliance is likely to break down in the *task* domain. Although therapist and client may have a good collaborative relationship (an effective bond) and may agree on the client's goals (shared goals), they disagree about the tasks that the client is prepared to do in order to achieve the therapeutic goals. Second, such overly persistent therapists serve as poor role models, as they tend to believe that clients *must* be "efficient" in their approach to therapy and *must* therefore do full-exposure assignments. Paradoxically, these therapists, by insisting that their clients execute certain types of homework assignments, are in fact being inefficient themselves. A breakdown in the therapeutic alliance often leads to therapeutic impasses, which in turn often lead to clients' dropping out of treatment.

In such cases, what should therapists preferably do? There is no need to return to therapeutic gradualism, for there is another alternative that allows therapists and clients to effect a working compromise. Whenever I encounter clients who steadfastly refuse to execute full-exposure homework tasks and who prefer gradual assignments, I explain this therapeutic compromise. I invite them to choose assignments that are sufficiently *challenging* to discourage reinforcement of their philosophy of low frustration tolerance, but that are not overwhelming for them. I explain their choices thus:

There are three ways that you can overcome your fears. The first is like jumping in at the deep end. You expose yourself straightaway to the situation you are most afraid of. The advantage here is that if you can learn that nothing terrible will happen, you will overcome your problems quite quickly. However, the disadvantage is that some people just can't bring themselves to do this and get quite discouraged as a result. The second way is to go very gradually. On the one hand, you do only something that you feel comfortable doing, and on the other, you don't really get an opportunity to face putting up with discomfort, which, in my opinion, is a major feature of your problem. Also, treatment will take much longer this way. The third way is what I call "challenging but not overwhelming." Here, you choose an assignment that is sufficiently challenging for you to make progress but not what you feel would be overwhelming for you at any given stage. Here, you are likely to make progress more quickly than with the gradual approach but more slowly than with the "deep end" approach.

I find that when clients are given an opportunity to choose their own rate of progress, the therapeutic alliance is strengthened. Most clients who refuse to execute full-exposure assignments choose the challenging-but-not-overwhelming approach; only very rarely do they opt for gradual desensitization therapy. When they do so, I do try to dissuade them and frequently succeed. In the final analysis, however, I have not found it productive to insist that clients choose a particular way of tackling problems that is against their preferences.

Case Example

Mary, a 23-year-old single woman, came to therapy for help in overcoming her anxiety about eating in public. Typically, she had both ego- and discomfort-anxiety-related beliefs (Ellis, 1979, 1980a), and in the early sessions, I helped her to identify and dispute such self-defeating attitudes as "I must not be anxious while eating"; "If other people see me leave my food, they will think I'm odd, and I need their approval"; "I am a shameful individual for having this problem': "There is something wrong with me because I have a small appetite"; and "I must not make a fuss and draw attention to myself."

Mary claimed that her anxiety would be at its peak if she were faced with the prospect of not finishing her food in a crowded, fashionable restaurant. However, although she was successful in verbally disputing both ego- and discomfort-anxiety-related beliefs about this hypothetical incident in therapy sessions, she could not initially conceive of putting this learning into practice in this particular setting, even though I presented the rationale for full-exposure homework assignments and emphasized the benefits that she would experience as a result. She literally could not imagine herself doing such an assignment (a good sign that such an experience would, in her terms, be "too" traumatic). She inquired whether there was not a painless method for overcoming her problems. I explained the dangers of such "painless" methods and introduced her to the idea of challenging-but-not-overwhelming tasks. She agreed, although with some reluctance, to select such an assignment. My hunch was that she would have terminated therapy if I had persisted in persuading her to expose herself fully to her anxieties. Over the following weeks, she set herself and successfully executed the following challenging-but-not-overwhelming tasks while disputing her salient irrational beliefs. These tasks were, in temporal order:

1. Eating two squares of chocolate in a public place.
2. Eating a meal of fish and chips on her own in a crowded restaurant, full of strangers.
3. Eating out in a snack bar with her boyfriend.
4. Eating out with her parents in a semifashionable restaurant.
5. Eating out with her boyfriend in a fashionable restaurant.
6. Deliberately asking for smaller portions in a fashionable restaurant.
7. Eating out with a large group of friends in a very exclusive restaurant, sending back any portions that were too big.

As I have said, each task was seen by the client as "sufficiently" challenging but not overwhelming, and Tasks 5, 6, and 7 were initiated by her in a planned break from therapy. This principle allows clients to take responsibility for their therapy quite early, once they have fully understood it and have experienced initial success. On follow-up, Mary was able to eat out in a variety of settings with a variety of people without anxiety.

Variations on a Theme

Although I have not used the challenging-but-not-overwhelming principle in planning a hierarchy of assignments before treatment begins, it can be used in this way. I have not found this necessary because what clients find challenging but not overwhelming changes over time, so that the initial hierarchy becomes redundant. Theoretically, therapists can also use Subjective Units of Disturbance Scale (SUDS) ratings of hierarchy and/or nonhierarchy items, although, again, I have not found this necessary.

Although I have used this principle mainly in helping clients set appropriately challenging tasks to overcome their anxiety problems, I have also used it successfully in helping depressed clients set appropriately challenging behavioral tasks. In so doing, I stress to clients the importance of defining what is challenging in personal terms in relation to their depressed state rather than in relation to their nondepressed state. The successful execution of small tasks deemed personally challenging by depressed clients when they are depressed is highly encouraging for such clients and make them more amenable to the subsequent use of more traditional cognitive change procedures (Beck, Rush, Shaw, & Emery, 1979).

Problems with Compromises

There are, of course, problems associated with the compromises outlined thus far:

1. Clients who succeed in changing negative inferences may later encounter events that realize their inferences. As they have not changed their irrational beliefs, they may make themselves disturbed about such events. Thus, the client of my colleague may later discover that her father, in fact, has been prying into her affairs, and my own client with social anxiety (Robert) may later encounter a group of people who will notice his anxiety and stare at him.

2. Clients who do change their behavior for the better may still encounter events that serve to activate their latent unchanged irrational beliefs. Thus, Sylvia, my client with examination anxiety, may in the future fail an important examination, and Mrs. Anderson's family may again make unreasonable demands on her.

3. Clients who change or remove themselves from problem activating events may later reencounter such situations, which again may activate their latent unmodified irrational beliefs. Thus, Mrs. Curran's family may later mistreat her and Mr. Brown's enthusiasm for the law may wane.

4. Finally, clients who overcome their problems by using challenging-but-not-overwhelming methods are still vulnerable to overwhelming situations.

Although I have described cases where productive changes in inferences, behavior, and situations have not led to belief change, other clients do later change their irrational beliefs after effecting such changes. And yet, although RET theory has emphasized the interdependence of ABC factors, I have wanted to show here that change, particularly at the level of beliefs (B) does not necessarily follow changes achieved at A or C.

The implications of this analysis for empirical study are clear. It would be helpful to research questions such as: (1) With what clients, at which stages of the therapeutic process, are belief change (inference change, behavior change, and situation change) methods appropriate? And (2) under which conditions do changes in inferences, behavior, and situations lead to belief change, and when do they not promote such change? Indeed, it would be interesting to discover how frequently RET therapists do, in fact, make such compromises in their daily clinical practice.

In summary, it is my contention that it is *insufficient* for therapists to practice RET in a way that is theoretically correct for effective therapy to occur. Rather, RET is made more effective, I hypothesize, when therapists also attend to the components of the therapeutic alliance outlined above, are prepared to intervene flexibly based on their understanding of such components, and are willing to make therapeutic compromises when appropriate.

CONCLUSION

Although, in this chapter, I have discussed separately the concept of the therapeutic alliance and the idea of making compromises in RET, these are, in reality, interrelated. For example, making compromises with "elegant" RET is sometimes an important way of sustaining the therapeutic alliance, which may be severely threatened if one dogmatically insists that an elegant therapeutic outcome be sought with particular clients. This, of course, is an example of flexibility—an idea both in keeping with the spirit of RET theory and, I would argue, a hallmark of its effective practice.

REFERENCES

Anchin, J. C., & Kiesler, D. J. (Eds.). (1982). *Handbook of interpersonal psychotherapy.* New York: Pergamon Press.
Beck, A. T., Rush, A. J., Shaw, B. F., & Emery, G. (1979). *Cognitive therapy of depression.* New York: Guilford Press.
Beutler, L. E. (1983). *Eclectic psychotherapy: A systematic approach.* New York: Pergamon Press.
Bordin, E. S. (1979). The generalizability of the psychoanalytic concept of the working alliance. *Psychotherapy: Theory, Research and Practice, 16,* 252–260.
Dorn, F. J. (1984). *Counseling as applied social psychology: An introduction to the social influence model.* Springfield, IL: Thomas.
Dryden, W. (1984). Rational-emotive therapy. In W. Dryden (Ed.), *Individual therapy in Britain* (pp. 235–263). London: Harper & Row.
Dryden, W., & Hunt, P. (1985). Therapeutic alliances in marital therapy: 2. Process issues. In W. Dryden (Ed.), *Marital therapy in Britain: Vol. 1. Context and therapeutic approaches* (pp. 144–168). London: Harper & Row.
Ellis, A. (1979). Discomfort anxiety: A new cognitive behavioral construct, Part 1. *Rational Living, 14*(2), 3–8.
Ellis, A. (1980a). Discomfort anxiety: A new cognitive behavioral construct, Part 2. *Rational Living, 15*(1), 25–30.
Ellis, A. (1980b). The value of efficiency in psychotherapy. *Psychotherapy: Theory, Research and Practice, 17,* 414–419.
Ellis, A. (1983). The philosophic implications and dangers of some popular behavior therapy techniques. In M. Rosenbaum, C. M. Franks, & Y. Jaffe (Eds.), *Perspectives in behavior therapy in the eighties* (pp. 138–151). New York: Springer.
Emmelkamp, P. M. G., Kuipers, A. C. M., & Eggeraat, J. B. (1978). Cognitive modification versus prolonged exposure in vivo: A comparison with agoraphobics as subjects. *Behaviour Research and Therapy, 16,* 33–41.
Golden, W. (1985). An integration of Ericksonian and cognitive-behavioral hypnotherapy in the treatment of anxiety disorders. In E. T. Dowd & J. M. Healy (Eds.), *Case studies in hypnotherapy* (pp. 12–22). New York: Guilford Press.

Lazarus, A. A. (1981). *The practice of multimodal therapy.* New York: McGraw-Hill.

Meichenbaum, D., & Gilmore, J. B. (1982). Resistance from a cognitive-behavioral perspective. In P. L. Wachtel (Ed.), *Resistance* (pp. 133–156). New York: Plenum Press.

Pinsof, W. M., & Catherall, D. R. (1986). The integrative psychotherapy alliance: Family, couple and individual scales. *Journal of Marital and Family Therapy, 12,* 137–151.

Safran, J. D. (1984). Assessing the cognitive-interpersonal cycle. *Cognitive Therapy and Research, 8,* 333–347.

Strong, S. R., & Claiborn, C. D. (1982). *Change through interaction.* New York: Wiley-Interscience.

6

A Rational-Emotive Model of Assessment

RAYMOND DiGIUSEPPE

Rational-emotive therapy has always been presented as an active, directive, efficient form of psychotherapy (Ellis, 1957, 1962, 1985, 1989a). It is often described as a no-nonsense, no-cop-out form of therapy because it advocates forceful, active disputing, challenging and confronting clients' irrational beliefs. An extensive RET literature has developed that explicates the theory (Bernard & DiGiuseppe, 1989; Ellis, 1962, 1973, 1985), specifies the application of RET to different populations and hypothesizes specific irrational beliefs likely to be held by various client populations (Ellis & Bernard, 1983, 1985; Ellis, McInerney, DiGiuseppe, & Yeager, 1988; Ellis, Sichel, DiMattia, Yeager, & DiGiuseppe, 1989), and details disputing strategies to be used with clients (Ellis, 1985; Ellis & Dryden, 1987).

The missing topic in the RET literature has been assessment. Most recent books on RET spend little time discussing assessment. The consideration of assessment in the RET literature is usually limited to one chapter focusing on discovering the client's As, Bs, and Cs, and on detailed hypotheses concerning which irrational beliefs probably underlie the problem in the client group being discussed. Few, if any, systematic procedures or comprehensive rationales for assessment are outlined in the RET literature. Rational-emotive theory and therapy appear to lack a conceptual statement on the place of assessment.

This state of affairs has probably emerged because of Ellis's attitude toward traditional assessment strategies in mental health services and his commitment to efficient intervention strategies. In my 15 years of teaching

RAYMOND DiGIUSEPPE • Department of Psychology, St. John's University, Jamaica, New York 11432, and Institute for Rational-Emotive Therapy, 45 East 65th Street, New York, New York 10021.

workshops and lectures on RET with Dr. Ellis he has repeatedly commented that most traditional psychological assessment is a waste of time and is highly inefficient.

Are all diagnostic judgments irrelevant in RET? Do RET therapists avoid treatment decisions based on the client's type or degree of psychotherapy or personality style? How does a psychotherapist using RET choose what to dispute? Many clinicians watch Ellis perform a demonstration of RET and wonder how he starts disputing so quickly. They fail to see anything that resembles assessment.

Ellis's professional history and list of publications (American Psychological Association, 1985) reveals that he is no stranger to psychological assessment. His doctoral dissertation investigated the psychometric properties of the Minnesota Multiphasic Personality Inventory (MMPI). He published several research reviews of personality inventories in the 1940s and 1950s. He was director of a statewide psychological assessment unit for many years. All of these accomplishments occurred before he initiated rational-emotive therapy.

It would be correct to say that Ellis has been dismayed by the inefficiency of traditional intake procedures in mental health settings. It would be correct to say that, as a result, Ellis's past and present clinical practice and his writings on RET eschew the traditional assessment strategies in mental health. It is correct to say that assessment has been underplayed in the RET literature. However, it would be incorrect to conclude that Ellis and other rational-emotive therapists do not have any assessment strategies. In fact, clinicians at the Institute for Rational-Emotive Therapy who work with Ellis frequently share stories concerning the amount of information he recalls about his clients, or how he uncovers important clinical information in just a session or two.

In this chapter, I propose that RET has a distinct approach to assessment and that RET's active-directive reputation is derived more from its assessment strategies than from its intervention strategies. Based on my work with Ellis for 15 years, having listened to hundreds of his therapy tapes and having discussed clinical and training issues with him, I attempt here to specify the rational-emotive approach to assessment. I compare the rational-emotive model of assessment on a number of assumptions with the traditional approach to psychological assessment.

OVERVIEW OF RATIONAL-EMOTIVE ASSESSMENT PROCEDURES

Clients who come for therapy at the Institute for Rational-Emotive Therapy in New York are typically told to come for their appointment about an hour early. They are asked to complete a four-page biographical information form, the Millon Clinical Multiaxial Inventory II (Millon, 1987), the short form of the Beck Depression Inventory (Beck & Beck, 1972; Beck, Rial, & Rickels, 1974), the General Psychological Well Being Scale (DuPuy, 1984), the General Health Questionnaire (Goldberg, 1972), the Satisfaction with Life Scale (Diener, Emmons, Larsen, & Griffen, 1985), and the Attitudes and Beliefs Scale 2 (DiGiuseppe, Exner, Leaf, & Robin, 1988). Usually, clients are not finished before the session begins, and the scales are completed after the first session. The scales are computer-scored on the premises and are usually available to the therapist by the second session. The brief version of the Beck Depression Inventory, the General Psychological Well Being Scale, the General Health Questionnaire, and the Satisfaction with Life Scale are repeated every four weeks so that therapists and clients can review their progress.

Although therapists at the Institute for Rational-Emotive Therapy do use standardized assessment instruments, diagnostic assessment is not the first task of the therapist. The first task is to develop a therapeutic alliance. Assessment is dynamic, not static. By *dynamic,* I mean that is ongoing. The therapist is always aware that diagnostic impressions are hypotheses and subject to change on attainment of new information. Also, ongoing assessment provides information on the effectiveness of the interventions, which subsequently helps to guide the therapist's clinical decisions.

RET assessment is hypothesis-driven. Rational-emotive theory rejects logical positivism and its emphasis on induction. It acknowledges that therapists are always creating hypotheses about their clients and postulates that it is best to test such hypotheses as quickly as possible.

RET assessment does not follow the medical model. Assessment is treatment-oriented. The most important aspects of assessment are those that lead to treatment decisions. The treatment utility of all assessment strategies guides the therapist.

RET versus Traditional Models of Assessment

It is proposed here that the traditional models of assessment in psychotherapy, psychiatry, and mental health are based on certain assumptions and models of psychopathology and epistemology. Typically, the medical model is contrasted with the behavioral model. Such a contrast usually compares a trait view of behavior with a behavioral or environmental view. RET appears to be a hybrid theory in this regard, in that it postulates traitlike irrational beliefs but also considers the role of the environment.

The traditional models of assessment appear to rest on the view that assessment and treatment are separate activities. Clinicians have traditionally perceived a clear demarcation between their role as diagnostician and their role as therapist (Blatt, 1975). The traditional models of psychopathology and epistemology that have guided assessment are, respectively, the medical model of mental and emotional disorder and the logical-positivist position of knowledge. In addition, the medical model of psychopathology leads to a medical model of assessment. This model, which assumes clients' willingness to self-disclose, fails to place priority on establishing a therapeutic relationship before assessment. Rational-emotive theory differs from traditional models of assessment because it takes different positions on these issues, as is discussed below.

MEDICAL MODEL OF ASSESSMENT

The medical model of behavioral disorders assumes that a complete diagnosis and a total assessment of the problem are necessary before any treatment begins. Mental health clinics and psychiatric hospitals are dominated by the medical profession. The result has been the adoption of the medical model of assessment as the primary paradigm in the mental health field. In medicine there is usually a specific treatment for specific disorders. One does not receive the same antibiotic regardless of the type of infection. The physician performs tests to diagnose the specific flora that have invaded one's body and then prescribes a medication designed to treat that infection. Based on the medical model, mental health treatment also requires a complete diagnostic assessment. This will include a social history, followed by a psychiatric or intake interview. Next, psychological testing may be done. Finally, the case is discussed at a clinical case conference, a diagnosis is reached, and a treatment plan is mapped out. At this time, the case is assigned to a therapist. After several weeks have gone by, the client has spoken with a number of professionals. There are three major criticisms of the traditional medical model of mental health assessment made here: (1) it interferes with developing the therapeutic alliance; (2) differential diagnosis does not lead to differential treatment; and (3) the inductive procedure fails to help clinicians disconfirm their hypotheses.

In private practice, where multidisciplinary teams are rarely used, therapists often perform the necessary tasks themselves, spending a considerable amount of time obtaining a psychosocial history, assessing clients' functioning in all areas of his or her life, and acquiring a full history of the symptoms. Does the client understand the purpose of the assessment? Does the process of delving into so much information, which may be viewed as irrelevant by the client, really enhance the therapeutic relationship? I would say not. And I would go so far as to suggest that, in addition to being inefficient and costly, the medical model of assessment often alienates clients. The problem with placing a priority on diagnostic assessment before therapy is the brief number of sessions most clients remain in therapy. Depending on the study and the population sampled, from 25% to 90% of clients terminate therapy by the fifth session. Up to

80% may leave by the eighth session (see review by Garfield, 1986). I would hypothesize that the high dropout rate in psychotherapy (Garfield, 1986) is partly due to the traditional intake process. Therapists may not have sufficient time to perform a diagnostic assessment before the client leaves.

A recent internal study at the Institute for Rational-Emotive Therapy of 731 clients who had terminated therapy revealed that RET is most often a brief therapy. The mean number of sessions was 16.5, the median was 11 sessions; 30% of the clients had had 5 sessions or fewer, 42% had had 8 sessions or fewer, and only 25% had had 23 sessions or more. Actually, RET ends up having somewhat longer session lengths because fewer people drop out in the first five or so sessions.

Clients come to us in psychological pain. They want help. They may perceive their being shuffled around to different professionals as being abandonment. They may perceive therapists' questions concerning their past, family, and other areas of their lives as voyeuristic and irrelevant. They may perceive the lack of an intervention as a sign of incompetency.

The medical model assumes that a diagnosis is necessary before any treatment can begin because specific disorders respond to different treatments. However, this practice is usually not the case in psychotherapy. Ask any therapist you know if she or he uses different treatments for different diagnoses. In fact, ask yourself if you would be more likely to use Gestalt approaches with one client, behavioral approaches with another, and psychoanalytic approaches with yet a different client. The answer clearly is no.

Psychologists have questioned the utility of diagnostic assessment before therapy. Several authors have concluded that therapists do not find the information revealed in a diagnostic assessment useful for treatment planning or for enhancing therapeutic effectiveness (Adams, 1972; Daily, 1953; Meehl, 1960; Moore, Bobbit, & Wildman, 1968). Clearly, the present diagnostic taxonomy and our present knowledge in psychotherapy do not yet lead to prescriptive psychotherapy (Beutler, 1989). The single best predictor of the type of treatment a client receives is the theoretical orientation of the therapist. All theoretical orientations in psychotherapy claim that their orientation is appropriate for all disorders. Decision rules in psychotherapy treatment manuals concerning which clients are unlikely to benefit from psychodynamic (Luborsky, 1984; Strupp & Binder, 1984), interpersonal (Klerman, Weissman, Rounsville, & Chevron, 1984), cognitive (Beck, Rush, Shaw, & Emery, 1979), and experiential therapy (Daldrup, Beutler, Greenberg, & Engle, 1988) are based on patients' motivation and acceptance of therapeutic philosophy and psychological-mindedness rather than on diagnostic judgments from the third edition of the *Diagnostic and Statistical Manual* (DSM-III; American Psychiatric Association, 1980). Reviews of comparative outcome studies with homogeneous samples have failed to indicate the different successes of specific therapies (Beutler, 1989; Beutler & Crago, 1987).

The best way to start therapy may be to ask the client what problem brought him or her to therapy. Cummings (1986) argued that it is best to ask what motivated clients to come when they did. This problem focus communicates to the client the therapist's willingness to help alleviate his or her pain. From the RET perspective, the assessment of the activating events, the emotional consequences, and the irrational beliefs (Dryden & DiGiuseppe, 1990) may be the most efficient use of the client's and the therapist's time. This kind of assessment helps the therapist apply his or her theoretical orientation to the problem that the client is most willing to present. This kind of assessment also helps the client evaluate the trustworthiness and competence of the therapist and gives the client a chance to evaluate the therapist's orientation. Applying the ABC problem-solving model to the first problem that the client raises also helps the client learn the model on a less difficult problem. As a result, it may be easier to apply RET to the most important issues when the client chooses to discuss them.

Although Ellis and his associates have eschewed assessment for diagnosis, the RET literature has focused on client behaviors and personality characteristics that may influence the course of therapy (Ellis, 1973, 1985; Ellis & Dryden, 1987; Walen, DiGiuseppe, & Wessler, 1980). As proposed by Hayes, Nelson, and Jarrett (1987), RET advocates that assessment focus on issues that are relevant to treatment. In addition to the activating events, emotions, and irrational beliefs, RET recommends that therapists assess clients' introspection, cognitive flexibility, social-problem-solving skills, the presence of secondary emotional reactions, and secondary gain.

There are a few diagnostic categories that may lead to different treatment. These are psychotic syndromes, organic brain impairment, and biologically based depression. All of these disorders may best be treated with medication. However, two points are worth noting. Although these disorders often do respond to medication, the patients often require or benefit from psychotherapy as well. Second, there is no reason why one has to perform the entire ritual of assessment to uncover these problems. Perhaps a more focused style of assessment would uncover these disorders efficiently. The process of identifying and challenging irrational beliefs provides the RET therapist with much information about the way the client thinks. Such cognitive processing information is more likely than a social history to suggest or corroborate the diagnosis of organicity or psychosis.

Therapists can pursue a hypothesis-driven assessment once they suspect one of these disorders. For example, certain things that the client says may suggest to the therapist the presence of a major depression or another diagnostic category that will respond to medication. Once a therapist develops such a hypothesis, she or he would construct questions to corroborate or disconfirm it immediately. This process is discussed in more detail in the next section.

Static versus Dynamic Assessment

The medical model of assessment and the medical model of psycho-pathology present assessment as static. Emotional and behavioral disorders are mental symptoms of intrapsychic diseases that are categorically diagnosed. They are present or absent at intake, as are irrational beliefs. The therapist performs an assessment first to formulate a diagnosis and then begins treatment.

The RET model assumes that assessment is an ongoing process, although we are still searching for stable traits. All diagnostic impressions are tentative. Therapists had better be prepared to shift their conceptualization of the client as new information is revealed throughout the progression of therapy. An attitude of ongoing assessment means that assessment is an integral part of all therapy sessions, as similarly stressed in behavior therapy (Wolpe, 1969). RET advocates the scientist-practitioner model (Barlow, Hays, & Nelson, 1984) of ongoing assessment to monitor the effectiveness of the therapy. If an intervention is not working, the case can be reformulated and a new strategy tried. Ongoing assessment means that the successful outcomes are assessed for the systemic effect that they may bring about (Freeman, 1986). For example, a depressed client may overcome his or her depression and behave in newly assertive and independent ways. These behaviors may be a threat to other family members, who will try to subvert them. The client may not have the skills to cope with the sabotage. The therapist who assesses for the potential of these possible outcomes can work either with the primary client on new goals or with the family members to help them adjust to the client's new behavior.

Therapeutic Relationships and Self-Disclosure

Ellis (1962, 1985, 1989a) has attempted to help clients identify the irrational beliefs causing their emotional difficulties as quickly as possible. He frequently engages in the disputation of an irrational belief in the first session, possibly 20–30 minutes into the session. RET assumes that clients may be reluctant to reveal their problems at the initial session. Ellis attempts to actively teach clients a process of resolving emotional problems to increase the clients' confidence in the efficacy of treatment.

The traditional model of psychological assessment gathers information to achieve a diagnosis before treatment begins. This strategy assumes that clients will reveal their deepest, darkest secrets, symptoms, thoughts, and emotions in the first couple of contacts with mental health professionals *before* a therapeutic *alliance* is established. I would argue that clients are likely to withhold shameful, important information about themselves or about their reason for seeking therapy until after they have established a therapeutic alliance. Such a therapeutic alliance involves trusting that the therapist will accept them regardless of their problems. A therapeutic alliance also requires confidence that the therapist is sufficiently skilled to handle a problem if the client does risk revealing himself or herself. Traditional mental health assessment is poorly designed to build a therapeutic relationship. Interviews designed to obtain all the information necessary for a psychosocial history and diagnosis require a significant amount of immediate disclosure, and to a professional whom the client does not know and may not see again. Also, the information requested in such an interview may not seem *relevant to the client*. If clients believe in a historical insight model of therapy, this information may seem relevant. However, many clients (as well as many therapists) do not perceive the relevance of the psychosocial history. The possible perception of irrelevance further detracts from the therapeutic alliance. Finally, clients usually seek therapy when they are in psychological pain. Rational-emotive theory postulates that a therapeutic alliance is best developed by offering the client some interventions as quickly as possible to demonstrate the therapist's willingness and ability to perceive the client's pain.

Recall, Recognition, and Private Thoughts

Traditional assessment strategies in psychology assume that clients are able to report their inner thoughts and feelings. It has long been established that the clients who are good candidates for psychotherapy have good verbal skills. The clients who benefit from therapy the most are termed *YAVIS clients*. This acronym stands for "young, attractive, verbal, intelligent, and successful." People who have poor verbal skills, or who are not psychologically minded or introspective, are considered poor candidates for the "talking cure." Even therapists who are not cognitively oriented seem to believe that clients are capable of verbally expressing their feelings. I would like to suggest that the reason that verbal skills have been considered such a prerequisite for psychotherapy is that therapy involves a translation process.

Bernard (1981) pointed out that irrational beliefs and other such private thoughts may not be readily accessible for verbal report. Research in cognitive psychology suggests that people are capable of expressing all of their cognitive processes (Nisbett & Wilson, 1977). Bernard suggested that cognitive approaches to clinical phenomena consider the relationship between thought and language suggested by Vygotsky (1962; also see Fodor, 1973). According to Vygotsky, thought and language are not synonymous. Children think before they develop linguistic abilities; therefore, people's thoughts are not encoded in the words of their spoken language. Once language is developed, thoughts can still be generated without language. Thoughts appear to be encoded in shorthand. A great many associations can be connected to a particular thought, and those associations can be experienced almost instantaneously. To communicate a thought to another, the person has to formulate the equivalent ideas in his or her native language. As an example, think of your mother—only for a second. How many different associations and ideas come to your mind? Now, try to imagine translating all of those associations into spoken English. Do all the thoughts and feelings have direct equivalents in our language? How much longer would it take to verbalize all the associations than it took to think them? Because it would take much longer to say them, you may struggle with which associations are most important. Because thought and language are not the same, Bernard suggested that clients may not always be able to express their irrational beliefs and, I would add, any other thoughts or feelings.

The relationship between programming and processing languages in computers may demonstrate the relation between thought and language. Information in a computer is encoded in a series of electronic impulses. The code used to derive meaning from these series of impulses is called *binary*. For the computer to communicate with the user, the binary code is translated into the programming language: Pascal, Basic, Fortran, or some other. There are limits on the information that can be communicated because of the limitations of any program language. There are limits on the speed with which the information can be retrieved depending on the hardware of the computer. Although I recognize that the computer is a poor model of human thought, this aspect of the computer demonstrates the importance of the translation process.

Thoughts are encoded in some physiological neural engram that science does not yet understand. In order for a person to share his or her thoughts with others, the thoughts have to be translated into the person's native language. Some languages are better suited to the expression of certain points than others, and some human hardware is better suited to the translation task than others.

Bernard suggested that another reason why private thoughts may be hard to recall is the distinction between linguistic and episodic memory. Memory of linguistic information and memory of information concerning events or episodes are organized separately (Tulving, 1972). Historic events and early experiences that may be associated with a disturbed emotion or evaluation of a class of stimuli would most likely be stored in episodic memory and easily accessible to linguistic recall.

Self-disclosure in therapy requires that clients go through two processes: (1) uncovering ideas that are organized in episodic memory and encoded in the neuronal coding system, which is dense with connections and (2) extracting the central idea and translating it into their native language. This could be a difficult task, as it involves the recall of information and expressive language. Most forms of psychotherapy rely on these expressive and recall processes. Clients have to recall their feelings and thoughts and then express the translation. Clients with proficient verbal skills are good at this task. However, the recall of information is always more difficult than recognition, and receptive language is always more difficult than expressive language. Clients who have not learned to be psychologically minded, or who have limited emotional vocabularies, or who have limited intellectual and verbal abilities, do less well. But we let them suffer through this process anyway.

Clients who have difficulty with the translation process may benefit from a recognition or receptive language task in therapy. This is precisely what occurs when the therapist offers interpretations or hypotheses. If the hypothesis formulated by the therapist is similar to an idea or feeling experienced by the client, the client recognizes it and affirms the hypothesis. If the hypothesis is off the mark, and the client does not recognize it as reflecting her or his own experience, the client disconfirms the hypothesis, and the therapist starts over again. I would argue that such hypothesis-driven assessment, as practiced in RET, is more effective—and is perceived as more friendly and less threatening by clients with poor insight and limited verbal skills. I would also hypothesize that clients with poorer verbal skills benefit more from therapy with hypothesis-driven assessment than those who are more verbal and who can benefit from self-discovery.

EPISTEMOLOGY

Another major difference between RET and traditional models of psychological assessment concerns the directiveness of the interviewer. Traditionally, assessment is thorough and comprehensive. Interviewers refrain from offering hypotheses about the client's behavior. After all the information is collected, the professional team sifts through the data looking for conclusions about the client. The assessment process in the mental health professions appears to follow the same epistemological model that psychology advocates for the process of science: logical positivism (Ayer, 1936; Cook & Campbell, 1979). Logical positivism in psychology has always placed a premium on inductive logic and reasoning. According to this model, scientists (or clinicians) collect as much data as possible and do so "objectively" and dispassionately. They then search for patterns of results present in the data. Following this model, the therapist asks questions in all areas of clients' lives and functioning, including the social, family, medical, academic, and vocational arenas. A complete history is taken in each of the above-mentioned areas. A good interviewer avoids any premature conclusions until all the data are collected. If the therapist has any hypotheses, she or he does not share them with the client.

Rational-emotive theory has rejected the logical-positivist approach to epistemology (Ellis, 1989a; Woolfolk & Sass, 1989) and instead posits a constructivistic, hypotheticodeductive view of epistemology based on the philosophy of science (Hempel, 1966; Lakatos, 1970) and Bartley's (1984) comprehensive critical rationalism (DiGiuseppe, 1986a; Ellis, 1989a,b; Ellis, Sichel, DiMattia, Yeager, & DiGiuseppe, 1989). Rational-emotive theory holds that humans can not help but make up theories. One tests one's theories by logically deducing hypotheses from the theory and empirically testing them. Although this model of epistemology has been applied to clients' irrational beliefs and has lead to identifying disputing strategies (see Chapter 7), its implications for therapist behavior have not been fully explored.

The primary reason why the philosophy of logical positivism is inappropriate as a model for clinical assessment is that therapists cannot collect data in the manner suggested by this philosophy. Therapists (and people) cannot dispassionately collect data and wait for an inductive, logically accurate conclusion (Polanyi, 1958). I propose that all therapists formulate hypotheses concerning clients' diagnoses within minutes of the interview. Ask yourself how long it takes you to have a working hypothesis the next time you see a new client. A novice therapist may take longer, but before the session is over, they will still have some hypothesis.

So why does human hypothesis formation pose a problem to the inductive model of reasoning? The answer follows from the way human memory works. Humans (and therefore clinicians) tend to remember confirmatory information more than disconfirmatory information (Achenbach, 1985). Let us suppose two clinicians are interviewing a client together. During the interview, they develop different hypotheses concerning the client's diagnosis. They stick to the structured, inductive way of asking questions concerning all of the areas mentioned above. They share their different impressions after the interview. Because of human nature, each clinician will claim that he or she is correct and will recall information from the interview to support his or her hypothesis. The two could discuss their differences and reach a consensus. In most interviews, there is another interviewer present to remember information that supports a rival hypothesis.

Another problem involves the possible distorting of the process of induction through the interviewer's influence on the data gathering. Once a clinician has formulated a hypothesis concerning the diagnosis (or other aspects of the client's personality), she or he is more interested in hearing confirmatory than in hearing disconfirmatory information. The interviewer may be inclined to show more interest when the client speaks about topics that confirm her or his hypothesis. This differential interest on the part of the therapist may be expressed in his or her facial expression, tone of voice, or body posture. The therapist's actions may reinforce the client to talk more about some topics than about others. The fact that such nonverbal, innocuous reinforcers can affect the responses of the interviewee has been well documented in behavioral psychology and is referred to as the *Greenspoon effect* (Greenspoon, 1965).

Achenbach (1985) argued that there are a number of such cognitive distortions in clinicians' judgments. His solution to the problem is the use of objective, standardized, normed questionnaires to collect data. Although I concur with Achenbach, there is an alternative solution. The solution to the problems of clinician errors in judgment is to change the model of science on which the assessment strategies are based. Rather than rely on an inductively driven model based on logical positivism, clinicians can base their interviewing strategies on a constructivist, modern, hypotheticodeductive philosophy of science.

Historians of science (Kuhn, 1970) have argued that science has not progressed by induction. In fact, scientists are not dispassionate, objective data gatherers (Polanyi, 1958). Scientists formulate hypotheses or theories and then develop deductions from their theories that are testable empirically (Hempel, 1966; Lakatos, 1970). Philosophers of science such as Popper (1962) have argued the importance of deduction from theories of testable hypotheses that can be falsified. Popper's method is important precisely because humans are apt not to give up their constructed hypotheses and theories.

The resulting interviewing strategy includes the following elements: (1) assessment is viewed as an ongoing process, not as an activity for the initiation of treatment; (2) it is acknowledged that clinicians formulate hypotheses quickly in any interview; (3) questions are developed in the interview with the intent of testing the theory about the client that the clinician has formulated; (4) attempts to disconfirm hypotheses are given as much importance as or more importance than attempts to confirm them; and (5) after a hypothesis is rejected, the information gathered to disconfirm the hypothesis is used to formulate new hypotheses.

HYPOTHESIS-DRIVEN ASSESSMENT

RET advocates training clinicians to develop hypotheses concerning their clients and to test them as quickly as possible. One must be careful not to confuse the two uses of the term *induction* and must discriminate between logical induction and psychological induction. The term *logical induction* refers to a form of testing the truth of a statement and involves drawing a conclusion of a general rule from observing all particular elements (Bachhuber, 1957). Psychological induction is a process of construing theories or hypotheses concerning things based on observations (Holland, Holyoak, Nisbett, & Thagard, 1989). The psychological induction used by a therapist (or a scientist) to develop a theory concerning a client does not imply that the theory or hypothesis generated by the therapist has been proved by the logical rules of induction. The therapist (or scientist) must develop ways to test the theory. I would argue that, because therapists develop theories about clients all the time, and because the traditional data-gathering strategies can foster the logical errors mentioned above, it is best for therapists to actively test their theories immediately. This can be done in several ways. First, they can deduce other facts that they would expect to be true if their theory is correct. Second, they can construct questions to ascertain if this hypothesis is correct. Third, the therapist can ask the client if the hypothesis is true. The client can provide a large amount of confir-matory or disconfirmatory evidence.

Consider this example. After listening to the client discuss the reasons for coming to therapy, a therapist learns that the client is fatigued, sleep-less, and unmotivated and does not enjoy life. The therapist develops the theory that this client is depressed. The therapist can let the client go on reporting and search her reports for more evidence of depressive symp-toms, or she can develop a set of questions that will help to rule in favor of or to disconfirm depression. The therapist thinks about what other symp-toms accompany depression. She decides to ask the client if he has the cognitive triad associated with depression (Beck et al., 1979). The client responds affirmatively. The therapist may ask for more data: "Do you feel extremely sad, or do you lack energy to complete activities?" The client responds yes. Now that the hypothesis is confirmed, the therapist's mind is still active. Based on the body posture and the way the client enters the room, the therapist wonders if the client's depression is biologically based. What would one expect if this were true? She recalls her knowledge of the difference between exogenous and endogenous depression. She then asks the client if there are any vegetative symptoms. He answers no. She is unsure yet what to conclude. If his depression is endogenous, it is less likely to be reactive to a particular event. So she asks, "Was there anything that happened to you that preceded your depression?" The client responds affirmatively and reports that the depression started when his wife left him and that he had never been depressed before. The therapist surrenders her notion of endogenous depression and hypothesizes that the client's main irrational belief leading to the depression is a demand for love and approval.

In this brief example, the therapist quickly creates a theory about this client, refers to a knowledge base from which to deduce a series of ques-tions that will help corroborate or disconfirm the theory, and develops questions based on this knowledge. The therapist also develops new ideas after each confirmation or disconfirmation of her hypothesis. This is an active-directive hypothesis-driven model of assessment. Therapists are constantly using their experience and knowledge to test and disconfirm hypotheses and, finally, to develop new hypotheses. Therapists avoid the errors of memory and leading the client.

Teaching Scientific Thinking

Hypothesis-driven assessment models scientific thinking for clients. RET teaches clients to think scientifically, that is, to evaluate their thoughts, and to test whether they are logically accurate and empirically consistent with reality. RET further emphasizes that one develops new ideas to replace ideas that have been proved to be false. This is exactly what the therapist is doing. Therapists demonstrate that they test their thoughts, give them up when data are wanting, and develop new thoughts in exchange.

Developing a Therapeutic Relationship

The hypothesis-driven assessment model is also helpful in establishing a therapeutic rapport. Once it is established, clients are more willing to reveal their true purpose for seeking help and to share more personal and possibly shameful information about themselves.

RET advocates that the best way to develop a therapeutic alliance (Ellis, 1985; Ellis & Dryden, 1987) is to attempt to solve the client's immediate problem. Usually, the therapist asks the client which problem he or she wishes to discuss. The therapist then interviews the client to identify the activating events, irrational beliefs, and emotional consequences in the problem identified by the client. The therapist does this for two or three sessions and then possibly suggests larger issues that the client may wish to work on. In this way, clients can reveal information at their own pace. They can see how the therapist uses the information they reveal, and they can develop a sense of trust and faith in the therapist's ability.

The client can see that the therapist not only is listening and empathizing with the client but is also actively thinking about the client and demonstrating his or her willingness to search for ways to understand and help the client. Offering hypotheses concerning the client's thoughts also demonstrates empathy. Not only does the therapist understand how the client feels, but the therapist also understands how the client is thinking. Cognitive therapy has always stressed the collaborative aspect of therapy and the importance of collaboration in building a therapeutic relationship (Beck et al., 1979). Asking the client directly for feedback on the accuracy of the clinician's hypotheses is the ultimate form of collaboration. The therapist's behavior demonstrates the importance of the client's cooperation in the process and the therapist's trust and respect for the client.

Limitations

Such a directive assessment strategy is not without its pitfalls, the most serious of which is narcissistic epistemology on the part of therapists. Therapist's hypotheses are what are normally referred to in psychotherapy as *interpretations*. Because interpretations result from the psychological induction of therapists, they can be wrong. Therapists have to be willing to accept that their brilliant hypotheses and interpretations may be false. If therapists continue to cling to false hypotheses, they not only pursue irrelevant lines of inquiry but may also impair the therapeutic relationship. A client's refusal to accept the interpretation of a therapist does not automatically mean that the client is resisting. The therapist may be wrong.

Testing hypotheses requires the feedback of the client. This can be honestly obtained only if the client perceives that the feedback is desired. To ensure that the client's participation will be forthcoming and to avoid the appearance (or reality) of closed-mindedness and authoritarianism by the therapist, it is recommended that hypotheses and interpretations be given in hypothetical language and not in declarative sentences: "Could it be that you're feeling . . . ?" or "I have an idea I would like to share with you. Could you . . . ?" or "Other clients with your problem also seem to experience X. Could that be true of you?"

ASSESSING IRRATIONAL BELIEFS

Assessing clients' irrational beliefs is the most important diagnostic task in rational-emotive therapy. Most therapists who come for training in RET usually attempt to discover the client's irrational beliefs by asking the client, "What are you telling yourself?" This seems to be an appropriate strategy because irrational beliefs are cognitions, and cognitions are conscious. However, most clients respond to the questions concerning their conscious thoughts that precede or coexist with their disturbed emotions with inferences or automatic thoughts and not irrational beliefs.

A closer examination of rational-emotive theory suggests that irrational beliefs are not as transparent as many therapists initially think. Irrational beliefs are subconscious or tacit (Ellis, 1962, 1989a). By the term *subconscious*, Ellis does not imply the Freudian concept of *libidinal urges*. Ellis (1962) originally thought of irrational beliefs as preconscious. By that, he meant that they were outside the client's immediate consciousness but readily available to consciousness.

Beck (1976) and his colleagues (Beck & Emery, 1985; Beck et al., 1979) have a similar conceptualization. They refer to irrational beliefs as underlying schema or assumptions and also describe them as tacit cognitive constructs. They posit that the negative distortions are readily available in consciousness and therefore call them "automatic thoughts." These cognitions are what RET theory refers to as "inferences" (DiGiuseppe, 1986a,b, 1989; Huber & Baruth, 1989; Wessler & Wessler, 1980). It is most important that therapists learn to distinguish between automatic thoughts and inferences, on the one hand, and irrational beliefs, on the other. Below are six strategies for uncovering clients' irrational beliefs.

Inductive Awareness

The first strategy that therapists may use to uncover the core irrational beliefs I have labeled *inductive awareness*. In this strategy, the therapist asks clients what they are telling themselves when they feel upset. Therapists' queries concerning clients' thoughts, self-statements, or beliefs that precede or are linked to the clients' disturbed emotions frequently uncover clients' automatic thoughts or inferences, and not their irrational beliefs. The therapist then disputes the automatic thoughts. Each session proceeds in this way. Eventually, the client becomes aware that an underlying theme permeates all the beliefs that she or he and the therapist have been disputing. This underlying theme will be a schematic irrational belief. After the client has discovered this underlying irrational belief, the therapist switches the focus to disputing the irrational belief. This strategy appears to be the most common among people who have been exposed to RET and cognitive therapy by reading and workshop attendance, but who have had no formal training and supervision. RET would find nothing harmful in this strategy; however, it appears to be very inefficient. Therapists spend most of their time disputing inferences. Although this maneuver may be cognitive therapy, it is not RET (Ellis, Young, & Lockwood, 1987). In fact, Dryden and DiGiuseppe (1990) identified the most common error of new rational-emotive therapists as disputing the first belief that clients report. This first belief represents the client's inferences, and therefore, in disputing the first belief, the therapist will not get to the underlying irrational beliefs.

Inductive Interpretation

A similar strategy involves the therapist's asking clients what they are thinking as they experience the disturbed emotion, thereby uncovering the inference, and subsequently disputing the inference. This strategy is followed for several sessions, perhaps 5 to 10. During these sessions, the therapist has to uncover numerous automatic thoughts or inferences that covary with the client's emotional disturbance. While examining these inferences, the therapist has been looking for a common theme among them. The therapist may collect more data before she or he is sure what the client's core schematic irrational belief is. Finally, the therapist shares with the client the underlying theme that appears to be a common thread throughout the automatic thoughts or inferences that the client has reported. If the client accepts the interpretation, the therapist starts challenging the validity of the core underlying theme.

This strategy is the one recommended by Beck and his colleagues (Beck & Emery, 1985). The decision to dispute automatic thoughts first, as a way to uncover core underlying irrational beliefs, versus immediately uncovering and disputing irrational beliefs appears to be the primary difference between general cognitive therapy and RET (DiGiuseppe & Linscott, 1990; Ellis, 1987). The inductive awareness strategy also appears inefficient for several reasons. First, the therapist probably has a hypothesis concerning the client's core irrational belief long before he or she gives the interpretation. Holding the hypothesis in abeyance while collecting more data inductively allows the therapist to make some of the logical errors mentioned above. Second, the inductive interpretation strategy is inefficient because both Beck (1976) and Ellis (1987) believe that the automatic thoughts or inferences are caused by the underlying schematic irrational beliefs. So why not get to the core cognitions and challenge them as quickly as possible?

Inference Chaining

As it is common for clients to report automatic thoughts or inferences when asked what they are thinking, one can take the information that they give and use it to uncover the underlying core irrational beliefs. In inference chaining, the therapist socratically asks the client to assume that the inference is true. Then, the therapist follows with questions concerning what would happen if the first inference were true. This process is followed repeatedly until the client reports a different kind of thought, usually a schematic rule or core irrational belief. The therapists' questions might be the following: "And if that were true, what else do you think would happen?" or "Let us suppose X were true. What would that mean to you?" or "If X were true, what would that mean about you?" In inference chaining, the therapist unravels layers of meaning that the client has connected to the automatic thought that first jumps into the client's consciousness.

Conjunctive Phrasing

Ellis has frequently been observed performing a variation of the inference chaining, which I have labeled *conjunctive phrasing*. In this strategy, Ellis asks his client what she or he was thinking when she or he got upset;

the client is likely to respond with an inference. At this point, Ellis responds not with a question or a challenge, but with a conjunction or a conjunctive phrase. Some typical responses are "and then . . ." or "and that would mean . . ." or "and if that were true . . ." or "and that means I would be . . ."

The conjunctive phrase does not challenge or dispute the inference. It partially confirms its truth and is an invitation for clients to finish their thought. An advantage of this method is that it keeps clients focused on their thoughts. The less a therapist says, the less clients have to respond to the therapist's words or attend to whether the therapist has understood them. The conjunctive phrase focuses clients on the meaning of their statements. This strategy appears to be the most elegant and the most effective strategy for uncovering irrational beliefs.

Deductive Interpretation

Inference chaining and conjunctive phrasing both involve some degree of self-discovery on the part of the client. Even though the therapist guides the inquiry, the clients examine their own unconscious thought processes and are helped to uncover their core scheme or irrational belief. However, many times, clients are unable to label their thoughts. As the therapist persists in asking open-ended or Socratic questions, clients feel frustrated by the long pauses and their inability to express their thoughts in words. Ellis almost always starts to assess clients' beliefs through inference chaining or conjunctive phrasing. It is best if clients can use self-discovery to become aware of their irrational beliefs. How long does a therapist pursue self-discovery and at what cost? How long does the therapist have to allow the client to explore and await self-discovery?

Usually, Ellis does not wait very long before he offers an interpretation, the interpretation being a hypothesis concerning what the client is thinking to cause his or her disturbance. Most clients respond to the early and frequent interpretation positively. They often comment that the therapist not only understands how they feel but also understands how they think. Although clients usually welcome therapists' hypotheses, they do not always accept them. If the therapist is off the mark, clients usually say this outright. More often, the hypothesis offered is close to, but not exactly, what the client is thinking. The interpretation may be close enough so that clients can put their thoughts into words themselves. On other occasions, therapists know that they are in the correct area and try to refine the hypothesis. This hypothesis testing frequently happens several times before the therapist and the client agree on the irrational belief that is underlying the client's emotional disturbance.

Disputing as Assessment

Once the client's irrational belief has been identified, the therapist usually moves on to disputing. However, clients' responses to the disputing questions may provide more information about the irrational beliefs that is at the core of their emotional disturbance. It is not uncommon for clients to respond to disputes of one irrational belief with another irrational belief to justify the first irrational belief. For example, a 38-year-old recently divorced man sought therapy for social anxiety about meeting women. He had identified his irrational belief as "I can't stand being rejected by women." After several attempts to dispute the client's LFT concerning female rejection, the therapist asked, "Why do you think you could not stand being rejected by women?" The client responded that he could not stand rejection because that would mean (to him) that he was an unlovable person. If this were true, he certainly would be worthless. Although there is no logical connection between these two irrational beliefs, there was a psychological connection for this client. The fastest way to get to the most core irrational belief may be to dispute. Thus, the line between assessment and treatment is a fine line and may involve the same questioning.

This chapter has attempted to provide a model of assessment in rational-emotive therapy. I hope it clarifies some of the misconceptions about how RET is done. This model could be described as directive, hypothesis-driven, deductive, and collaborative. It is my hypothesis that the general effectiveness and the short-term nature of RET result as much from this model of assessment as they do from the active disputing of irrational beliefs.

References

Achenbach, T. (1985). *The assessment and taxonomy of child and adolescent psychopathology.* Newport Beach, CA: Sage.

Adams, J. (1972). The contribution of the psychological to psychiatric diagnosis. *Journal of Personality Assessment, 36,* 561–566.

American Psychiatric Association. (1980). *Diagnostic and statistical manual of mental disorders* (3rd ed.). Washington, DC: Author.

American Psychological Association. (1985). Professional contributions to psychology as a profession—1985: Albert Ellis.

Ayer, A. J. (1936). *Language, truth and logic.* New York: Dover.

Bachhuber, A. (1957). *Introduction to logic.* New York: Appleton-Century-Crofts.

Barlow, D., Hayes, S., & Nelson, R. (1984). *The scientist practitioner.* New York: Pergamon Press.

Bartley, W. W., III. (1984). *The retreat to commitment* (2nd ed.). New York: Knopf.

Beck, A. (1972). *Depression: Causes and treatment.* Philadelphia: University of Pennsylvania Press.

Beck, A. (1976). *Cognitive therapy and the emotional disorders.* New York: International Universities Press.

Beck, A., & Beck, R. W. (1972). Screening depressed patients in family practice: A rapid technique. *Postgraduate Medicine, 52,* 81–85.

Beck, A., & Emery, G. (1985). *Anxiety disorders and phobias: A cognitive perspective.* New York: Basic Books.

Beck, A., Rial, W. Y., & Rickels, K. (1974). Short Form of Depression Inventory: Cross validation. *Psychological Reports, 34,* 1184–1186.

Beck, A., Rush, A., Shaw, B., & Emery, G. (1979). *Cognitive therapy of depression.* New York: Guilford Press.

Bernard, M. (1981). Private thought in rational emotive therapy. *Cognitive Therapy and Research, 5*(2), 125–142.

Bernard, M., & DiGiuseppe, R. (Eds.). (1989). *Inside rational-emotive therapy: A critical appraisal of the theory and therapy of Albert Ellis.* Orlando, FL: Academic Press.

Beutler, L. (1989). Differential treatment selection: The role of diagnosis in psychotherapy. *Psychotherapy, 26*(3), 271–281.

Beutler, L., & Crago, M. (1987). Strategies and techniques of psychotherapeutic intervention. In R. E. Hales & A. J. Frances (Eds.), *Annual review of psychology,* Vol. 6 (pp. 378–397).

Blatt, S. J. (1975). The validity of projective techniques and their research and clinical contribution. *Journal of Personality Assessment, 39,* 327–343.

Cook, T. D., & Campbell, D. T. (1979). *Quasi-experimentation design and analysis issues for field settings.* Boston: Houghton Mifflin.

Cummings, N. (1986). The dismantling of our health care system. *American Psychologist, 41,* 426–431.

Daily, C. A. (1953). The practical utility of the clinical report. *Journal of Consulting Psychology, 17,* 297–302.

Daldrup, R. J., Beutler, L. E., Greenberg, L. S. & Engle, D. (1988). *Focused expressive psychotherapy: A Gestalt therapy for individuals with constricted affect.* New York: Guilford Press.

Diener, E., Emmons, R. A., Larsen, R. J., & Griffin, S. (1985). The satisfaction with life scale. *Journal of Personality Assessment, 49,* 71–75.

DiGiuseppe, R. (1986a). Cognitive therapy for childhood depression. *Psychotherapy and the Family, 2*(3/4), 153–172.

DiGiuseppe, R. (1986b). The implications of the philosophy of science for rational-emotive theory and therapy. *Psychotherapy, 23*(4), 634–639.

DiGiuseppe, R. (1989). Cognitive therapy with children. In A. Freeman, K. Simon, L. Beutler, & H. Arkowitz (Eds.), *Comprehensive handbook of cognitive therapy.* New York: Plenum Press.

DiGiuseppe, R., & Linscott, J. (1990). *Philosophical differences among cognitive behavioral therapists: Belief in rationalism, constructivism, or both?* Manuscript submitted for publication.

DiGiuseppe, R., Exner, T., Leaf, R., & Robin, M. (1988). The development of a measure of rational/irrational beliefs. Poster session presented at the World Congress on Behavior Therapy, Edinburgh, Scotland.

Dryden, W., & DiGiuseppe, R. (1990). *A rational therapist's primer.* Champaign, IL: Research Press.

DuPuy, H. (1984). A measure of psychological well-being. In N. K. Wenger, M. E. Mattson, C. D. Furberg, & J. Elinson (Eds.), *Assessment of quality of life* (pp. 353–356). New York: Lecajq Publishing.

Ellis, A. (1957). Rational psychotherapy and individual psychology. *Journal of Individual Psychology, 13,* 38–44.

Ellis, A. (1962). *Reason and emotion in psychotherapy.* Secaucus, NJ: Lyle Stuart.

Ellis, A. (1973). *Humanistic psychotherapy: The rational-emotive approach.* New York: McGraw-Hill.

Ellis, A. (1985). *Overcoming resistance: Rational-emotive therapy with difficult clients.* New York: Springer.

Ellis, A. (1987). A sadly neglected cognitive element in depression. *Cognitive Therapy and Research, 11,* 121–146.

Ellis, A. (1989a). Comments on my critics. In M. E. Bernard & R. DiGiuseppe (Eds.), *Inside rational emotive therapy: A critical appraisal of the theory and therapy of Albert Ellis* (pp. 199–233). New York: Academic Press.

Ellis, A. (1989b). Is rational-emotive therapy (RET) "rationalist" or "constructivist"? Keynote address to the World Congress of Cognitive Therapy, Oxford, England, June 29. Also in W. Dryden (Ed.). (1989). *The essential Albert Ellis.* New York: Springer.

Ellis, A., & Bernard, M. E. (Eds.). (1983). *Rational emotive approaches to children's problems.* New York: Plenum Press.

Ellis, A., & Bernard, M. E. (Eds.). (1985). *Clinical applications of rational-emotive therapy.* New York: Plenum Press.

Ellis, A., & Dryden, W. (1987). *The practice of rational-emotive therapy.* New York: Springer.

Ellis, A., Young, J., & Lockwood, G. (1987). Cognitive therapy and rational-emotive therapy: A dialogue. *Journal of Cognitive Psychotherapy: An International Quarterly, 1*(4), 204–256.

Ellis, A., McInerney, J., DiGiuseppe, R., & Yeager, R. (1988). *Rational emotive therapy with alcoholics and substance abusers.* New York: Pergamon Press.

Ellis, A., Sichel, J., DiMattia, D., Yeager, R., & DiGiuseppe, R. (1989). *Rational emotive couples therapy.* New York: Pergamon Press.

Fodor, J. (1973). Some reflections on L. S. Vygotsky's thought and language. *Cognition, 1,* 83–95.

Freeman, A. (1986). Understanding personal, cultural and family schema in psychotherapy. *Journal of Psychotherapy and Family Therapy, 2,* 79–99.

Garfield, S. L. (1986). Research in client variables in psychotherapy. In S. L. Garfield & A. Bergin (Eds.), *Handbook of psychotherapy and behavior change.* New York: Wiley.

Goldberg, D. P. (1972). *The detection of psychiatric illness by questionnaire: A technique for the identification and assessment of non-psychotic psychiatric illness.* Oxford: Oxford University Press.

Greenspoon, J. (1965). Learning theory contributions to psychotherapy. *Psychotherapy: Theory, Research and Practice, 2*(4), 145–150.

Hayes, S., Nelson, R., & Jarrett, R. (1987). The treatment utility of assessment: A functional approach to evaluating assessment quality. *American Psychologist, 42,* 963–974.

Hempel, C. G. (1966). *Philosophy of natural sciences.* Englewood Cliffs, NJ: Prentice-Hall.

Holland, J., Holyoak, K., Nisbett, R., & Thagard, P. (1989). *Induction: Processes of inferences, learning, and discovery.* Cambridge: MIT Press.

Huber, C., & Baruth, L. (1989). *Rational-emotive family therapy.* New York: Springer.

Klerman, G. L., Weissman, M. M., Rounsville, B. J., & Chevron, E. S. (1984). *Interpersonal psychotherapy of depression.* New York: Basic Books.

Kuhn, T. (1970). *The structure of scientific revolutions* (2nd ed.). Chicago: University of Chicago Press.

Lakatos, I. (1970). Falsification and the methodology of scientific research programs. In I. Lakatos & A. Musgrave (Eds.), *Criticism and the growth of knowledge* (pp. 91–196). London: Cambridge University Press.

Luborsky, L. (1984). *Principles of psychoanalytic psychotherapy: A manual for supportive-expressive treatment.* New York: Basic Books.

Meehl, P. (1960). The cognitive activity of the clinician. *American Psychologist, 15,* 19–27.

Millon, T. (1987). *Manual for the MCMI-II.* Minneapolis, MN: National Computer Systems.

Moore, G. H., Bobbitt, W. E., & Wildman, R. W. (1968). Psychiatric impressions of psychological reports. *Journal of Clinical Psychology, 24,* 373–376.

Nisbett, R. E., & Wilson, T. D. (1977). Telling more than we can know: Verbal reports on mental processes. *Psychological Review, 84,* 231–259.

Polanyi, M. (1958). *Personal knowledge: Towards a post-critical philosophy.* Chicago: University of Chicago Press.

Popper, K. R. (1962). *Objective knowledge.* London: Oxford.

Rorer, L. G. (1989). Some myths of science in psychology. In D. Cicchetti & W. Grove (Eds.), *Thinking clearly about psychology! Essays in honor of Paul E. Meehl.*

Russell, B. (1945). *A history of Western philosophy.* New York: Simon & Schuster.

Strupp, H. H. & Binder, J. L. (1984). *Psychotherapy in a new key.* New York: Basic Books.

Tulving, E. (1972). Episodic and semantic memory. In E. Tulving & N. Donaldson (Eds.), *Organization of memory.* New York: Academic Press.

Vygotsky, L. S. (1962). *Thought and language.* Cambridge: MIT Press.

Walen, S., DiGiuseppe, R., & Wessler, R. (1980). *The practitioner's guide to rational emotive therapy.* New York: Oxford University Press.

Wessler, R. L., & Wessler, R. A. (1980). *The principles and practice of rational emotive therapy.* San Francisco: Jossey-Bass.

Wolpe, J. (1969). *The practice of behavior therapy.* New York: Pergamon Press.

Woolfolk, R., & Sass, L. (1989). Philosophical foundations of rational-emotive therapy. In M. E. Bernard & R. DiGiuseppe (Eds.), *Inside rational-emotive therapy: A critical evaluation of the theory and therapy of Albert Ellis.* Orlando, FL: Academic Press.

Comprehensive Cognitive Disputing in RET

RAYMOND DIGIUSEPPE

Disputing irrational beliefs has always been at the heart of RET. However, my 13 years' experience in teaching therapists to do RET has revealed that disputing is the art of the science and the hardest thing about RET to teach. Most new therapists learn how to identify the activating event, the emotional consequences, and then the irrational belief. Once the client reveals his or her irrational belief, the therapist asks, "Where's the evidence?" The client looks confused and says, "I guess there is none." And the therapist assumes that the client has "got it" and responds, "What other problem would you like to discuss?" As therapists develop more experience, they spend more time disputing. They somehow develop a guide to all of the possible disputes that are available to use with a specific type of problem or a specific irrational belief.

Experienced RET therapists spend most of their time in therapy disputing clients' irrational beliefs. New therapists always appear perplexed by this fact and are not sure how one can spend so much time disputing. This confusion appears explainable if one examines the RET literature. Until now, most RET texts, (e.g., Bard, 1980; Ellis & Dryden, 1987; Grieger & Boyd, 1980; Maultsby, 1984; Walen, DiGiuseppe, & Wessler, 1980; Wessler & Wessler, 1980) have attempted to teach disputing by providing specific disputational arguments that can be used to challenge specific irrational beliefs. Although such writings have been helpful, they do not provide a blueprint for the *process* of disputing, which allows therapists to generate new disputes.

RAYMOND DIGIUSEPPE • Department of Psychology, St. John's University, Jamaica, New York 11432, and Institute for Rational-Emotive Therapy, 45 East 65th Street, New York, New York 10021.

This chapter attempts to expand and specify the possible disputing strategies that can be used in RET. First, I present an expanded model of an emotional episode, discuss the difference between what has been referred to as *philosophical* and *elegant disputing* versus *empirical* and *inelegant disputing*, and then focus on expanding the strategies that therapists can use in challenging and reconstructing clients' thoughts. The disputes are organized by four factors, each factor having two or more levels. The model allows therapists to move across levels of a factor and across factors. The factors are (1) the nature of the evidence—logical, empirical, heuristic, and so on; (2) the rhetorical style of the argument—didactic, Socratic, metaphorical, and so on; (3) the level of abstraction of the argument; and (4) the centrality of the client's irrational belief (i.e., disputing both the core and the derivative irrational beliefs).

AN EXPANDED MODEL

Originally, Ellis (1958, 1962) presented his well-known ABC model. Wessler and Wessler (1980) expanded the original version. In their model, the B consists of two elements: inferences, which are statements, predictions, and conclusions about the world; and evaluations, which are the appraisals and meanings that people apply to the world. DiGiuseppe (1986) further revised the model to include an even finer distinction between different aspects of the B. According to this model, when clients encounter an activating event they produce inferences about the world; then, they evaluate the inferences that they have made. However, the evaluations and inferences that clients create are readily generated because of their core underlying personal paradigms or schemata. Irrational beliefs are of two types: evaluations of events or inferences, and core paradigms or schemata through which the client construes the world. Thus, the new model divides the beliefs into three components: inferences, evaluations, or appraisals, and core paradigm irrational beliefs.

DiGiuseppe (1986) theorized that irrational beliefs do not lead to disturbed emotions in a linear model; rather, he suggested that human beings think in a hypothetically deductive fashion. The inferences or automatic thoughts that one experiences are limited to those that are consistent with the underlying schema or worldview that one has. Kuhn (1970) argued that people draw only the inferences that they are prepared to make from their paradigm. Similarly, the evaluations one makes are logically derived from the same schema or worldview: the core irrational beliefs.

Disputing in RET is the process of challenging the truth of a client's beliefs and reconstructing new beliefs. Disputing follows a complicated, involved set of arguments that follow from the epistemological position taken in rational-emotive theory by Ellis. Most forms of cognitive-behavior therapy do not specify their epistemological assumptions. Beck's cognitive therapy (Beck, Rush, Shaw, & Emery, 1979; Beck & Emory, 1985) appears to rest on an empiricist or logical-positivist view of epistemology that posits that knowledge is accumulated by logical induction from empirically demonstrable facts. Most of the cognitive distortions that Beck and his colleagues believe lead to disturbed emotion are false inductions made from inadequate data. The approach in cognitive therapy of empirically testing automatic thoughts seems to this author to be a logical outgrowth of an unstated but implied epistemological position in favor of radical empiricism.

RET, however, is much clearer about its epistemological assumptions than cognitive therapy or most other forms of psychotherapy (Woolfolk & Sass, 1989). Ellis (1989a,b; Ellis, Sachel, DiMattia, Yeager, & DiGiuseppe, 1989) has put forth the notion that all humans think in a constructivist, hypotheticodeductive manner. People cannot help but create theories of the world, of their interpersonal relationships, and of themselves. These theories, schemata or paradigms may guide the person to cope adequately with the environment or may lead to poor coping and psychopathology.

Ellis has theorized that people think in a constructivist, hypotheticodeductive way and has posited that RET is based on a similar model of epistemology. Ellis (1962, 1973, 1985, 1989a,b) has stated that RET is based on the scientific outlook and that disputing helps the client to think scientifically. However, he has not specified how such an assumption influences the disputing of clients' irrational beliefs. DiGiuseppe (1986) suggested that RET formally adopt a model of disputing that is based on a similar epistemological view. I propose here that Kuhn's model (1970) of scientific paradigms and his historical account of the types of evidence that lead scientists to forsake theories are helpful guides to disputing in psychotherapy to help clients relinquish their personal theories.

Kuhn's model suggests that scientists work from theories or paradigms that are broad schemata. A paradigm not only explains important variables but organizes one's view of the world, suggests which data one is prepared to select, suggests which inferences one is prepared to draw from the data, and suggests how various inferences will be evaluated. Kuhn indicated that scientists do not give up their paradigms easily. They do so only when either one or all of the following types of arguments are presented: (1) when there are considerable empirical data to suggest that the inferences that are deduced from the paradigm are false; (2) when there is considerable logical inconsistency within the paradigm; (3) when the paradigm lacks heuristic value, in that it fails to solve important problems; and finally, (4) when there is an alternative paradigm that is better at accounting for empirical findings and solving problems than the existing paradigm.

DiGiuseppe (1986) proposed that Kuhn's model (1970, 1977) of scientific thinking is generally accurate about human thinking and that the

Kuhnian model of scientific epistemology can be considered a model of human epistemology.

The adoption of Kuhn's philosophy of science as a model of cognitive functioning has several advantages. First, it suggests that some specific relationships exist between different types of cognitive structures. For example, core schemata determine automatic thoughts and the type of evidence the person notices to support them. Second, we can look at the types of arguments and evidence that help humans change their thinking. Most of the criteria that Kuhn outlined as criteria that scientists use to evaluate theories correspond to the definitions of rational beliefs. Both Ellis (1962) and Maultsby (1972) have defined beliefs as irrational if they are (1) illogical, (2) inconsistent with empirical reality, and (3) inconsistent with reaching one's goal (not functional or heuristic).

THE TARGET OF THE DISPUTE

The most frequent error made by new rational-emotive therapists is disputing the inference instead of the irrational beliefs (Dryden & DiGiuseppe, 1990). This happens for two reasons. First, most other forms of cognitive therapy specifically recommend that therapy begin in this manner (Beck et al., 1979). Second, clients often respond to therapists' inquiries about what they are thinking with inferences. Beck (1976), in fact, referred to inferences as automatic thoughts because they are quick to emerge into human consciousness. RET (Ellis, 1962, 1973, 1989a,b; Ellis & Dryden, 1987; Walen et al., 1980) has always recommended that disputing of the inferences be a secondary goal. Disputing inferences has been referred to in RET jargon as *empirical* or *inelegant disputing*, whereas disputing the irrational beliefs has been referred to as *philosophical* or *elegant disputing*.

My supervisory experience over the years has suggested that the appellation *empirical disputing* for disputing the inferences has confused trainees. The term *empirical disputing* uses a description of a type of argument to refer to the object or target of the dispute. This is confusing because, as I point out below, one can and often does use empirical arguments directed at the irrational beliefs. Trainees and critics of RET are justifiably confused when they observe an empirical argument directed at an irrational belief and hear it referred to by Ellis as elegant and philosophical when Ellis at the same time refers to empirical arguments as inelegant. That confusion can be avoided if rational-emotive theory develops a consistent and organized way of categorizing the disputes used in therapy. Disputes can be labeled first by the target at which they are directed and, second, by the type of argument used in the dispute. Therefore, disputes leveled at the inferences or automatic thoughts of a client should be referred to as *inferential disputes.*

Disputes targeted at the irrational beliefs or underlying schemata of the client should be referred to as *philosophical disputes* to communicate that they are leveled at the client's core underlying philosophy.

Inferences themselves can be challenged on both logical or empirical grounds. Beck (1976) provided an extensive list of the types of cognitive distortions that usually account for the erroneous nature of inferences or automatic thoughts. If one studies this list it becomes evident that most of the cognitive distortion processes that Beck mentioned are errors of induction. A negative inference such as "Because my spouse did not kiss me when I came home, my spouse does not love me" may be an error of false induction. Here, the client may be making an overgeneralized conclusion on insufficient data. Erroneous inferences can be challenged in a variety of ways. First, one can dispute the inference logically. Here, the therapist points out to the client that there are insufficient data to draw the conclusion she or he has reached. Second, one can search for more empirical data that will bear on testing the inference that the client reports she or he is thinking. The therapist could ask the client to search her or his memory for other examples of information relevant to the inference in question. Or the therapist can ask the client to collect specific data between sessions that can be a basis for testing the inference.

The point to be stressed here is that empirical disputing is a process or type of argument, not a target of an argument. Irrational beliefs or core schemata can also be disputed empirically, philosophically, or in other ways that are discussed below. Both inferences-automatic thoughts and irrational beliefs-core schemata can be disputed with the same types of arguments. Separating the target and the process of the dispute by the way we refer to them will make RET clearer and facilitate learning for new therapists and for clients.

The Nature of the Dispute

As I have suggested above, disputing can follow the model of paradigm change outlined by Kuhn (1970, 1977) in his philosophy and history of science. Kuhn suggested that scientists (and I would add people in general) change for several reasons: first, there are logical inconsistencies in the theory; second, substantial empirical evidence is accumulated that is inconsistent with the theory; third, the theory can not solve important problems and loses its practical or heuristic value; and finally, there is an alternative theory that is better. Since 1988, the fellows at the Institute for Rational-Emotive Therapy and I have been listening to Ellis's therapy tapes in an attempt to devise a content-analysis scoring system to determine what he actually does. Our informal impressions suggest that the disputing processes that Ellis uses correspond to the categories of evidence proposed by Kuhn.

General Considerations

Disputing strategy puts the responsibility on clients to prove that what they are thinking is correct. Often, there is no actual evidence for the irrational belief (that is why the beliefs are irrational). If left to dwell on this fact, clients may begin to become uncomfortable with their inability to defend what they are thinking. When clients cannot answer and hence feel uncomfortable, novice therapists usually rescue them from their discomfort and provide answers. This is fine. Clients may be motivated to think through the problem if they are uncomfortable about it. However, it may be more convincing for the client to continue to struggle to search for a proof and fail to find one.

Personal Epistemologies

Disputing clients' irrational beliefs involves teaching the client for the first time that humans usually have reasons for believing what they think. All people have some implicit epistemology for holding beliefs. The call for evidence helps clients become aware of what their personal epistemology may be. If the client does provide some sort of a rationale for the particular irrational belief, it is best for the therapist to take this rationale seriously, to attempt to evaluate its adequacy with the client, and if it is incorrect, to point out why.

As clients attempt to answer, the therapist's disputing questions may reveal the clients' implicit epistemology. That is the criterion the clients use to decide what to believe. We have noticed that clients may hold certain epistemologies that make it unlikely that they will cooperate or benefit from disputing because their epistemology is different from the scientific view inherent in RET.

Some examples of personal epistemologies are the following:

1. *Authoritarian epistemology.* Some clients believe that knowledge comes from a higher source, either spiritually or socially. A family member (i.e., a parent or a spouse) or a social or religious institution is believed to be the oracle of truth.

2. *Narcissistic epistemology.* Some clients believe that things are true just because they thought of them. That is, they take an extreme constructivist position and believe that whatever pops into their head must be true. This view may be held because the clients arrogantly believe that they are so

smart that they must be correct, or because they have never evaluated why they believe things.

3. *Constructivist epistemology.* Some clients believe, like many constructivist social scientists (Mahoney, 1976, 1988; Polyani, 1966), that all views of reality are equally valid and that they are therefore entitled to believe what they think because it is right for them, even though the therapist has demonstrated that it is illogical.

Whenever clients hold any of these epistemological positions, it is advisable first to dispute the validity of the epistemology and convince them of the advantage of advocating a scientific epistemology before attempting to restructure any of their specific irrational beliefs.

Logical Disputing

The first criteria of rational thinking is that it is logical, and irrational beliefs usually do not meet this criterion. Clients can be shown that their beliefs are unsound on logical grounds. Logical arguments may focus on whether the irrational belief logically follows from the reasoning that the client uses to defend it. For example, when most clients are asked, "Why must the world be the way you say it must be?" they proceed to explain that it would be more desirable for them if the world were the way they wanted it to be. Ellis's classic dispute points out that something's being more desirable does not logically lead to the *nonsequitur* conclusion that the world must be constructed in a desirable way. Desirability and reality have no logical relation to each other. Other disputes may focus on the logical inconsistency of different aspects of a client's belief system. For example, a client who condemns himself or herself for not accomplishing a specific goal or aspiration may be asked if he or she would condemn others for either failing to reach that goal or failing to reach some other goal important to the person. Clients often respond "no" to such a question. "How," one can ask, "is it logical to condemn one person for a failing and not another?" The logical inconsistency of clients' evaluations can be repeatedly stressed.

Reality Testing of Irrational Beliefs

Irrational beliefs can also be challenged on empirical grounds. As noted above, therapists often miss this point because "empirical disputing" in the RET literature has referred to disputing the inference. But one of the criteria of rational beliefs has always been that they are consistent with empirical reality. If a client's personal paradigm is correct, logical deductions from the paradigm will be consistent with reality. Just as scientists empirically test hypotheses that are logically deduced from their scientific paradigms, so, too, therapists can test the veracity of clients' personal paradigms by making deductions from the clients' paradigms and testing them against empirical reality. These are empirical disputes aimed at clients' irrational philosophies.

For example, suppose a client is angry at his spouse because he believes that she must love him and in fact she no longer does. The client's anger is generated by the irrational belief, "She must love me." The therapist could dispute this belief by pointing out to the client that, if his belief is correct his wife would in fact behave lovingly toward him. Then, the therapist and the client can review the evidence regarding her present or recent behavior. Failure to find loving behaviors by the wife toward the client disconfirms the prediction deduced from the irrational belief. Most demanding beliefs can be shown to be inconsistent with reality. No matter how strongly the client believes that the world "must" be the way he or she wants it to be, the universe usually does not change to match the "must."

Our content analysis of Ellis's tapes indicates that he often uses this argument. He asks clients what reality is and then points out that it is not consistent with their "must." They have avoided noticing the reality and instead have clung to their demands.

Empirical disputes can also be constructed against the other three irrational belief processes. For example, clients who endorse low-frustration-tolerance beliefs can be shown that, even though they think that they can not stand the occurrence of an activating event, they have, in fact, stood it over and over again. Also, catastrophizing beliefs can be challenged with the argument that the activating agent did not result in a totally, 100% bad outcome. Self-downing beliefs can be challenged empirically by pointing out that an assessment of a person as totally worthless is almost always incorrect because all people do some things well and have some worth to some other people, even though that worth may be based on values that are very different from one's own.

Heuristic Disputing

The next criterion of rational beliefs is that the belief should help one attain one's goals. Scientists have always evaluated theories and beliefs on their heuristic or functional value. That is, does a particular idea help solve major important problems? Does it assist in accomplishing desired goals? Such functional disputes have long been advocated in RET (Walen *et al.*, 1980). Clients can be asked to evaluate the consequences of holding their irrational beliefs. What are the emotions that the irrational beliefs elicit? What good do these emotions do? If the feelings are undesirable or troublesome, why would one want to hold a belief that makes her or him feel miserable? What are the behaviors that usually follow the irrational thoughts? Do these behaviors bring good or bad consequences? Do these behaviors help clients reach their long-term goals?

It is possible that heuristic disputes are the most influential, as they are the most closely linked to the behavioral notion of reinforcement. Heuristic disputes may help clients conceptualize or become aware of the actual reinforcement of holding irrational beliefs.

Constructing Rational Beliefs

Challenging irrational beliefs is not sufficient to change them. People frequently hold on to beliefs that they know are logically flawed and do not lead to accurate predictions of reality, but no alternative ideas are available to replace the flawed idea. The history of science is filled with such examples. People do not give up ideas, regardless of the evidence against the idea, unless they have an alternative idea to replace it.

Many forms of psychotherapy are based on consciousness raising alone (Prochaska & DiClemente, 1984). Consciousness-raising models of therapy assume that, once clients become aware of what their problem is or why they behave the way they do, their human potential for self-actualization will lead to their choosing an adaptive way of responding. In psychoanalysis, one becomes aware of the early conflicts that have led to one's development, and once this insight is conscious, the person will choose more adaptive behavior. In client-centered therapy, the therapist unconditionally accepts the client, so that the client becomes aware of and surrenders her or his conditions of worth. Again, once this is accomplished, it is assumed that the self-actualization drive will lead the individual to adjustment. Also, with Gestalt therapy, the therapist's role is to confront clients so that they become aware of their suppressed feeling and the "phony" roles that they are playing. Again, consciousness raising is assumed to be sufficient for change, and it is assumed that the insight into one's emotions will free one to choose an adaptive life.

RET does not state that insight is sufficient for change. It is not sufficient to have the insight that one has irrational beliefs that are causing one's emotional disturbance, nor is it sufficient to have the insight that a particular irrational belief is irrational. Unless clients have new ideas to replace their old irrational beliefs, they are likely to cling to their irrational beliefs even though they are aware that the ideas are incorrect. Several lines of research support the importance of restructuring alternative rational beliefs. Wein, Nelson, and Odom (1975) compared two forms of cognitive restructuring. In one treatment condition, clients were made aware of the reasons why their thinking was irrational, and in a second treatment condition, clients were taught alternative ideas. The second group improved significantly over the first. Also, DiGiuseppe, Leaf, Exner, and Robin (1988) constructed a scale of both irrational and rational ideas. They found that although the irrational belief subscale significantly distinguished between disturbed clients and normal college students, the disturbed and normal groups differed more on the rational belief subscales than they did on the irrational belief scores. The authors concluded that, although disturbed groups do appear to endorse irrational beliefs, they are much less likely to endorse rational beliefs. This finding suggests that clients will not get better by just reducing their endorsement of irrational beliefs; they must also increase their endorsement of rational beliefs.

Even when clients become aware of the disputing arguments, which RET predicts will take both insight and lots of practice, clients have to learn new adaptive styles of thinking. For example, people are not always quick to come up with a self-accepting philosophy once they realize that their self-worth beliefs are irrational. Our content analysis of Ellis's therapy tapes indicates that he frequently suggests to clients that their irrational beliefs are wrong and that the rational alternative is better. New therapists frequently forget this part and dispute without emphasizing the new rational belief.

RHETORICAL DISPUTING STYLES OF THERAPISTS

Clients are not convinced only by the nature of the evidence against their irrational beliefs. Their beliefs are influenced by more than logic. The manner of presentation of the arguments is as important as the dispute itself. Ellis (1985, 1989a) has frequently argued that clients change when he disputes forcefully and vigorously. We have identified four different rhetorical styles that therapists can use in disputing irrational beliefs. They are didactic, Socratic, metaphorical, and humorous.

Didactic and Socratic Styles

By far the most noticeable rhetorical strategy is the didactic dispute. When therapists observe Ellis performing one of his frequent demonstrations of RET, they notice that he teaches his client the difference between irrational and rational beliefs in a direct, didactic manner. RET has always been presented by Ellis (1962, 1973, 1985, 1989a,b) as a psychoeducational intervention. As a result, the RET therapist frequently does a lot of direct education about the therapy, its theory, where emotions come from, and the reason why specific beliefs are irrational.

In addition to the direct, didactic presentation of material, RET therapists frequently use the Socratic method of questioning to help clients learn to dispute their irrational beliefs themselves. The term *Socratic questioning* comes from the Socratic Dialogues written by Plato of the conversations of the Greek philosopher Socrates. Socrates believed that people are more intelligent than they get credit for. He thought that the best way to teach people is to try to draw information out of them through a series of directive questions. In one of the most famous of the Socratic dialogues, the philosopher teaches a slave boy a geometric principle by asking questions.

Socratic disputing is probably the mainstay of interventions among most RET therapists. The therapist asks clients questions to get them to see for themselves that there is no evidence for their irrational beliefs. Some Socratic disputes are "How does it follow logically that your spouse must love you because you really strongly desire her to?" or "Can you tell me how it has helped you to think that your spouse must love you?" or "Is there any evidence that your spouse behaves lovingly to you when you demand that she must?" These are examples of the logical, heuristic, and empirical disputes using the Socratic style.

Didactic and Socratic interventions are the major strategies that RET therapists use in verbal disputing of clients' irrational beliefs. Some therapists prefer one over the other, but I suggest that each has its limitations and strengths in certain contexts.

Didactic disputing is probably essential to some degree for all clients in the initial sessions of therapy or when the therapy focuses on new problems. However, remaining in a didactic rhetorical mode can be inefficient. Although didactic interventions teach clients the arguments against their irrational beliefs and what the new rational beliefs are, didactic strategies do not involve the client in the actual *practice* of the disputes themselves. A therapist who relies too much on didactic intervention is doing all the work. The client is coasting. Once clients have learned some of the information from didactic interventions, they can put their skills to work by Socratic disputing and practice on their own.

Many therapists prefer Socratic disputing almost exclusively. They believe that knowledge is better acquired through self-discovery. The idea that learning occurs best through self-discovery has been a popular notion in American educational thought. It was probably best promulgated by the educational philosopher John Dewey and was strongly advocated by many progressive educators in the 1960s. Many therapists seem to take the preference for self-discovery learning to an extreme and believe that self-discovery is necessary for learning. Most forms of psychotherapy and counseling (except for behavior therapy) appear to share this view. It is frequently stated in the therapy and counseling literature that interpretations should not be given until clients have almost reached the same conclusion by themselves (Cormier & Cormier, 1986). Rational therapists do believe that Socratic dialogue is helpful and may even be preferable. But it is not the only way people learn.

Some clients of limited intelligence, limited creativity, or extreme emotional disturbance may not come up with an appropriate answer to a Socratic question. Letting them suffer because they have not thought of the solutions to their problems seems unnecessary or even unethical. It is recommended that therapists try Socratic questioning early in the session.

However, if a client does not seem to be able to answer the questions after 5–10 minutes, the therapist can revert to the didactic style.

Another problem frequently encountered in therapy supervision is responding too quickly to clients' inability to answer Socratic questions. Socratic questioning requires clients to *think* about their answers, and Socratic disputing requires clients to defend their irrational beliefs. Because clients may never have thought through the issue in question and because their irrational beliefs may be indefensible, they may take some time to respond with an answer. Therapists frequently become impatient with the silences that occur while the client is thinking. Silences in social conversations are awkward events, and people often try to fill such pauses. Therapists are no different. They start talking to fill the pause and to rescue the client from the discomfort of this awkward social situation. This would be a mistake in therapy, as it interrupts the client's thought processes and disrupts the purpose of the Socratic question. There are several reasons that it may be better to let the pauses remain. First, clients often have nonlogical psychological reasons for holding irrational beliefs. For example, a client may believe that his wife must love him. When asked for the evidence for why she must love him, he responds that he needs a significant other in his life because he believes that he cannot stand to be alone. This is a psychological and not a logical reason for holding the irrational belief. Filling the pauses that occur in response to Socratic questions does not allow clients to search for, formulate, or explore the psychological reasons that support their irrational beliefs. In this way, Socratic disputing becomes a primary assessment strategy for uncovering clients' irrational beliefs.

If the client has already discovered his or her core irrational beliefs, it is also good to let the pauses remain. In that case, the client may be searching for the logical reasons for holding his or her irrational beliefs. And because the beliefs are irrational, there often is no good reason to hold the belief. This is not immediately apparent to the client, and he or she does not know that there is no evidence to support the core irrational belief. The experience of searching for the support and not being able to find it leads to some discomfort. This discomfort helps create cognitive dissonance with the irrational belief. It is wise to let the client feel the discomfort. Thirty seconds or so of silence in a therapy session may seem like an eternity, but it may be time well spent.

Clients often respond to Socratic disputes with illogical reasons for maintaining their core dysfunctional ideas. It is important for the therapist to know what the client is thinking so that these illogical reasons can be addressed. Finally, clients may be unable to answer Socratic disputes. They may feel discomfort about being unable to do so. However, they may not conclude that the reason they have failed to formulate an answer is that there is none. The therapist may have to interpret the client's failure to muster any evidence to support the irrational belief as stemming from the lack of support for the irrational belief.

Both didactic and Socratic interventions are used over the course of therapy and over the course of a session. As a general rule, didactic strategies are used more in the beginning of therapy and when the focus is switched to a new problem. Socratic questioning is used more as therapy progresses and as the therapist prepares clients to function more independently and to dispute on their own.

Metaphorical Disputing

RET has always advocated the use of metaphorical disputing strategies that work to shift clients' thinking (Walen et al., 1980). Metaphors and parables are part of the RET therapeutic armamentarium. Metaphor use is extremely popular in psychotherapy and many therapists report using metaphors in therapy. Although metaphors are popular among therapists, there appears to be no well-developed theory or explanation of how metaphors operate in bringing about change. Most of the literature on metaphor use in psychotherapy has been generated from the work of Milton Erickson (see review by Muran & DiGiuseppe, 1990). Several problems emerge in following the metaphorical strategies recommended by the Ericksonian camp. The first problem is the assumption that the therapist need not (and had better not) communicate the meaning of the metaphor to the client. Muran and DiGiuseppe argue that this practice comes from a long theoretical history in psychotherapy dating back to Freud and Jung. Both of these seminal thinkers in psychotherapy believed that symbols had shared meaning among humans. This view, the foundation of Freud's theory, was based on a Lamarckian view of genetics and appears to be unfounded (Gould, 1988).

The contemporary theory that reflects the shared-meaning hypothesis is the work of Milton Erickson. The Ericksonian use of metaphor is subtle. The therapist does not teach the client how to use the metaphor, does not explain the metaphor, and assumes that the client understands the metaphor unconsciously.

DiGiuseppe and Muran (in press; Muran & DiGiuseppe, 1990) proposed that none of the hypotheses assumed in the Ericksonian use of metaphor are valid. They proposed that metaphor is a standard yet powerful form of language. One function of metaphor in psychotherapy is memory consolidation. Clients may not remember all of the things that go into the disputing process. Such information would include all the reasons why the irrational belief is erroneous, the new rational belief, the reasons why the rational belief is more correct, and the instructions that help to rehearse the disputing. When all this information is new and fresh and more difficult to recall, the metaphor may well function as an organizer. When the metaphor is recalled, all of the information consolidated around it is more accessible to memory.

DiGiuseppe and Muran (in press) provided guidelines for using metaphors in cognitive psychotherapies. The first step is for the therapist to clearly identify the idea they wish to communicate to the client. Next, the therapist explores a topic that the client is familiar with (e.g., art, literature, film, or sports). Then, the therapist searches for a concept in the content of the schema system that is analogous to the concept that the therapist wishes to teach. This analogous concept serves as the metaphor. The therapist then presents the metaphor to the client. Because it can not be assumed that the client will automatically (or inherently) see the analogous content in the metaphor, the therapist didactically or socratically explores the client's understanding of the metaphor. Finally, the therapist asks clients how they can use the metaphor to help them dispute their irrational beliefs. Clients can be instructed to recall the metaphor when they experience emotional disturbances, and the metaphor can remind them to dispute.

Humor

Another rhetorical style of disputing is the use of humor. Ellis (1977) has long advocated the use of humor, and he usually considers it an emotive intervention (Ellis, 1985). A full theoretical discussion on the mechanism whereby humor leads to attitude change is beyond the scope of this chapter. Humor has long been ignored as both a psychotherapeutic intervention and a strategy of persuasion. At the Institute of Rational-Emotive Therapy, we try to teach all therapists to use humor. If the supervisors are bored listening to a therapy session, we assume that the client may be bored as well. In order to use humor effectively, there are only a few rules that the therapist can follow. Never make fun of a client; joke only about the client's behavior or thoughts. Ellis frequently isolates the thought that he is disputing before the humorous comment. He does this by careful use of pronouns to ensure that the target of the joke will always be clear and that no one could infer that the target is the client.

LEVEL OF ABSTRACTION

Irrational beliefs can be stated in varying levels of abstraction. For example, if Ralph is angry at his spouse over her not behaving as he thinks she "should," several irrational beliefs can be identified as leading to his anger: (1) "My wife must make dinner when I want her to make it"; (2) "My wife must do chores the way I want her to do them"; (3) "My wife must do things the way I want her to do them"; (4) "Family members must do things the way I want them to do them"; (5) "People in my life must do things the way I want them to do them"; (6) "All people must behave the way I want them to behave"; and (7) "The world must be the way I want it to be." These beliefs vary across a dimension of abstraction and generalizability. Fewer activating events would lead to emotional disturbance if the client believed only irrational belief Number 1. Successively, more activating events would be capable of activating emotional upset as the abstraction of the beliefs increases. The same also holds for rational beliefs: the more abstract the rational belief, the more activating events it can be associated with, and the more elegant and useful belief will be in helping the client to avoid emotional disturbance. The less abstract a belief is, the more it applies in a concrete, specific situation, and the more it resembles a self-statement than an unspoken philosophy.

Clients may be more likely to identify the concrete versions of the irrational beliefs in their therapy sessions. If we ask Ralph, "What were you thinking the last time you got angry at your wife?" he is most likely to have thought the concrete version (1). Therefore, the concrete irrational belief will be the one that he most clearly experiences, is more ready to admit he is thinking, and is more motivated to change.

When therapists hypothesize clients' irrational beliefs or when they use didactic disputing strategies, they usually suggest abstract beliefs such as Number 5 or Number 6, rather than concrete irrational beliefs like Number 1. Again, the most abstract dispute is seen as the most elegant and the most likely to generalize to the widest number of stimuli.

Ellis (1962, 1973, 1985, 1989a,b) has always credited general semantic theory and the work of Korzybski (1933) as providing some of the philosophical foundations for RET. Korzybski and other general semantic theorists have postulated the notion of the ladder of abstraction. They have posited that almost all words can be placed on a continuum of abstraction. As one goes up the ladder of abstraction, words express more general, abstract meaning and provide less information about specific cases. For example, we could refer to a specific client as Ralph, as a certain macho personality type, as a male humaniodae, as a primate, a mammal, or a vertebrate. Each step up the ladder of abstraction includes more cases under it, yet provides less information about Ralph. The general semanticists argue that communications are more clearly understood if the speaker goes up and down the ladder of abstraction. Communications that stay at only one level of abstraction are unclear. A communication including words only at the concrete level provides lots of specific information. However, listeners may fail to transfer the learning to new situations because they may not have grasped the abstract principle. Communications including only words at the top abstract level of the ladder may be able to express the abstract rule, but clients may fail to learn to apply the rule to specific situations, or they may never have seen (or heard) a specific application of the rule and may therefore misconstrue it.

The solution to this problem is to ensure that communications designed to teach or change attitudes include both concrete and varying levels of abstractions. Specifically, the therapist should move up and down the ladder of abstraction during the dialogue.

A question that needs more theoretical and research attention in RET is the relationship between the irrational beliefs held at one level of abstraction and those endorsed at another. Could a client lightly believe a concrete belief and more strongly hold an abstract one? I would think not. Holding an abstract irrational belief cannot lead to emotional upset unless the client holds the specific irrational belief associated with an activating event.

In supervision, we frequently hear therapists who provide elegant disputations of the most abstract version of the client's irrational belief, but the client does not appear to comprehend the point. The therapist has failed to present a concrete example that the client understands. Another problem can emerge if the therapist disputes only at the abstract level. Clients may verbally report that they comprehend the disputation but there is no resulting change in their emotion or behavior. These clients have not *applied* the change in their abstract belief to the particular irrational belief that they think when faced with the most provocative and/or frequent activating event. Other therapists dispute only the specific, concrete, irrational belief that the client presents when confronted with the activating event. Although clients may respond to treatment and not get upset when the same activating event occurs again, they become just as upset when a new troublesome activating event emerges on the horizon.

When disputing Ralph's irrational belief, it is recommended that therapists start disputing at the most concrete level with "My wife must make dinner when I want her to." By starting here, Ralph is likely to get some control over his emotions in the situation that offers the most problems. This strategy will provide some reinforcement for disputing and for continuing in therapy. Next, the therapist may want to teach Ralph that he tends to be demanding about other things as well and that the world does not have to be the way he wants it to be. By moving up and down the ladder of abstraction, the therapist ensures that Ralph will learn to deal with specific activating events, that he will be able to apply the RET solution to other similar events, and that he will understand the rule behind the reasoning and will be able to apply it to future aversive stimuli.

MULTIPLE IRRATIONAL BELIEF PROCESSES

Ellis (1958, 1962) originally identified 11 common irrational beliefs that he observed in his clients' thinking. Most research and writing in RET tended to center on these 11 irrational beliefs as the core of the theory and the therapy. Critics of RET (see Ellis & Whitely, 1979) thought that the 11 irrational beliefs were too content-specific. They argued that RET was over-concerned with the content of what clients thought. Beck (1976) in particular thought that the content of clients' dysfunctional beliefs is idiosyncratic in each case. He and other cognitive therapists thought it more helpful to focus on the process of clients' thinking. As rational-emotive theory has progressed, there has been more focus on such irrational thinking processes. Walen *et al.* (1980) categorized the 11 irrational beliefs into five process categories: demandingness, need statements, human worth statements, awfulizing, and low frustration tolerance. Later, Campbell and his associates (Burgess, 1990; Campbell, 1985) collapsed demandingness and need statements and proposed that all irrational beliefs fall within a four-by-three grid with four process variables (demandingness, human worth, awfulizing, and low frustration tolerance) and three content levels (approval, achievement, and comfort).

Ellis (1985, 1989a,b) has gone on to hypothesize that demandingness is the core irrational belief that is responsible for human emotional disturbance. The newest version of rational-emotive theory posits that demandingness is always present in cases of emotional disturbance. Irrational beliefs concerning awfulizing, human worth, and low frustration tolerance are psychologically or logically deduced from holding a core demanding belief (Ellis, 1985, 1989a,b). At issue is the number of irrational belief processes that the client may endorse around one content area.

Ralph could have any of four concrete irrational beliefs when he gets himself emotionally disturbed: "My wife must make dinner when I want her to do it"; "My wife is a worthless person when she does not make dinner when I want her to do it"; "It is awful if my wife does not make my dinner when I want her to do it"; or "I cannot stand it when my wife does not make dinner when I want her to do it." If Ralph endorses one of these irrational beliefs, what is the likelihood that he will endorse them all? More important, if Ralph does endorse one or more of them, does his changing one automatically lead to change in the others?

Therapists in RET training often naively believe that clients have only one irrational belief. After all, it is an ABC model. Therefore, they forget to dispute all the irrational beliefs that clients think while they are getting upset. If a therapist fails to dispute the "must" or demandingness belief and disputes only the derivative irrational belief that the client reports, the theory states that the client may remain upset and may deduce more beliefs from the core "must."

Our research experience suggests that, although therapists trained in RET may quickly and reliably differentiate between the four irrational belief processes, clients may experience them as similar (DiGiuseppe, Robin, Leaf, & Gorman, 1989). When DiGiuseppe *et al.* (1989) created items for a new irrational belief scale, they wanted a separate subscale for each of the four irrational belief processes. Definitions were written for each of the four processes, and items were written to match the definitions. An item was used only if 13 psychologists, either staff or fellows at the Institute for Rational-Emotive Therapy, agreed that the item matched the definition. Although the resulting subscale yielded adequate internal consistency, clients who completed the inventory complained that the items were redundant; that is, they experienced the items as having the same meaning. A factor analysis of the scale did yield a very strong major general factor. Several other studies have found similar results. DiGiuseppe and Leaf (in press) found one general factor in Burgess's irrational belief scale (1986), and Demaria, Kassinove, and Dill (1989) found a large general factor in another measure of irrational beliefs (Kassinove, 1986). One could take this factor analysis literature to suggest that the four irrational belief processes are psychologically, if not logically, related. It seems that endorsing an item containing one of the irrational thought processes is related to endorsing items for all four processes.

We do not yet know whether disputing or changing thoughts about one irrational thought process will logically or psychologically cause change in the other irrational processes. There is always the possibility that the beliefs, once established, have functional autonomy. Allport (1955) suggested that personality constructs may persist well after the factors that created them cease. Traits take on a life of their own, so to speak, and continue even though the reasons for their emergence are no longer present.

The practical implications of the multiple irrational belief processes were spelled out by Dryden and DiGiuseppe (1990). They pointed out that, if Ellis's model is correct, clients usually have more than one irrational belief associated with an activating event for each emotional episode, that is, a core demandingness belief and one or more derivative irrational thoughts. Therapists cannot assume generalization across belief processes. If we successfully dispute Ralph's demandingness about his wife's behavior, there is no reason to assume that he has changed his low frustration tolerance beliefs about his wife's behavior. Dryden and DiGiuseppe argued that it is best to dispute all of the irrational thoughts that a client endorses. Therefore, the therapist would dispute the core "must" and any other derivative irrational beliefs that have been assessed. In this way, they argued, generalization of change from disputing one irrational belief process to another is not assumed but planned for.

Although Ellis's new theory that demandingness is the core irrational belief remains to be confirmed, the advice by Dryden and DiGiuseppe (1990) remains sound whether Ellis's hierarchy is confirmed or not. Regardless of which irrational belief is found to be core, or of whether each client has his or her own core and derivative beliefs, it remains important to dispute all the irrational belief process that the client endorses. The factor-analytic data mentioned above strongly suggest that if a client holds to one irrational belief process, she or he will hold to another.

COMPREHENSIVE COGNITIVE DISPUTING IN RET

The model presented above describes four factors in disputing strategies: the nature of the dispute, with four levels; the rhetorical style, with four levels; the level of abstraction, with at least two levels but probably more; and the number of irrational processes that the client endorses with up to four levels. That gives at least 128 disputing statements that one can make to a client. Clearly, there is no reason for aspiring RET therapists not to have enough to say when the time comes to dispute!

It is recommended that, whenever possible, a therapist go through as many disputing strategies as possible. Kuhn (1977) suggested that scientists change their paradigms only when there is considerable challenge of their theory. If we are correct in believing that good scientific thinking results in mental health, should we not expect that clients will require just as much disputing of their paradigms before they surrender them? If people change their paradigms or belief systems only when considerable evidence has accumulated to show that the paradigms are not working, disputing only one factor or only one level of disputing may not be sufficient to move a person to change. Each of us may be susceptible to persuasion through different types of challenging strategies. Until we have a theory of personality or cognitive style that can predict which type of argument will be most influential with a particular client, it may be best to go systematically through the matrix of disputing strategies provided here to get clients to change.

Therapists can use the model systematically, starting in one cell of the matrix and working their way through as many cells of the model as possible. Having such a model in mind may remind new therapists to create disputes in cells that they have not covered yet. Experienced therapists can use the model to remind them to cover all disputes. Although this may sound like a mechanical recommendation for doing therapy, it is likely to force therapists to use all of the disputing strategies until they are familiar with them. It will ensure that considerable evidence will be mustered against clients' irrational belief systems and will ensure that clients will learn different rational beliefs to replace the irrational ones.

For an example, let us return to the client Ralph and show how the model can be applied. Once we are ready to dispute his irrational thinking, we would start with the concrete, core irrational belief: "My wife must make dinner when I want her to do it." We could also start with Socratic disputing. So what follows are Socratic, concrete, core disputes varying along the dimension of the nature of the evidence:

1. *Logical.* "How does it follow, Ralph, that just because you want your wife to make dinner at a certain time, or that it would be more convenient for you if she made dinner at a certain time, she must behave in the way that would be to your liking?"

2. *Empirical.* "It seems that you have told your wife when you want her to have dinner ready and you keep believing that she must do it when you want her to, but do we have any evidence that she has had to or has actually done what it is you demand of her?"

3. *Heuristic.* "How has your marriage, or your home life, or your life in general benefited from believing that your wife must make dinner when you want her to?"

4. *Construction of a new rational belief.* "Ralph, if you agree that your wife does not have to make dinner just when you want her to, what idea or thought could you tell yourself instead?"

If Ralph is unable to answer any of these Socratic disputes, the therapist can switch to didactic disputes. After the didactic interventions, the therapist can return to disputing socratically to see if Ralph has incorporated the disputes or understood them.

As therapy progresses, the therapist may want Ralph to generalize his disputing to other areas because it has been revealed that Ralph is just as demanding of his wife in many other areas. One possible strategy for generalizing the error of demandingness is to stay with the core "must" belief and to dispute it at all possible levels of abstraction and then down the ladder again to all possible specific events that it is linked to:

1. *Didactic, abstract, logical dispute.* "Ralph, there is no law of physics that says that your wife must do what you want her to do."

2. *Didactic, abstract, empirical dispute.* "You are frequently upsetting yourself about the fact that your wife *does not* do what you want her to do. That proves that she does not behave the way you want her to just because you decreed or demand it."

3. *Didactic, abstract, heuristic dispute.* "From the evidence that you have given me, it appears that your demanding philosophy toward your wife has resulted in several negative consequences for you: you feel depressed and angry when your wife does not behave as you demand; you have behaved obnoxiously toward your wife and as a result have reduced the goodwill between you and the pleasant parts of your relationship; and your kids are afraid to be with you because they fear your yelling. So you have lost many of the pleasures of your relationship with your family."

4. *Didactic, abstract construction of an alternative rational belief.* "Perhaps you can think instead, 'I would like my wife to always do what I want, but there is no law of the universe that says that she must behave as I want nor that she should even want to behave as I want her to. She is her own person with desires of her own.'"

Once the therapist has finished these didactic disputes she or he can do the Socratic version of each, again to assess whether Ralph has understood or incorporated them. If he has not, more time can be spent in the area of difficulty in a didactic mode. If Ralph does seem to understand the dispute on an abstract level, it is wise to test this out in a concrete mode: "OK, Ralph, you seem to understand that neither the world nor your wife has to be the way you want them to be. Let us see if you can apply this new way of thinking to another problem. You said that you also get yourself upset when your wife talks on the phone with her friends. Now, what belief are you thinking then?" The therapist can then find the concrete belief and progress with Socratic or didactic concrete disputes along the nature-of-evidence dimension.

After disputing the core irrational beliefs that underlie Ralph's emotional disturbance, the therapist can also dispute the derivative beliefs that are deduced from the "must." Ralph has two such beliefs: first, that he cannot stand not to have things the way he wants them (low frustration tolerance; I can't stand it when my wife does not do things I want her to do) and, second, self-downing ("I am not a real man and therefore a worthless person if I can not command my wife").

The therapist can start on Ralph's LFT and first dispute using didactic, concrete disputes for all levels of the nature of the evidence. Then, the therapist can follow with Socratic concrete disputes for all types of evidence. The next step is abstract Socratic disputes for all types of evidence. Once all these interventions have been tried, the therapist can move on to the same sequence for the derivative irrational belief of self-downing.

The sequence of disputes used above is not mandatory. This is an actual example of a real therapy case. A therapist could have used a different sequence. For example, one could have started with concrete, core, didactic disputes and then moved on to concrete didactic derivative disputes. There are no rules about the sequence of moving through the model. However, I maintain that the more the cells in the model that the therapist follows, the more likely the client is to change.

Although the model provided here applies to verbal disputation strategies, there is no intention to downplay the use of imagery or emotive or behavioral intervention in RET. When one adds these interventions to the number of disputational interventions presented here, the therapist has a large armamentarium to choose from.

REFERENCES

Allport, G. (1955). *Becoming: Basic considerations for a psychology of personality.* New Haven, CT: Yale University Press.

Bard, J. (1980). *Rational-emotive therapy in practice.* Champaign, IL: Research Press.

Beck, A. (1976). *Cognitive therapy and the emotional disorders.* New York: International Universities Press.

Beck, A., & Emory, G. (1985). *Anxiety disorders and phobias: A cognitive perspective.* New York: Basic Books.

Beck, A., Rush, A., Shaw, B., & Emery, G. (1979). *Cognitive therapy of depression.* New York: Guilford.

Burgess, P. (1986). Belief systems and emotional disturbance: An evaluation of the rational emotive model. Unpublished doctoral dissertation, University of Melbourne, Parkville, Victoria, Australia.

Burgess, P. (1990). Towards resolution of conceptual issues in the assessment of belief systems in rational-emotive therapy: Some preliminary results. *Journal of Cognitive Psychotherapy: An International Quarterly.*

Campbell, I. (1985). The psychology of homosexuality. In A. Ellis & M. Bernard (Eds.), *Clinical applications of rational-emotive therapy.* New York: Plenum.

Cormier, W., & Cormier, L. S. (1985). *Interviewing skills for helpers: Basic skill and cognitive behavioral interventions.* Monterey, CA: Brooks/Cole.

Demaria, T., Kassinove, H., & Dill, C. (1989). Psychometric properties of the survey of personal beliefs: A rational-emotive measure of irrational thinking. *Journal of Personality Assessment, 53*(2), 329–341.

DiGiuseppe, R. (1986). The implications of the philosophy of science for rational-emotive theory and therapy. *Psychotherapy, 23*(4), 634–639.

DiGiuseppe, R., & Leaf, R. (in press). Endorsement of irrational beliefs in a general clinical population. *Journal of Rational-Emotive and Cognitive-Behavior Therapy.*

DiGiuseppe, R., & Muran, C. (in press). The use of metaphor in rational-emotive therapy. *Psychotherapy in Private Practice.*

DiGiuseppe, R., Robin, M., Leaf, R., & Gorman, B. (1989, June). A discriminative validation and factor analysis of a measure of irrational/rational thinking. Poster session presented at the World Congress of Cognitive Therapy, Oxford, England.

DiGiuseppe, R., Leaf, R., Exner, T., & Robin, M. (1988, Sept.). The development of a measure of irrational and rational thinking. Poster session presented at the World Congress of Behavior Therapy, Edinburgh, Scotland.

Dryden, W., & DiGiuseppe, R. (1990). *A primer on rational-emotive therapy.* Champaign, IL: Research Press.

Ellis, A. (1958). Rational psychotherapy. *Journal of General Psychology, 59,* 37–49.

Ellis, A. (1962). *Reason and emotion in psychotherapy.* Secaucus, NJ: Lyle Stuart.

Ellis, A. (1973). *Humanistic psychotherapy: The rational-emotive approach.* New York: McGraw-Hill.

Ellis, A. (1977). Fun as psychotherapy. *Rational Living, 12*(1), 2–6.

Ellis, A. (1985). *Overcoming resistance: Rational-emotive therapy with difficult clients.* New York: Springer.

Ellis, A. (1989a). Comments on my critics. In M. Bernard & R. DiGiuseppe (Eds.), *Inside rational-emotive therapy: A critical appraisal of the theory and therapy of Albert Ellis.* San Diego, CA: Academic Press.

Ellis, A. (1989b, June). Is rational-emotive therapy "rationalist" or "constructivist"? Paper presented at the World Congress of Cognitive Therapy, Oxford, England.

Ellis, A., & Dryden, W. (1987). *The practice of rational-emotive therapy.* New York: Springer.

Ellis, A., McInerney, DiGiuseppe, R., & Yeager, R. (1988). *Rational-emotive therapy with alcoholics and substance abusers.* New York: Pergamon Press.

Ellis, A., Sichel, J., DiMattia, D., Yeager, R., & DiGiuseppe, R. (1989). *Rational-emotive couples therapy.* New York: Pergamon Press.

Ellis, A., & Whitely, J. (1979). *Theoretical and empirical foundations of rational-emotive therapy.* Monterey, CA: Brooks/Cole.

Gould, S. J. (1988). Freud's phylogenetic fantasy. *Natural History.*

Grieger, R., & Boyd, J. (1980). *Rational-emotive therapy: A skills-based approach.* New York: Van Nostrand Reinhold.

Kassinove, H. (1986). Self-reported affect and core irrational thinking: A preliminary analysis. *Journal of Rational-Emotive Therapy, 4*(2), 119–130.

Korzybski, A. (1933). *Science and sanity.* San Francisco: International Society for General Semantics.

Kuhn, T. (1970). *The structure of scientific revolutions* (2nd ed.). Chicago: University of Chicago Press.

Kuhn, T. (1977). *The essential tension: Selected studies in scientific tradition and changes.* Chicago: University of Chicago Press.

Mahoney, M. (1976). *The scientist.* Cambridge, MA: Ballinger.

Mahoney, M. (1988). The cognitive sciences and psychotherapy: Patterns in a developing relationship. In K. Dobson (Ed.), *Handbook of the cognitive behavior therapies* (pp. 357–386). New York: Guilford.

Maultsby, M. (1984). *Rational behavior therapy.* Englewood Cliffs, NJ: Prentice-Hall.

Muran, C., & DiGiuseppe, R. (1990). A cognitive formulation of the use of metaphor in psychotherapy. *Clinical Psychology Review, 10*(1), 69–88.

Polyani, M. (1966). *The tacit dimension.* New York: Doubleday.

Prochaska, J., & DiClemente, C. (1984). *The transtheoretical approach: Crossing traditional boundaries of psychotherapy.* Monterey, CA: Brooks/Cole.

Walen, S., DiGiuseppe, R., & Wessler, R. (1980). *The practitioner's guide to rational-emotive therapy.* New York: Oxford University Press.

Wessler, R. A., & Wessler, R. L. (1980). *The principles and practice of rational-emotive therapy.* San Francisco: Jossey-Bass.

Wein, K., Nelson, R., & Odom, J. (1975). The relative contribution of reattribution and verbal extinction to the effectiveness of cognitive restructuring. *Behavior Therapy, 6,* 459–474.

Woolfolk, R., & Sass, T. (1989). Rational-emotive philosophy. In M. Bernard & R. DiGiuseppe (Eds.), *Inside rational-emotive therapy: A critical appraisal of the theory and therapy of Albert Ellis.* New York: Academic Press.

8

RET and the Assertive Process

Paul A. Hauck

Two Types of Problems

The term *cognitive-behavioral therapy* refers to an important relationship, in simple terms: the relationship between reasoning and action. It also refers to the relationship and the differences between intrapsychic and interpsychic conflicts. Intrapsychic problems are problems we have only with ourselves, as we might on a desert island, or over failing to discipline ourselves enough to stay on a weight control program. Interpsychic problems are those we have because others frustrate us. This is an important distinction to bear in mind because each type requires very distinct applications to reduce the consequent discomforts.

Intrapsychic problems are managed best in most instances with cognitive techniques, especially RET. Interpsychic problems, however, almost invariably require cognitive *and* behavioral techniques. Thus far, RET has placed most of its attention on the ABCs of emotional disturbance, that is, on the cognitive side of this equation. A coherent, rational, and systematized method for understanding the fundamentals of the behavioral part of the equation is imperative in dealing with interpersonal problems.

I maintain that such a conceptual framework has not been complete enough to be of great help to therapists guiding couples over marital hurdles, employees in conflict with employers, or parents and children trying to live harmoniously. This chapter, hopefully, offers a more comprehensive system so that we counselors will have a better idea of how to proceed when dealing with difficult interpersonal problems, how to know just where the participants are as their struggles escalate, and what options we

Paul A. Hauck • 1800 Third Avenue, Suite 302, Rock Island, Illinois 61201.

can offer our clients, knowing full well that we will usually be on target and can predict with enviable accuracy what is likely to happen when a particular option is chosen.

In the final analysis there are essentially three objectives in having a relationship with anyone, such as marriage and family relationships, employer–employee relationships, friend-to-friend relationships, and even huge bodies of people, such as communities, states, and nations. What we all want from each other are three things: cooperation, respect, and love (Hauck, 1984).

We ask for cooperation from those people who provide some of our most fundamental and daily services. The cab driver is hopefully a courteous person. We are not interested particularly in his respecting us or loving us, but we do hope that he will charge us fairly, that he will get us to our destination without adding on many miles for his own profit, and that he will help us with our luggage.

We also want respect from those people with whom we have a deeper degree of involvement. Our employers will hopefully recognize our contributions and promote us accordingly. Our banks will take into consideration our good credit rating and extend us a loan, knowing that we have earned their trust and respect. This degree of involvement is certainly more than mere cooperation, as the consequences are often more serious, and as respect is an item that generally has to be earned, not merely given because one happens to be in frequent contact with others.

And last, we want love from those people whom we devote our lives to and who are capable of satisfying our deepest desires and needs. These include the members of our family, our spouses, and our very closest friends.

It is not difficult to predict that the intensity of the frustration caused us by a problem in any one of these three types of relationships depends entirely on which category the frustration comes from. Having someone cut in front of us in a movie line causes a mild frustration to most of us, whereas being dismissed from a job causes us much more displeasure. The greatest degree of suffering, of course, comes from the loss of a loved one through abandonment, divorce, or death.

To alleviate the sufferings in each of these three categories requires slightly different strategies for keeping these relationships in good balance, as many of the frustrations that involve lack of cooperation can often be safely ignored, whereas those that involve a betrayal of respect and love call for the most stringent methods to correct.

It behooves the therapist, therefore, to make a quick assessment of the nature of the problems early in therapy so that an appropriate plan can be offered to deal with these problems of varying frustration and disturbance (Dryden, 1987; Hauck, 1980).

The Two Principles of Human Interaction

It is not enough to help our clients understand that they create their own emotional disturbances. What is also needed is to make them fully aware of the fact that they play a vital role, although an indirect one, in the creation of emotional problems in others. They are often puzzled by the unfair treatment they receive at the hands of their families, fellow workers, and friends. And with some bewilderment and justification, they pose the question repeatedly of why they are being treated in these very frustrating ways. It is at this point that the RET therapist uses her or his knowledge of behaviorist principles (Skinner, 1953) and educates her or his client about precisely why these events happen.

There are two principles of human interaction: (1) *We get the behavior we tolerate;* and (2) *if we want to change someone else's behavior, we must change ours first.*

The first principle tells the client that behavior exists because it is reinforced (Skinner, 1953). A husband neglects his wife because he gets away with it. Children are lazy around the home and don't help with chores because mother tolerates that behavior. Pushy workers at the office impose themselves on weaker workers and ask for excessive favors from the client because she simply does not stop that behavior. We get the behavior that we reward.

Our clients had better understand that the frustrations that they object to are often not accidental; they are the result of much reinforcement to those people who are doing the abusing. Behavior cannot exist without being reinforced, and despite what clients say, if the behavior is continuing, we must make the assumption that someone in that relationship is doing the reinforcing. Clients often resist this interpretation and insist that they have talked about this to the people who are annoying them time after time and that, therefore, they couldn't possibly be responsible for reinforcing the behavior. Or they protest that they have sometimes left their home and spent the night at a motel to penalize their partner. Or they have taken the bicycle away from their son, expecting him to modify his behavior and to assume more responsibility. In short, they point out that they have already done what you are suggesting, that they have not tolerated these behaviors, and that, still, very few changes have resulted. Therefore, another explanation must be offered.

In countering these objections, I stoutly maintain that the behavior is caused and reinforced, fed, rewarded, and nourished, if not by my client, then by somebody. And who might that person be? Is there a grandmother reinforcing this behavior? Is it the spouse? Are there any other children at home whom we don't know of who could be doing this? Is there a cat or dog at home who is reinforcing this behavior? Or is it the man in the moon?

And of course, the client quickly comes to the realization that, if anyone is doing the reinforcing, it is probably the client.

I then try to show clients that, although they have attempted to discourage unacceptable behavior, they may very well continue to receive it simply because they are very inefficient in trying to discourage it. I then teach them how they are missing the essential ingredients to get the results they want.

At this point, I also make sure to remind the client that he or she is not responsible for the other person's annoying behavior even though the client is unwittingly supporting it. The frustrating person whom my client is dealing with is the one who is ultimately fully responsible for his or her own behavior, and my client is only 49%, at the most, *indirectly* responsible for the trouble that is arising between the two of them. I clarify that point further by saying that, although they can't make the other people behave unacceptably, my clients are such tolerant people that it is easy for others to act unfairly in their company. In other words, my clients set up an atmosphere in which abuse can take place very readily, and the irresponsible people causing the problems know this. They don't have to do that, but most people are immature enough to take advantage of any indulgence that is offered to them.

I then briefly describe the nature of reinforcement itself. When an act is rewarded, it tends to be strengthened. If an act is not rewarded, it tends to become extinct (Skinner, 1953). If an act is rewarded intermittently, the behavior tends to be powerfully reinforced. Therefore, it is extremely important to be consistent and not to lapse into occasional reinforcement in the belief that, as it happens only infrequently, it cannot have much of an effect on the target behavior. Clients grasp these principles readily. Almost all of them seem to comprehend the fact that giving people bonuses for their behavior tends to encourage that particular behavior.

I then explain the second principle of human interaction, which says that, if other people are to change, the client must change first. Why and how? Because the offender will usually change only when he or she is made sufficiently uncomfortable with a particular behavior to want to stop that behavior.

Recent research by Bernard (1988) and Bernard and Laws (1988) reports that children in particular are made upset by two irrationalities: that people should let them do as they want (referred to as *demands on others*), and that people should not have to obey all rules (*nonconforming attitudes*). These attitudes, not reinforcement principles alone, account for children's misbehavior.

In the final analysis, these problems usually require the dual application of both the disputation of these irrationalities and the penalizing of the unacceptable actions.

At this point, to make RET more powerful, I show them how they can become more assertive by giving them a fuller understanding of the dynamics of assertion, the sequence in which the steps should be followed, and what options they have if the steps don't work.

To Be or Not to Be Assertive: The JRC Principle

I believe we should do something about our frustrations when we are less than just reasonably content. If we are below this level for any period of time, we feel psychological and physical stresses that are unmistakable and that are symptom-producing. The Just Reasonably Content level (JRC) is that point below which we are starving for emotional and psychological satisfactions. It is equivalent to the point where we are consuming fewer calories than we are expending. For example, a person who needs 1,000 calories a day to maintain a barely acceptable level of health but is receiving only 900 calories a day will eventually starve to death.

If we need 10 strokes a day and are receiving only 9, psychological stress will be the inevitable consequence. It can be forestalled only by our lowering our expectations and thereby deciding that 9 strokes is all we really need; otherwise, we must protest so vigorously against those who are denying us that minimal level of satisfaction that our satisfactions are brought up to the JRC.

Living up to the JRC bothers some people because they have to be self-interested and put their interests for a time completely ahead of those of others. They interpret this as selfishness, immaturity, and greed. It is none of these. To bring oneself up to a point where one is barely getting by is hardly greed or selfishness; it is simply a healthy degree of *enlightened self-interest*. Just as we spend time daily in showering, brushing our teeth, dressing nicely, and feeding ourselves so that we can get through the day acceptably, so we had better also not allow ourselves to be taken advantage of by the people who borrow money and don't repay it, or who undertake tasks with us and then don't do their share of the work.

The JRC is the point where the wisdom of the body begins to respond and gives signals that something is seriously wrong. And its messages are almost infallible. How do we know when we are thirsty? The body tells us so. How do we know when we are tired, hungry, need sleep, or need not sleep? The body tells us so. How do we know when we are being taken advantage of? Our bodies tell us. We get an internal message when we know we are being manipulated, threatened, seduced, and in general treated unfairly.

Clients must learn to respect the messages that come from within, and these are sufficiently uncomfortable, they had better learn to pay attention and decide which option they want to use: lower their expectations, get away from the problem, or change the nature of the frustration through protest.

If we listen to our bodily reactions and use that orientation to guide us in the decision-making process, we fare better than we do when we ignore our deepest feelings. This is an internal compass that can guide us if we are attuned to it. It tells us when we've had enough of people's nonsense and what to do about it; when to protest in a marriage or to get out of it; and when to tolerate a situation or to fight it. Our clients don't have to ask us if they need to protest; all they need do is note if they are not sleeping well or not eating well, if their hearts are racing, or whether their bowel movements are regular. All these and a multitude of other bodily and psychological manifestations can tell our clients in a moment whether what they are about to do is or is not to their liking.

And what if they don't listen to their JRC? What happens when they live below the JRC over an extended period of time? Three consequences almost inevitably follow:

1. They will be unhappy and probably also emotionally disturbed.
2. They will begin to fall out of love.
3. They will want to end the relationship.

Happiness comes from not being painfully frustrated for long periods of time. Granted, some frustration gives us a challenge and stimulates us. But the painful frustrations that come from conflict and that are ever-present, such as grinding poverty, are bound to leave the sufferer in an unhappy mood; he or she will eventually develop feelings of inferiority, low self-esteem, anger, obesity, anorexia, and a host of other typical symptoms.

The second consequence of living below the JRC is that one will gradually fall out of love with the people who are causing the frustrations. The vows one made at the altar will weaken once one's partner turns out to be an impossible person and one is not getting any of the reasonable benefits from a relationship that he or she dreamed of. One's feelings will change toward that person if one has any common sense at all. He or she may not want to reject that person, but it is going to be hard not to. At the very least one will certainly dislike that person, and whatever feelings one once had will gradually change into indifference or even hatred.

And, again, why not? Love, as I have shown in my book *Marriage Is a Loving Business* (1977), is the feeling one has for someone who has, is, or will satisfy one's deepest desires and needs. Not satisfying deep desires and needs leads almost inevitably to the loss of feelings of love. When one is below the JRC and is not getting even the most meager of satisfactions from one's partner, then what is there to love? Love is reciprocity. We love people for what they do for us. Technically, we don't love people themselves. When we say we love someone, that is actually only a convenient way to express the idea that a particular person understands our desires and needs and satisfies them to a high degree. For practical reasons we aren't inclined to say, "I love my partner's considerateness, friendliness, and helpfulness around the house."

The third consequence of living below the JRC for an extended period of time is that people eventually want to leave or end the unsatisfactory relationship.

And why not? Anyone in his or her right mind would leave an over-heated room. Anyone in his or her right mind would stop working in order to eat if he or she hadn't had anything for three days. Anyone in his or her right mind would leave a job in which the boss was treating him or her unfairly and didn't offer advancement or show appreciation for efforts made. So why should it be any different in a marriage? This doesn't mean that people should necessarily run to a divorce lawyer when they are seriously frustrated. But I think it does mean that they had better do something about it if they know that those feelings of separation are growing.

For those people who cannot consider a divorce for religious reasons, I strongly recommend a separation. And the separation should be for only a day or two at first, but if this does not correct the inequities within the relationship, then I would recommend leaving for weeks or months. Eventually, if the marriage does not improve, the separation may be permanent.

THE THREE RULES OF ASSERTION

Rule 1 is that if somebody does something good to you, you should do something good to them (Madsen & Madsen, 1980). This is the way we show appreciation, and this is the way we reinforce behavior. If our positive responses approximate the strength of the positive responses in those we are dealing with, we tend to come to an increasingly satisfactory balance of benefits. Frustrations are continually eliminated or reduced when we follow this schema. This rule is fundamental and is nothing less than the reinforcement principle of operant conditioning (Skinner, 1938). It certainly needs no elaboration from me.

Rule 2 is that if people do something bad to you and they don't realize they are behaving badly, you should turn the other cheek, go the extra mile, forgive them by getting over your anger, tolerate their thoughtless-ness, and reason with them on two separate occasions (Hauck, 1984). Ther-apeutic effectiveness is increased when we limit the number of times we talk to people about their misbehavior, as talking itself has a reinforcing effect. When we discuss misconduct with others, we are actually tolerating the misconduct. The toleration becomes a reinforcement itself. The person has generally not been made sufficiently uncomfortable by a lecture to achieve changes, and thus it is imperative that we not spend many occasions (more than perhaps two), during which we reason with them not to behave as they do. Otherwise, we find ourselves in the same position as the mother who is continually warning, scolding, and threatening, all the while actually unwittingly reinforcing the very behavior she is condemning. It is for this reason that I recommend we discuss misconduct no more than twice. If we suspect that one lecture or explanation is sufficient, there is no need to go into a second. What do we expect to say the third or fourth time that we haven't said the first or second?

This turning of the other cheek and going the extra mile is nothing more than a philosophy of tolerance of rudeness, selfishness, and inconsiderateness. Those groups, especially from religious persuasions, who would argue that one must always turn the other cheek and go the extra mile, that we must forgive 70 times 7, are confused and quite imprecise in their advice.

I fully agree that we should not get angry with people who bother us and that we need to forgive them. But what is forgiveness? Operationally defined, forgiveness exists only when we can truthfully say that (1) we are no longer angry with the person who has offended us; (2) we do not think he or she is a bad person; and (3) we are not going to seek revenge because we think that person is bad. That is forgiveness. However, most people equate forgiveness with tolerance. That is the essential error that some religions make and why we have so much difficulty in our interpersonal relationships. Forgiveness is one thing; tolerance is another. I maintain that we should forgive every injustice (never be angry at anyone over anything), but that we should become *intolerant* after we have been forgiving, and then we had better penalize the negative behaviors.

It has been my observation that there are only two kinds of people who can be reasoned with. The first are those who are mature, and the second are those who are emotionally untroubled. When we talk to these people and appeal to their sense of fairness and justice, they listen and understand and make the necessary accommodations in their behavior to achieve justice. Straight RET works wonders for them.

This is not the case when we are dealing with (1) immature or (2) disturbed people. When we reason with them two times and they still have not made an effort to change, we are creating a self-defeating situation for ourselves and for them if we lecture to them a third or fourth or fifth time. They are often too immature or too disturbed to benefit by the reasoning process. Therefore, we had better stop after the second time because immature and disturbed people think their behavior is quite acceptable. Therefore, they will not change, as their behavior is being reinforced.

The absence of change can now serve as a definition of maturity or disturbance: if we reason with people twice and they don't seem to under-stand the fairness and the correctness of our arguments, we're dealing with immature or disturbed people, at least from our point of view, and there is no sense in wasting our time trying to reason with them further. At that point it is important to move on to Rule 3 because RET can be quite ineffective if we concentrate on clients' intrapsychic problems using only rational persuasion as an intervention when the problem is clearly interpersonal.

Rule 3 is that, if people do something bad to you and reasoning with them two times has not helped, do something equally annoying, frustrat-ing, or discomforting to them; however, you must do it without (1) anger, (2) guilt, (3) other-pity, (4) fear of rejection, (5) fear of physical harm, and (6) fear of financial harm.

People correctly remind me that the use of Rule 3 (aversive conse-quences) will only bring out more resistance and can, therefore, hardly be a recommendation for therapeutic change.

In the short run, this objection is absolutely valid. Things get worse before they get better, especially after applying Rule 3. Because people dislike changing their long-standing habits as much as children dislike washing their faces, we must be prepared for this resistance.

Rule 3 works when we make people uncomfortable and when we do it without (1) being angry and (2) while at the same time applying Rule 1 (positive consequences). When we learn to be firm *and* kind in dealing with people whom we want to influence, we will have the maximum effect on them.

Not to eliminate anger and not to praise or reward the offending person for decent behavior will lead to certain failure to bring about desired changes.

The six conditions listed above must not be ignored if one is to become an assertive person by using Rule 3 and can be taught in classical RET style. The first I have already elaborated on, namely, that when we reward nega-tive behavior with negative behavior, it must be done without *anger*. The second is that it must be done without *guilt*. If we try to become firm with people but feel we are bad and unworthy people for what we are doing, we are obviously not going to stick to our beliefs and our tough-love process for very long because our strategy will crumble like a house of cards.

The same is true of the third condition for being assertive. *Other-pity* also weakens our resolve to the point where we simply will not stand up for our rights and will find ourselves tolerating unacceptable actions be-cause our hearts are breaking over the discomforts we are putting others through. When we think of firing a poor employee, we are not going to get our task accomplished if we feel very sorry for that person.

The fourth condition to observe is *not to fear rejection*. Those who fear rejection, even though they may usually assert themselves without anger, without guilt, or without pitying others, can still spoil the best of intentions if they begin to fear losing the affection and approval of those people who are taking advantage of them. Fear of rejection is one of the strongest of all the fears normally experienced by a civilian population and is something I have elaborated on in my book *Overcoming Worry and Fear* (Hauck, 1975).

The fifth condition is *fear of harm*. If we are afraid of being physically attacked, we had better either learn to box better, get lessons in kung-fu, do muscle-building exercises, or train ourselves to run swiftly. Calling the police and using body guards are other practical solutions.

The sixth condition to avoid is *fear of financial harm*. Women in particular have often been subject to great control by men because of the economic advantage they have over their wives. Among the better things that have happened since the women's movement is that females have been able to find employment and are able to support themselves in greater numbers than ever before. This circumstance has given them freedom from fear of financial harm and has brought about many separations and divorces that were clearly called for. But if a person is under unavoidable financial control, he or she simply has to accept the fact that a bad situation must be tolerated because the economics of the problem are so potent that they cannot be ignored.

There we have the six conditions that all of us want to overcome if we are to be assertive people.

THE FOUR OBJECTIONS

The belief that, when people do bad things to us, we should do bad things to them sound very much like an eye for an eye and a tooth for a tooth. This position offends those who follow the biblical teaching that such behavior falls within the province of God and no one else. Such objections are well taken because, if this actually were an act of revenge, I would agree with that viewpoint completely.

What must be clearly understood in following Rule 3 is that this is not revenge; it is an act of correction. It is an act of love because it dares to confront immoral, cruel, inconsiderate, and neurotic behavior in the strongest possible terms needed to correct such behavior. Those who care a great deal for the persons to whom they are applying such measures are showing love when such stringent actions are used. It takes courage to be so intolerant of the immaturities and irresponsibilities of those we care for to stand up to them nose to nose and simply apply whatever energies we can to get them to cease behaving self-defeatingly or antisocially. Following Rule 3 is nothing like revenge; it is the last opportunity to demonstrate the deepest love that parents can show their children, or that one person can show another. Instead of letting people believe that they are being wicked or inconsiderate when they stand up to immoral or wicked behavior, we should instead applaud the courage and the sacrifice being made at such times when confrontations alone will cure or contain violence and disrespect.

Revenge always means that, when we react to people, we are doing so with a desire to hurt them—not to teach them or help them in anyway, but simply to punish them severely because we think they are evil and undesirable people. That is revenge, and it is not what I am referring to when I suggest that we return bad behavior for bad behavior. That is why I list the absence of anger as one of the six conditions that we must learn to overcome if we are to become efficient at being assertive people. I am teaching my clients the very important distinction between aggression and assertion. I define *aggression* as standing up for one's rights *with* anger, and I define *assertion* as standing up for one's rights *without* anger. Only in the case of self-defense, as when one is being attacked or raped or is at war, is actual violence called for.

The second objection is that we have to lower ourselves to the unseemly behavior of others if we use this method. I'm afraid that is sometimes unavoidable. Let us always remember that we tried not to have to do equally frustrating things to those who offend us because we first explained ourselves to them and let them know quietly and rationally why we considered some of their behavior off-color and unacceptable. When such an approach is ignored, we have every right to give up what seems not to be working and to resort to something else. That may very well bring us to using some of the same negative behaviors used against us. In other words, if a teenager lies to his mother repeatedly, I sometimes tell the mother to lie to the teenager. And when the child discovers that his mother has not been truthful, I tell her to admit to the youngster that she did lie. If he can do it, so can she. If a toddler goes around biting people or kicking their shins and has been warned not to do this on two separate occasions, I then suggest that the parents put the youngster in time-out. This is always to be done, however with a feeling of "I'm not angry with this person. I don't like her behavior, and I think enough of her so that I want the behavior changed. Reasoning has not helped, but by penalizing her, I will be helping her stop this behavior."

RET is often only half as effective as it might be if it were accompanied more often by action. Action is highly recommended in marital situations. For the man or woman whose partner leaves the house in disarray, I often recommend making a mess twice as bad. A woman should have no trouble curing such problems if she has the courage to leave the kitchen dishes in the sink, the bathroom unwashed, the clothes lying on the floor, and so on. She may very well have to endure some discomfort when she practices such uncomfortable behavior, but if it cures the problem in the long run, it will be well worth it.

The third objection is that two wrongs don't make a right. Of course, two wrongs do not make a right, but we must not look on our frustrating others, when we are trying to help them, as a wrong. What we are getting from others is thoughtless and inconsiderate behavior with no thought for our welfare. When we are doing similar things to them, we are hopefully trying to teach them that what they are doing is wrong and that they would get along better with all concerned if they would change their behavior.

It is not the act itself that determines whether it is moral or immoral; it is the intention behind the act. If a thug comes at you with a knife to harm you, that is a wrong. If a surgeon uses a knife to remove a tumor, that is a good.

The fourth objection is that this is too much like playing games. It is playing games only if the issues involved are trivial. And if they are trivial, then there is no point in making a serious issue over them. Who wants to get into serious altercations, confrontations, and yelling matches if an issue is a piddling one? Quite the contrary, one must determine in one's own heart that what she or he is protesting is a serious issue and that it must be dealt with.

WHEN RET IS ESPECIALLY CALLED FOR

Rational-emotive principles are clearly called for in applying all three of the rules mentioned above. To return one positive action with another positive action and thereby express appreciation calls for overcoming our anger, and allowing ourselves to become intimate. People who are afraid of rejection and of getting close to people find it very difficult to implement Rule 1. A father who loves his son but cannot show his love because he thinks tenderness is sissy stuff is going to have a hard time rewarding good behavior. He will have to be taught that rejection is not painful, only inconvenient, and that others cannot upset him without his cooperation. Giving children praise or hugs or giving our spouses and friends or employees a pat on the back and pointing out their good performance requires overcoming one's shyness or perhaps one's fear of being phony. Some people find it as hard to be tender as others find it to be tough. Straight RET therapy is required for people with these emotional blocks related to intimacy.

Rule 2, also, is not workable for individuals who have psychological impediments to turning the other cheek and going the extra mile. They need to learn how to control their anger, how to be completely forgiving, how to be patient and understanding of people's frailties, and how never to hate anybody for anything. They must become completely acquainted with and convinced of the rationality of the idea that we do not have to be perfect in order to be acceptable human beings. Those who do not understand this idea and who have never worked it through in their own minds simply cannot practice Rule 2 and be forgiving and patient human beings.

RET is also crucial in the implementation of Rule 3. As already stated, anger is again important to the third rule because, if we return negative behavior for negative behavior and do it with anger, we will not invite cooperation, respect, and love; we will invite resentment, bitterness, and opposition instead. This is why wars start, either at the domestic level or at the international level. Unless people know the psychology of anger, how it is created, and how it can be overcome, they are simply not going to pass the very first test of implementing Rule 3.

The second, third, and fourth conditions (guilt, other-pity, and fear of rejection) are also clearly normal and everyday psychological occurrences for the RET counselor. Unless these emotional disturbances can be clearly contained, the crucial third rule will seldom work. And if people allow themselves to be totally dominated by a fear of physical harm or financial harm, they will not come into their own as strong and capable people but instead will allow fear to dominate their lives.

It should be clear at this point that the cognitive and the behavioral meet very intricately in the application of these three rules. Unless the cognitive is mastered, the behavioral will not be achieved. But to know only the cognitive does not necessarily mean that the behavioral will change. It is not enough for us simply not to be angry or to be guiltless or fearless in dealing with others, we must know what to do about other people's negative behavior once we have ourselves under fine control. And that, of course, is where the behavioral techniques come clearly into question, and that's what this chapter is all about.

The Four Options

Assuming that you have applied Rule 3 for a reasonable period of time and you find that it does not work, what do you advise your clients to do? I tell them that there are four options to consider, not only in this instance, but in nearly every instance where a problem or frustration faces us.

Option 1: Tolerance without Resentment

Most frustrations can be tolerated if we so choose. They may be inconvenient and unfair, but they are not unbearable or catastrophic, as we repeatedly remind our clients. There are, unfortunately, some situations that all of us find ourselves in from time to time that will not change, and we had better learn to live with them. If the breadwinner in the family cannot provide a lifestyle that the wife or the children want, that circumstance simply has to be tolerated. If we have a job we don't like and can't find a better one, then we had better learn to lump that gracefully. If a woman is exceedingly possessive and wants to account for her husband's every move and he cannot divorce her, he will simply have to learn to tolerate her without resentment.

It is possible to tolerate almost anything if we decide to do so.

Option 2: Protest

I call this *cold war* or *strike*. If using the third rule (returning annoying behavior with annoying behavior) does not work, then let us increase the discomfort of our offenders. If the family is not helping with the dishes, instead of preaching *ad nauseum* simply let everything sit and do not cook in the kitchen again until the dishes are done.

If the family are not picking up their clothes but are dropping them wherever they take them off, pick them up and put them in a garbage bag. If that doesn't work, charge them a small price to have each item returned. If that doesn't work, give the garbage bag full of clothing to the Salvation Army.

Rule 3 states that we must return annoying behavior with behavior as intense as the behavior that we received. Therefore, as our efforts to stop others from abusing us continues, our frustrations with them increase as well. This additional discomfort justifies our getting equally annoying and difficult with them until one of us decides to compromise. Deliberate annoyance is the whole strategy behind a labor strike. The point of such an exercise is to frustrate the other party to such a degree that an agreement seems better than the continued confrontation. The same applies in a marital situation or in a family struggle between parents and children. *We want to create a crisis,* to create more and more tension until finally somebody is willing to make a compromise and stop the negative behavior. The time for reason has passed. Effective therapy calls for *action*.

Who usually gives in in such a situation? The party who cares the least about the relationship will win the power struggle. Therefore, if we want our marriage to improve but certain changes need to be made first, and the marriage is extremely important to us, we'll find ourselves giving in before the partner does. The one who cares about the marriage the least is the one who is going to hold out the longest and who will also usually win these struggles. Therefore, in order to be victorious more often in these struggles, I would suggest advising your client not to make any relationship too important because, the moment it is, that's the time when he or she will compromise the most in order to preserve the relationship.

Advise your client not to give in too quickly in using Rule 3. Simply because one tactic has not worked does not mean that it will not work if we increase the pressure. However, if escalating a particular strategy does not work, then let us alter the strategy and go to something else that may be more affective. For example, a wife who gave her husband the cold shoulder because he simply refused to communicate with her did not change him until she finally left the house whenever he did not respond to her overtures to talk. At first, she left the home overnight, but that did not work. She then took off two nights, then three nights, and so on, until he finally realized that, if he wanted his wife home, he would have to communicate with her at length.

Option 3: Separation or Divorce

When actions seem not to work at all and reasoning has also failed, one usually has the option of leaving a relationship or divorcing one's spouse. We can quit our jobs, break up with our friends, move away from a neighborhood, send the children off to grandmother, or get a nonbinding or a legal separation. For those people whose religion forbids divorce, there is always the option of a separation. If a separation is not possible, one can always live in a house as brother and sister, even though it may be very uncomfortable.

If one decides that separation is too drastic and does not want to break up a potentially good relationship, one then goes back to Option 1, tolerating the situation without resentment.

When an option needs to be selected, it is imperative that the therapist not choose for the clients. The clients must choose, as they are the ones who will live with the consequences. Do not allow yourself to make decisions like this for other people if you want to sleep soundly.

The first three options listed above are the only sensible ones, as they all have the potential for relief. It is the fourth option (toleration *with* resentment) that I do not recommend but that is selected by almost everyone. It is the only one that guarantees more discomfort rather than less.

Option 4: Toleration with Resentment

Let us not forget that we act neurotically when we make bad situations worse. This is precisely what happens when we put up with situations we resent but also allow. Because of the internal inconsistency of this process, when it is carried on long enough all manner of emotional disturbances result, such as symptoms of depression, intermittent explosive episodes, anxiety attacks, marital and family strife, substance abuse, infidelity, and physical abuse.

Even though this is obviously a clearly unwise option to choose in facing our difficulties, it is unquestionably one of the most frequently chosen. It forms the backbone of our psychotherapeutic practices. Without Option 4, we would all be out of business in short order.

MAKING A CHOICE

When clients ask us what they can do about their frustrations, the answer is simple and straightforward. They can choose to (1) resign themselves to the frustration without bitterness; (2) become intolerant of it until it changes; or (3) get away from the problem. Those are the three sensible choices. If people don't use one of these three, they can always use Option 4, tolerate the thing and magnify the suffering.

As simple as this process seems, it sometime meets with surprising resistance. Clients protest that they can't possibly put up with the situation for any number of reasons. I then agree with them that they may certainly be correct, but not to despair. There is the second option: they can make waves and go on strike until some healthy changes are made. To this, they protest that they don't want any more confrontations, that they can't stand the yelling and the fighting, and that Option 2 is clearly out of the question. Well enough. I then remind them that they can always leave their jobs, move to another neighborhood, separate from their partners, and if the issue is serious enough and their religion does not forbid it, they can always get a divorce.

But they protest against this, too. How can they leave a marriage of 25 years? And what will that do to the children? How can they leave one job when they don't have another one? And so on and on.

So I tell them that they can tolerate the situation with resentment, and of course, they completely refuse that suggestion, as they don't want to be depressed or to start drinking again.

I then bring them around to the first option again and tell them that they can tolerate it without resentment and, lo and behold, they turn that suggestion down, too.

This little exercise makes it quite clear to clients that *all* of the options are uncomfortable. Some are less so than others; nevertheless, it is the clients' responsibility to decide which of the four choices is the least painful.

The therapist then has to use standard RET techniques to help clients achieve relief by whatever method they have chosen. If they decide to tolerate the situation without resentment, they will have to learn not to demand events in their lives just because they would like them. Life is not fair, and they don't have to have everything they want. Also, they need to be reminded repeatedly that nothing upsets them except themselves, and if they learn to challenge their belief that the world makes them upset, they can make Option 1 work quite nicely.

Option 2 calls for the use of Rule 3, but this time more vigorously. When clients are frustrated a second time, they are generally more uncomfortable than they were when they were frustrated the first time. Each frustration adds to the discomfort. Therefore, when our clients protest what they regard as unfair behavior, we instruct them to become increasingly intolerant every time they respond.

It is for this reason that I caution my clients that, if they undertake Option 2, they must brace themselves for the storms ahead. There will be fights, arguments, and bad feelings of all kinds. And they are cautioned that the tougher they get, the tougher the partners usually become also. People generally do not change unless they are extremely uncomfortable. The tough love movement (York, 1980) is nothing less than Option 2 using Rule 3: protest by returning negative behavior with negative behavior.

Again, standard RET therapy is clearly called for in giving people the strength to face their unfair partners. They need to learn to be calm as the storm broods. They had better not feel guilt or other-pity as they go through this process, or they will fail. They need to be reminded of the rational idea that they do not *need* love or approval and that rejection is painless unless they make it hurt. And they also need to be reminded repeatedly that facing difficult tasks is easier in the long run than it is to avoid them.

These are all standard cognitive and RET techniques. Clients are cautioned that, if they find the situation getting too hot, they can always return to Option 1 and tolerate the situation without resentment. Or they can accept Option 3 and simply separate themselves from the problem by leaving it. Standard RET practices are also required when we are advising our clients to get a separation or a divorce because of all the trepidation they have in changing the direction of their lives so drastically, such as being out in the world alone, or having to face certain financial insecurities. They are imperfect and will do badly at times, but that is not a reflection on themselves. As Ellis and Knaus (1977) and Hauck (1976) have pointed out in their books on self-discipline, it is better to do the best one can than to do nothing at all.

WIDER APPLICATIONS

If what I have offered is a sensible description of human interaction at the individual level, the same principles ought to apply when they are addressed to individuals at a collective level. Greater understanding can then be gained of why we are having difficulties in our country and throughout the world in the academic arena, in social programs, in our political dealings with other nations, in the judicial system, and in our religious institutions. These are, after all, valid human activities, and I believe they are governed by essentially the same principles that individuals function by. Let us therefore study these five sectors of our society and see how we may influence them with these concepts.

Academics

Our school systems look very different today from the way they did 50 years ago. What seemed unthinkable in the past is routine today. Children are truant in great numbers and think that there is nothing wrong with truancy. Students are showing enormous disrespect for their teachers, being unruly in class, swearing at teachers, and at times being openly belligerent to school staff.

These behaviors, I contend, are the result of the same basic principles of human interaction that I enunciated previously: (1) we get the behavior we tolerate, and (2) if we want to change the behavior of others, we must change first.

These rebellious actions by grade-schoolers and adolescents must obviously be reinforced in some way or they wouldn't be present. But who is reinforcing such behavior? It is clearly the school system, the state, the parents, and the teachers who have tolerated these behaviors. If the staff cannot make students uncomfortable when they don't seat themselves in class on time, or when they are truant, or when they are rude and disrespectful, then how can we expect anything but that same behavior? If we reward such actions, they are precisely what we will get, and if we want students to change, we have to change first. We can do this by being less tolerant of such behavior and by making students increasingly uncomfortable when they behave badly. But clearly, our laws prohibit this form of action. Therefore, I fully predict that we are not going to get any significant change in the schools until we analyze precisely how we are teaching these youngsters to behave disrespectfully and what we can do to make them so uncomfortable with these actions in the future as to stop them.

Social Programs

All kinds of serious mistakes are being made by governments all over the world in attempts to help their disadvantaged populations. Some are so thoroughly socialistic that they unwittingly reward people not to work. Who in their right minds would get up in the morning and go to a job when their mortgage is being paid, and they are getting medical help and funds for food and heating if they are unemployed? This is nothing short of returning good behavior for negative behavior.

Would it not be better to give these forms of assistance contingent on performance that indicates learning how *not* to be dependent? No modern society needs to allow its people to starve and perish on the streets, but neither should an advanced society pay people not to contribute in some way. It seems to me that it has taken governments a long time to realize that healthy people should not be given anything for nothing, unless it is those who are seriously handicapped.

Politics

Rule 3 works in the political arena just as it works in the classroom, in the factory, or in the home.

When the Russians expel a few British diplomats, the prime minister instantly expels a few Russian diplomats and sends them back to Moscow.

Is this sensible behavior? Of course it is. There is no sense going to war over such political chess moves, but one has to make a statement nevertheless. When Gorbachev dismissed more British diplomats, Margaret Thatcher did the same. Eventually, this tit-for-tat behavior ceased, the lines were drawn, and no further diplomats were dismissed. And that's exactly the way it ought to work. Discomfort was created, each side went on strike for a time, and when they realized that things were getting too bad, they eventually stopped sending each other's diplomats home.

The trade wars between nations are another case where Rule 3 must obviously apply. If one country puts heavy embargoes on another country, it must anticipate that, eventually, the same will be done to it. If we allow other countries to heavily tax the goods that we export to them, but we don't tax their products coming into our country, we are simply rewarding taxing behavior. In the past, Japanese have done so to us because we tolerated it. Again, we get the behavior we tolerate. If we want that behavior to change, we must change.

But isn't it possible for these situations to lead to war? Regrettably, yes, but only if people forget Rule 3 and don't realize that they cannot be assertive and hostile at the same time. When parties are hostile, they are aggressive, and aggression is the first step toward a war.

I have never advocated violence in an attempt to deal with other people unless one is being attacked. The first condition of Rule 3 says that we must be firm with people and return negative behavior with negative behavior, but *without anger*, guilt, other-pity, fear of rejection, or fear of harm. When we use Rule 3 with violence, however, we are not following Rule 3; we are starting a war.

The Judicial System

The court system in this country is in trouble simply because we now allow plea bargaining. The criminals know it, they don't fear the consequences, they settle for less than their crimes would ordinarily get them, and they have less fear of breaking the law. As a result, our court systems and our jails are frequently revolving doors that do not create enough discomfort for the inmates to cause them to stop their behavior. If the behavior does not stop, we have to assume that the rewards of crime are satisfying enough to risk a few months or a few years in jail. If the discomfort does not exceed the pleasure, we can anticipate that the behavior that causes the pleasure will continue despite our protests or weak penalties.

Corporations that receive money from the government have been known to use those funds in illegal ways, especially simply to help their corporations with their pet projects. When these offenses are discovered, the corporation is simply told that it spent so many millions of dollars in a manner for which the money was not intended and, therefore, will have to return those funds. There you see it again—absolutely ridiculously tolerant behavior. No one is fined. No one is sent to prison. They are simply asked to return the money that was misspent. If that isn't inviting corruption, what is?

Religious Institutions

The theology of passivity has done great harm to the religious community. Instead of helping the faithful become strong and self-respecting persons, religion has often encouraged self-doubt, inferiority, and guilt. How could it be otherwise when we see how thoroughly they are trained to be sickeningly tolerant of all kinds of unacceptable behavior?

What the religious community has thought of as forgiveness is, in fact, tolerance. As a result, the most devout among them are often the most abused.

It is now time that religions appreciated the difference between forgiveness (the absence of anger) and tolerance (rewarding negative behavior). I insist that we want to forgive everything and forget nothing, as I wrote in Overcoming Frustration and Anger (1974). But why should we put up with just anything? To turn the other cheek endlessly is to train people to be manipulative, spoiled, and ruthless.

Organized religion also needs to be shown that its adherence to the notion of sin is destructive. Mental health professionals have earned very comfortable livings from millions of clients who feel depressed, guilty, inferior, or jealous as a result of religion's failure to separate behavior from person. Perceiving themselves as sinful or wicked persons rather than as imperfect persons has probably created more serious neuroses than any number of other conditions.

Effective RET can do wonders for these guilt-ridden masses, these millions of unhappy and passive people who seek salvation by denying themselves modest degrees of enlightened self-interest. The cognitive-behavioral techniques described in this chapter are sadly unknown or neglected by the religious community.

A Case Study

Tim, a 27-year-old single man, complained to me of his fiancée's possessiveness and jealousy. For months, he had been trying to reassure his friend that her suspicions were ungrounded, but these efforts never quieted her for long. With a mixture of anger and depression, he sought me out for help in coping with this unyielding pattern of hers.

In feeling him out about which option he preferred, I sensed that he did not want to tolerate such behavior any longer, but that he was not ready to end the relationship. This left him with Option 2: protest.

To make her uncomfortable enough to keep her nagging to herself, he decided not to answer any of her accusations, and if that did not work, he would leave her company instantly for the remainder of the day or evening.

She sensed the change in his strategy and rebelled immediately. Her insinuations became more vitriolic and persistent. Tim occasionally fell back into his old pattern of defending himself and made matters worse by saying nasty things in return. The strain on the relationship left him uneasy about its survival and depressed as well.

In taking an inventory of the conditions he had failed to meet to achieve Rule 3, I discovered that he was failing in his goal because he was using anger, guilt, other-pity, and fear of rejection in response to her complaints and tears. Unless these four conditions were eliminated, or at least reduced, he would be unable to persist in penalizing her negative actions.

It took three hours of therapy to teach him the basics of the psychology of anger, guilt, other-pity, and fear of rejection. Unless he had a modicum of control over these emotions, he had little chance of getting her cooperation, respect, or love by counteracting her insecurities.

Tim was a fast learner. Once he understood the ABCs of emotional disturbance and had practiced them diligently for several weeks, he was ready for Rule 3. With relative ease, he was able to stop defending himself. He changed the conversation to neutral subjects first, and when this failed to quiet her, he simply refused to converse further.

She began to change, but only sporadically. Several times, he left her for the night, even once before dinner. With a kiss on her cheek, he walked out of the apartment.

Finally, when she was pressuring him particularly vehemently, he gave her the ultimatum: Stop this behavior for good or he would leave for good.

He had played his hand very well. Nice to her in every way, and using Rule 1 throughout this ordeal (he rewarded most of her positive behavior), he was consistent in applying Rule 3, to the point where she had to believe him when he threatened to separate.

Because he had followed Rule 1 ("If people do something good to you, do something good to them"), it was easier for her to accept his firmness. Thus, when she let up, he became more loving, and led her to want to cook and clean for him as she never had before.

The young man was astonished at these changes. "I can't believe what's happened to us. It's incredible," he said several times when we held our session on the phone. The thought that, by being less giving, he was making her love him more was totally strange to him.

When I last heard from them they were getting along fine.

In retrospect, it is apparent that reason alone would not have achieved these results unless Tim was willing to tolerate her behavior without resentment. Because he wanted *her* to change, it was imperative that he change also, in particular, not to be so tolerant.

Teaching him to create a crisis, to risk the relationship at the cost of losing it, and to do this always with kindness and with the intention of helping her grow were the strategies I used to achieve these results. As the therapist, I was comfortable throughout the program and knew always what to expect and where we both were in moving toward our goal.

The judicious use of behavioral techniques along with rational procedures proved highly efficient over reliance only, or even primarily, on the latter. This case is only one of many examples of how psychotherapy has become highly efficient since the days when I was a graduate student and used psychoanalytic methods. RET in particular has been for me *the* indisputably most efficient system of psychotherapy available today.

REFERENCES

Bernard, M. (1988). *Teacher irrationality and teacher stress.* Unpublished manuscript.
Bernard, M., & Laws, W. (1988). *Childhood irrationality and mental health: Development of a scale.* Unpublished manuscript.
Dryden, W. (1987). *Counseling individuals; The rational-emotive approach.* London: Taylor & Francis.
Ellis, A., & Knaus, W. (1977). *Overcoming procrastination.* New York: Institute for Rational Living.
Hauck, P. A. (1974). *Overcoming frustration and anger.* Philadelphia: Westminster Press.
Hauck, P. A. (1975). *Overcoming worry and fear.* Philadelphia: Westminster Press.
Hauck, P. A. (1977). *Marriage is a loving business.* Philadelphia: Westminster Press.
Hauck, P. A. (1980). *Brief counseling with RET.* Philadelphia: Westminster Press.
Hauck, P. A. (1984). *The three faces of love.* Philadelphia: Westminster Press.
Madsen, C. H., & Madsen, C. K. (1980). *Teaching/discipline: A positive approach to educational development.* (3rd ed.). Boston: Allyn & Bacon.
Skinner, B. F. (1938). *The behavior of organisms: An experimental analysis.* New York: Appleton-Century-Crofts.
Skinner, B. F. (1953). *Science and human behavior.* New York: Macmillan.
York, P., & York, D. (1980). *Toughlove.* Doylestown, PA.

9

Depression and RET
Perspectives from Wounded Healers

Susan R. Walen and Mary W. Rader

> I want to register a complaint about the word *depression*. . . . Melancholia, as opposed to depression, would appear to be a far more apt and evocative word for the blacker forms of the disorder, but it was usurped by a term with such a bland tonality that it lacks any magisterial presence, used indifferently to describe an economic decline or a rut in the ground, a true wimp of a word for such a major illness. . . . for 75 years the word has slithered innocuously through the language like a slug, leaving little trace of its intrinsic malevolence and preventing, by its very insipidity, a general awareness of the horrible intensity of the disease when out of control. As one who had suffered from the malady *in extremis*, yet returned to tell the tale, I would lobby for a truly arresting designation. "Brainstorm," for instance, has unfortunately been preempted to describe, somewhat jocularly, intellectual inspiration. But something along these lines is needed. Told that someone's mood disorder had evolved into a storm—a veritable howling tempest in the brain—which is indeed what a clinical depression resembles like nothing else—even the uninformed layman might display sympathy rather than the standard reaction that depression evokes, something akin to "So what?" or "You'll pull out of it" or "We all have a bad day."
>
> Styron, 1989

Overview

The main point of this chapter is to share, as fellow professionals and "wounded healers" (Rippere & Williams, 1985), what we have experienced with our own depressive illnesses and, more important, what we have learned from them. Certainly, as therapists, we had seen depressed pa-

---

Susan R. Walen • Department of Psychology, Towson State University, and Baltimore Center for Cognitive Therapy, 6303 Greenspring Avenue, Baltimore, Maryland 21209.   Mary W. Rader • The Kennedy Family Center, 1235 East Monument Street, Baltimore, Maryland 21202.

tients and read a great deal about depression, but until we experienced depression firsthand, we felt we had never received as rich an introduction to the pain of this illness nor appreciated the fortitude of the patient who has it.

Our outline for this chapter is as follows: We begin with some self-disclosure—how it feels to write this chapter and "go public" with our story, the phenomenology of the depression, and our treatment experiences. Then we share some of our learning about depressive illness and biological psychiatry and discuss some conceptual issues about the interplay between biology, psychology, and the environment. Finally, what we have been through has had some important implications for our work as cognitive therapists, in diagnosis and treatment. We share some of these new appreciations in the form of "clinical tips" for working with patients who suffer depressive illness.

THE SELF-DISCLOSURE PART

Writing This Chapter

We are both a little nervous about presenting this material. First, this chapter represents a "shame-attacking assignment" for us (Ellis, 1973). Although we each know other cognitive therapists who suffer depression, they do not openly or publicly talk about it. They suffer in silence and do not "come out of the closet," largely because of shame, the same shame we continue to experience occasionally despite all our attempts at "rational thinking." Typically, they share our belief that, somehow, if we were just sufficiently stoic, cooperative as psychotherapy patients, or gifted enough as therapists, then we would have been able to decimate this illness by our enlightened thinking. The shame is thus based on the irrational but compelling perfectionist belief that we should be strong enough to take care of the problem ourselves.

There is also the very real stigma associated with "mental illness," even—perhaps especially—among mental health professionals. After all, we all grew up in the same phrenophobic society and shared the cultural stereotypes about patients and "shrinks." There seems to be evidence of a double prejudice when a healer suffers an illness. In an anonymously published account of his depression, one British psychiatrist described his plight as follows: "God, how I longed then that my depression be magically changed into a decent, straightforward physical ailment! The psychiatric hospital is intolerant of weakness in its staff. Compassion is for patients; for 'them' not 'us'" (Rippere & Williams, 1985, p. 15). Dr. Norman Endler is a noted Canadian clinical psychologist who wrote a small book describing his bouts of depression (*Holiday of Darkness*, 1982). He was en-

BEARSPAW
PLUMBING & HEATING
COCHRANE, AB.
932-3740

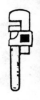

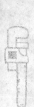

couraged by his colleagues to leave town for treatment and hospitalization and was discouraged by others from preparing his manuscript: "After I had recuperated and had thought of writing this book on the chance that it might help others who are depressed, I mentioned the possibility to a psychiatrist (not the one I was seeing). He said 'Norm, don't do it. You'll ruin your career. Wanting to write this book shows poor judgment on your part'" (p. 20). Another psychologist was warned by her sister (also a psychologist) not to let other clinicians know of her affective illness: "They'll *never* refer patients to you again," she was told. The stigma continues.

Another reason why preparing this chapter was difficult is that, at some point, we need to put the depression behind us as part of the recovery.

> *Sue:* When I began to feel better, I wanted others to learn from my experience. But at the same time, I didn't want men I was just starting to date to know about it. So I had a very mixed reaction, wanting to talk about it a lot and wanting to hide it a lot. In either case, though, the depression was the most important, most salient thing about me.

When first understood and treated, the depression seemed very central to our identities. With treatment, the symptoms began to remit, and we began to learn to live with and accept depressive illness as a *chronic recurrent condition*. Now we find that it is a less important part about us, something normative, a fact of reality, and not something we feel compelled to talk about as frequently. So it seemed important to us that we write about our experience while it's still fairly fresh, because at some point we will want to put it away and not make a career out of being depressed people, even though we may never be "cured."

Thinking about this chapter also generated some fear.

> *Mary:* Sue wrote me a note of invitation to discuss our experiences, and after the first time we talked, I was having some very "heavy" kinds of feelings. I realized it was because, for the previous year, I had really functioned well—had come to experience myself as a healthy person. And all of a sudden, we were bringing back all of this stuff, and it was very difficult and a little bit scary because I wondered if delving back into it was going to put me into a slide again.

One of the things that we have discovered during our recoveries is that we are again able to do difficult tasks, handle serious losses, cope with life crises, and feel sadness and grief—yet *not* become depressed. We have been learning that there is a very real and extremely important difference between these moods and depressive illness, a point on which we will elaborate later.

Another reason why it is hard to write about what we have been through is that, in some ways, we cannot truly reexperience it. Perhaps it is like childbirth: women remember the experience intellectually, but affectively or somatically, they dissociate from it. We remember the experience of depression, but without the full affective loading, which may be a result of a natural, protective, psychological repression process. Alternatively, our inability to fully re-create the experience of depression may be because memory is often state-dependent. The affective pain may not be encoded for memory retrieval in a nondepressed state. Nonetheless, we have tried to re-create from our diaries and our discussions the phenomenology of the illness, for *it is the internal experience of the patient that is crucial in understanding affective illness.*

The Phenomenology of Our Depressions

When we got together to discuss our experiences with depression, we discovered that each of us had kept a journal and thus had records of our illness. We have decided to share some of these diary entries to give a portrait of our internal states, both cognitively and physiologically. Throughout the chapter, when we are speaking "in our own voice" or from our personal experience, we will first identify the speaker.

THINKING: RUMINATIVE THOUGHTS

Sue's journal: My thoughts are very obsessional about TJ today. Going over and over the same stuff . . . different angles, but same stuff. *Comment:* I drove people around me to distraction because I wanted to talk about the same topics over and over again and I couldn't put them away. At one point, my teenaged son tearfully told me I was frightening him because I kept asking him the same questions repeatedly (e.g., "Do you think I made a mistake? Acted too hastily?"). I immediately tried to stifle my verbalizations, but the ruminative thinking went on unchecked and uncheckable.

SUICIDALITY

Sue's journal: I want to die, and today, I got to the point of laying out plans. . . . Lots of thoughts about death today. Pictures of myself hanging in the basement . . . with details like whether I will be nude or not, whether I should spread plastic out under me in case I crap, etc. Wondering how others have died . . . . Then, what happened was that I started thinking about suicide immediately. Moved the date up . . . next fall, if A. goes to live at his father's house, there will be no need for me to stay alive any longer and I can close it all up. I'm no longer an effective teacher. Not needed as a mother. Belong to no one. My folks will last only a little while longer, and then, they won't be there for me. There's no one I can depend on for care and love. So why live? The thinking is back again. I can't think of any reason to stay alive! *Comment:* There were days when most of my mental activity consisted of trying not to kill myself, because the imagery of suicide came up so clearly and automatically. Although most of the time I did not really want to kill myself, I could not help seeing my death, and it took a great deal of energy to keep distracting myself from this unwanted and unbidden set of images and thoughts.

Mary's journal: Suicidal feelings and plans resumed. On hold this evening, but time, method, *et cetera* decided, and that feels good. I'm tired of feeling unwanted, incompetent, undesirable. Sometimes, I can tell myself there are worthwhile things I can do and should do, but then, it always turns out I do more harm than good. I'm not interested in being a liability to the world. It will be good to be gone. [Other journal entries were just as despairing:] Depression, the desire to withdraw, longing to cease to exist, become oblivious is still very strong. I feel like eliminating all traces of myself from the world. My perception is that I am cursed, a curse, and have been from birth. I should not be trying to help others, should avoid contact with others as much as possible to keep from hurting them. This is my reality. A sense of competence is only wishful thinking, a fantasy born out of my desire to be worth something. It's better to simply accept that I'm nothing; that's the way it is. *Comment:* The last sentence was my feeble attempt to do elegant RET and accept the worst!

Aloneness

Sue's journal: I have a sense of being a speck in the void. . . . There is a huge gulf between me and all others. . . . My reality is that I live alone—and I always will. . . . I can't feel connected. *Comment:* Aloneness was particularly striking and was probably the most painful part of the depression for me. There was a terrifying sense of being totally alone in the universe and existentially isolated from all of humanity. I was unconnected with my children, my parents, friends, and even from my psychiatrist. No one was in the same plane of existence as I. I was totally in a vacuum and left floating in the universe, horribly alone.

Mary's journal: . . . experienced deep feeling that there is no place for me—that the world is "closed up" and I'm left out in the cold, peering in but never a part of what's going on.

Mood

Sue's journal: This doesn't feel quite the same as the trapped despair I felt when I was unhappily married, although I sure was sad then. Nor like the intense sadness and longing when R. and I parted, although I certainly sobbed plenty then. This feels *sick! Comment:* Obviously, the mood was very sad, but the sadness had a unique feel to it. It had a depth that was difficult to describe ("I have a sad, sad core") and was often mixed with a welter of other emotional states ("Very very sad again. Distracted, and guilty, and anxious"; "I'm getting scared"). More pointedly, I was unable to shift my mood, no matter what techniques I used, for more than a few moments at a time ("My conversation is filled with depressing talk, and it's like I can't stop it"; "I cannot sustain my mood with CT!").

CRYING

Sue's journal: Wept for about an hour today. I can talk aloud to myself about it and dry up my tears, but within a minute, they're back again. *Comment:* The crying I did was unlike crying spells I'd ever had. I had always cried quietly and privately. Now, when I cried, I was racked with sobs. I would frequently cry through the course of a day. Often, at midday, I would have an unexplained crying spell, not tied to any environmental happening. At those times, I would weep for hours. My emotional lability was astonishing to me.

Mary: I cried a lot at times, but often I was unable to cry. I felt a huge knot in my stomach and chest, and pressure in my throat, but tears would not come. It felt as if I had a heavy weight bearing down on me.

MASKING

Sue: Except for a few days when I was at the nadir, I could "put the symptoms away." I could say to myself, "I'm now going to stop crying, and I'm going to make dinner." I could do that, but as soon as I slowed down and stopped distracting myself, the crying was back.

PAIN

Sue: I had had patients say that the pain of depression is worse than any physical pain they'd experienced, and now I can truly understand what they meant. Living through that depressed period, feeling very ill before medication began to have an effect, was perhaps the most painful time of my life. The suffering seemed worse than any prior suffering. It is difficult to express how intense an experience it was.

The Pulitzer prize-winning author, William Styron (1989), who also suffered a bout of depressive illness, has spoken and written eloquently on the experience; yet despite his amazing descriptive powers, he states that "depression's exquisite torment can never really be communicated" (p. 214) and "my days were pervaded by a gray drizzle of unrelenting horror. This horror is virtually indescribable, since it bears no relation to normal experience" (p. 214).

Physiological Aspects of Depressive Illness

Although we both experienced many of the vegetative signs of depressive illness (e.g., appetitive change in the need for sleep, sex, and food; fluctuations in energy; and diurnal variation in mood), Sue experienced far more of the physiological symptoms than Mary. These and other indicators suggest to us that we probably have different "forms" of the illness of depression.

Sue: What was most shocking was the experience of the physiology of the depression. At one point, I was so sick that I was unable to do anything except keep nursing notes on myself. About every 10–15 minutes, I wrote in my journal about what I was experiencing and later organized these entries into symptom clusters.

Eating

Sue's journal: Literally couldn't eat a bite of dinner or dessert. . . . Can't eat anything but bagels; food looks nauseating to me! . . . Tried to eat, but later had terrible stomach distress and explosive bowel movement. . . . Stomach sour. . . . Lots of belching/farting. . . . My stomach is making so much noise! *Comment:* I had never in my life had no appetite or been unable to eat, yet I could not eat anything or even think about eating. I experienced a mild yet chronic nausea accompanied by a feeling of bloatedness. Yet, like a Jewish mother, I urged myself to have some chicken broth, and immediately, I was very sorry. I finally understood that my digestive system had just shut down.

Mary: I had seldom had much appetite, and during the depression, I lost what little I had. The thought of food was nauseating, and I could hardly choke down even a bite or two. It felt as if my throat had literally closed up. I had about a 15% weight loss, and my worried husband teased me gently that he didn't like my looking like a 14-year-old boy!

Sleeping

Mary's journal: Half-images, half-dreams the last three nights: being attacked, flesh torn from my bones by a huge bird with monstrous talons and beak. . . . being engulfed by flames, each limb flaming separately. . . . in a raging torrent of water, sinking into a whirlpool. *Comment:* My dreams were horrifying and vivid. A particularly disquieting dream of my death woke me violently ("A piece [me] torn out of the middle of a photograph, thrown into a toilet full of feces and flushed away"). Early wakening—often at 2 or 3 A.M.— was also a problem. I would be suddenly wide awake, my thoughts repetitive and totally negative.

Sue's journal: Woke before the children's alarm. Lots of dreams about depression. . . . Vivid dreams last night; twice, about being robbed. . . . Didn't sleep last night till after 4:30 A.M.. . . . For two nights running, I've had lousy sleep. Night before last, I went to sleep at 10 and was awake at 10:45! Yesterday, I was so groggy I could barely work or drive. *Comment:* The quantity and quality of my sleep was quite unusual for me. I wakened many times in the course of a night and had early-morning wakening. I always awoke with a startle response ("Eyes snap open again with a squirt of adrenalin").

Feeling Ill

Sue's journal: I feel shaky and racing inside. I am comforted only when I carry the doll A. brought me clutched to my chest. . . . like a mad woman. . . . just want to stay in bed; I feel so sick. . . . my muscles feel achey. . . . Draggy. . . . more and more as the evening wore on. *Comment:* I was certain that, if I held out my hands, they would tremble and shake, but to my surprise, they remained quite steady; the sensation was an internal one and was very distracting to me. My blood pressure went up, apparently a common physiological response in depression. I found I could feel these blood pressure changes, experiencing them as "swells." My rod (night) vision seemed to deteriorate. I was feeling very tense and was aware that my teeth were continuously clenched. I had a sense of frenzy, crankiness, and illness.

TEMPERATURE REGULATION

Sue: My internal thermometer seemed to be out of whack. I was alternately shaking with chills or feeling "hot." I kept taking my temperature, feeling so sick at one point that I was sure that what I had was a very rare flu with a high fever, but my temperature always registered in the normal range. The cold was felt very keenly in my extremities, especially in my hands and feet.

THINKING

Sue's journal: Concentration only fair. . . . undercurrent of thinking is constant ("I've made a bad mistake in love"; "I'll never experience love"; "I'll never feel better"; etc.). . . . Feeling spacey. . . . Having trouble concentrating. My thoughts drift off into reveries, fantasies, longings, etc. . . . My head feels as if it's stuffed with toilet paper. . . . Woolly headed and shaky. . . . Somewhat hard to read and concentrate. *Comment:* I had a mild, chronic headache, or sense of pressure, and a "buzzing" sensation in my head. My thinking felt fuzzy. I experienced a dullness of my intellect. My memory, especially in the retrieval system, was significantly impaired.

Mary: I had particular difficulty looking up telephone numbers. I couldn't remember them for the short time it took to glance from the directory to the telephone dial. Concentration was also a problem, especially when I tried to *back* out of a parking place. I had to force myself to look carefully enough to see if the road was clear, and often, I couldn't remember from one side to the other whether it was or not! I compensated by parking only in spaces where I could pull out frontward.

The Treatment Experience

Therapists' Responses to Depression

Many therapists seem to be threatened by the patient's experience of depression or the pain of that experience.

Mary: For example, at one point I went to a behavior therapist who seemed to be uncomfortable discussing any feelings at all. The therapist doggedly focused on trying to get me to eat more, convinced that if my weight increased, the depression would be ameliorated. As it turned out, gaining 10 pounds did not lift my mood and, in fact, only provided increased ammunition to turn back on myself: "You don't deserve to eat. What makes you think you have a right to food? You should be ashamed." The therapist (rightly) told me how dysfunctional my thinking was. Because I was already convinced that I was defective and a bad person and had brought all this misery on myself, I was willing to accept that proposition and to berate myself even more.

The most helpful stance for both of us was for the therapist to "be there" and to provide a sense of fully understanding our experience. A few empathic words went a long way.

> *Sue:* The most comforting thing my psychiatrist did was to murmur repeatedly, "Listen . . . I know . . ."

We were often so overwhelmed by the illness, so numbed with fatigue, that the simple experience of having someone sit with us and communicate understanding was most valuable and cannot be underestimated.

The following quotation is from Ann MacKensie (1985), a general practitioner in England, who also suffered depressive illness. She described her anxious thoughts before her first psychiatric consultation:

> I had anticipated a dismayed five minutes now and then, during which I was advised to "keep on taking the tablets." What I got was friendship, concern, and support. Perhaps I would have got better anyway with proper therapeutic doses of antidepressants, but it was so much easier with support. As soon as I knew that I had someone to go to if problems overwhelmed me, the problems got less. For months I got through each day to a litany of "never mind, it'll be all right on Friday."

MacKensie's experience parallels our own: *Supportive* psychotherapy is what is needed, in addition to medication. This combined treatment has been shown to be more effective in facilitating recovery and preventing relapse than medication alone (e.g., Belsher & Costello, 1988).

Medication and Its Side Effects

Finding the right medication is often a long, dismaying course of trial and error, exacerbated by the reluctance of many physicians to prescribe medication. Joyce and Paykel (1989) noted that, when medication is prescribed, it is often at too low a dosage for too short a time, or the patient is kept for too long a time on a regimen that has no benefit. Goethe, Szarek, and Cook (1988) also noted a significant difference in recovery between patients who were treated "vigorously" and those whose physicians made only tentative or limited use of medications. A National Institute of Mental Health (NIMH) study found that, in 1982, only 1 in 3 depressed persons received antidepressants and only 1 in 10 received adequate doses (Regier, Hirschfeld, Goodwin, Burke, Lazar, & Judd, 1988).

Perhaps nowhere in treatment is the need for a "collaborative empiricism" (Dryden & Golden, 1986, p. 74) between patient and therapist—a hallmark in RET and cognitive-behavioral therapy (CBT)—more pressing. Some physicians we encountered were clearly uncomfortable receiving input from the "ill" member of the team.

> *Mary:* Some therapists wanted to tell me what I needed without soliciting information from me. Questions, suggestions, or requests from me were viewed as more proof that I was noncompliant or controlling. The caregivers who not only listened but sought feedback from me were the most helpful, partly because my trying to be an accurate observer of the illness enabled me to come out of my "dark hole" to some degree.

It is important to take the patient's medication experiences seriously. In order to find the drug or the drug combination that will be most effective, it is essential to listen carefully to the patient. Often, when there is depressive illness in family members, the relative's experience on medication may provide useful hints for the physician.

> *Mary:* Fortunately, I had a physician who was gracious enough to listen to me when I pointed out that imipramine had worked with a close family member who had also had problems with depression. He was receptive when I said, "I think it might work for me. Can we try it?"

Not only is the patient battling the illness, the frustration of waiting for delayed medication effects to appear, and the worry that there will not be a positive response to the drug, but in addition, the drugs have side effects, many of which are quite debilitating and frightening to the already traumatized patient. We found that physicians were sometimes cavalier about our discomfort, rather glibly assuring us that we should get used to the side effects and work at not distressing ourselves about them. Our hunch is that if physicians personally experienced the discomforts, especially when in a debilitated state of mind, they might be more sympathetic in discussing side effects. Perhaps denying the patient's discomfort eases the discomfort in themselves. The battle against low frustration tolerance (LFT)—in a patient who feels so ill—had better be done with sensitivity and caring.

> *Mary:* I have been on an array of medications, with various side effects. Amitriptyline (Elavil) did not alleviate my depressive symptoms and wiped out what little bit of sex drive I had left and made the achievement of orgasm almost impossible. The bloating it caused—I looked as if I was five months pregnant—increased my self-loathing. Dry mouth, a very common side effect of the tricyclics, doesn't sound so terrible until it goes on for six months or

more. Some medications, such as amoxapine (Asendin), caused ataxia. I had trouble walking down stairs, and if I leaned over to throw something in the wastebasket, I nearly fell in myself. At one point on imipramine, my balance was so poor that, when I stumbled on a sloping walkway, I was unable to recover, fell flat on my face, and broke my nose. While I was on Trilafon, the akathisia made it almost impossible for me to sit through a therapy session with one of my clients. I felt as if I was going to crawl out of my skin, that I could not possibly sit still, and that I had to get up and move around or I would explode.

Sue: I was first put on a tricyclic (nortriptyline) and had—luckily, I now think—an almost immediate reaction. Within a week I had itching, stinging pustules, like wet hives, all over my body. (*Journal entry:* I think I'm having an allergic reaction. I've got hives, crusty skin, deepened and reddened wrinkles around my neck, itching, stinging, very dry and painful tongue, and constipation.) I was a mess, and my psychiatrist consulted with me by phone and told me to stop the pills immediately. Shortly after, I began to feel extremely good. Within a few days, I was feeling great! I felt myself to be terrific in the classroom and dynamite in my consulting room. (*From my journal:* I did not sleep *at all* last night. It's now 12:35 the next night and I'm still not feeling sleepy. Perhaps I'll never sleep again. My energy level is up today, thinking is clearer, not obsessional much at all. My classes went very well and I was able to be articulate and focused throughout, and at 11 P.M., when I presented that complex case to the consultant, he said it was a superb introduction. I also ate heartily today. Very thirsty, however. And a certain ringing in my ears. Skin is about 85% recovered. Getting excited about upcoming trip. Want to exercise tomorrow, but there clearly won't be time!) Within the week, I bounded in to see my psychiatrist, passing everyone in the corridors and feeling full of energy and pep. I was convinced that the depression had mysteriously lifted and I was experiencing relief. The psychiatrist, however, diagnosed this state as a hypomanic reaction to the sudden withdrawal of the tricyclic, and sure enough, within two days, I was deeply depressed again.

We discussed various other drug options—another tricyclic, lithium, lithium plus other medications, and so on—and I received the "informed-consent" talk about each. The potentials for harm sounded so serious and the side effects so malicious, that I decided that I could probably muddle along the way I was.

My mental image of the "shape" of my course of illness was like that of a condom with a reservoir at the tip. I felt I had slid down rather precipitously to the bottom but, once there, had dipped into and out of the well of the reservoir in about a week's time. Then, while I was still depressed, I felt that I was beginning to climb up the other side of the "condom," but I overestimated the degree of my recovery. (*From my journal:* I'm about 80% functional now, and that's not so terrible. I can make it like this. If this is where I'm stuck, I can manage this. I'll just use all my good cognitive therapy tools and my stoicism, and I'll manage this way.) It was another cognitive therapist whom I saw in consultation who suggested that it was not necessary to struggle so hard and that it seemed clear that I did not have a solid affective footing under me. If I started to cry, I would often be unable to stop for many hours, despite distractions, changes in the environment, and attempts at self-control. This cognitive therapist suggested that I discuss the use of a mono-amine oxidase inhibitor (MAOI) with my psychiatrist.

Other entries from Sue's journal and comments: "I have asked Dr. K. to try me on Parnate and we've been increasing the dose to the usual clinical level, 30 mg." On Day 13 of this dose, I woke up feeling different. ("I think I've had my first good day in a while. My Beck Depression Inventory (BDI) would be <10. I was active, happy, interested in people, etc.") By the fourth day on that dose, I knew what it was. I was no longer feeling sick. I was feeling good. ("Fourth day of a damned good recovery. I'm not labile any more! Appetite back [too bad], sex drive back [just had first orgasm in months], concentration better, obsessions and suicidal thinking virtually gone. Still sleepless and have lower energy and that pressure in my head and chest area . . . but these may be Parnate side effects, and they're not too terrible at all.") I was so grateful for this medication. I had that floor back under me. I would cry at things that struck me as sad, and particularly at things that reminded me of the recent past, but I could stop crying in a "normal" amount of time.

One of the realizations I had, after the Parnate began to work, was that I had probably been depressed (although less seriously) for years, without recognizing it. A marker for me was my end-of-year reports. For the previous four years, when I had taken time to gather my papers together for the tax accountant, I would spend some time writing about what I had done that year, about my children's activities, my professional life, and so on. And I always closed with the same essential idea: Although the year had been a pretty good one, I really didn't care if I died the next day. These "annual reports" reflected a joyless living of my life that I now believe was not "characterological," but a prolonged mild depression. During the year of this major depression, the medication effect had begun by Christmastime, and when I sat down in January to write my year's report I realized that my usual ending paragraph was no longer true. I was vigorously looking forward to the next year, very curious about what it might bring for me, excited to be around, and very happy to be venturing forth into my life. (*Journal entry:* Now I normally close with a report that I don't care if I die or not. Just makes me wonder how long I've been depressed without using that label as a meaningful diagnostic word [meaning requiring treatment of some sort]. Right now—today—I have no interest in dying. In fact, I want to hang around to see if I can meet my last life goal: to live with, perhaps even marry, a man I truly love. I have a good feeling about next year!)

Mary: I was walking down the hall at the community college where I was teaching, after I had been on imipramine for about four weeks, when I sud-denly realized that I was walking briskly and with my head held up. I realized that I hadn't walked that way for a very long time. I knew that something was different, and that I was at the beginning of the physiological remission. Other symptoms took longer: the horrible sinking feeling on awakening in the morning, lack of interest in anything, inability to think of something to say in a conversation, memory, concentration—all normalized at different times, slowly over about a year and a half. After I had felt better physically for about three months, I asked to discontinue imipramine because of the ataxia.

Although I had regained physical energy, I now recognize that other symptoms may have remitted more quickly if I'd continued on the medication. I was trying to be strong and stoic. I thought I had to conquer this thing myself, with as little help as possible.

The Experience of Hospitalization

Mary: I was hospitalized four times during a two-year period in which I was not yet effectively medicated. During one of the most awful periods, I was placed in seclusion. I was assured that when the new shift came on duty and got things settled, I would be taken out of seclusion because someone could be with me on the ward. But not enough people arrived on that shift, so they left me to sit on the floor in the seclusion room to do nothing except to try to keep myself together. For the next five hours, I couldn't move because I was afraid I would beat my head against the concrete walls. I was afraid that if I asked for help to keep myself safe, they would put me into restraints, and the thought of that seemed more than I could bear.

The utterly despairing, hopeless, helpless outlook of depression and the fear of self-harm may make hospitalization tolerable. Admitting that one cannot care for oneself and turning a major part of that responsibility over to hospital staff can be deeply humiliating, however. Concerned, nonpunitive, understanding caregivers make the experience more humane despite the unavoidable discomforts involved.

Mary: I can still remember waking up in the hospital the first morning and realizing I couldn't get out. I recall standing at the window with my head against the panes, thinking that I was in prison and I was being punished. It wasn't fair: I hadn't done anything. The depersonalization and the dehumanization of the experience were truly awful, often serving to deepen my despair. Standing in line for every meal, standing in line for medication, standing in line to be herded into a van to go on an activity took away whatever sense of competence or self-esteem that might have been left. Although I had entered voluntarily, I was very anxious that I would never get out and was unable to reassure myself. I felt utterly helpless to influence the system in any way. The staff had all the power. The patients were totally dependent on the staff's altruism.

Few people would want to be placed in a mental hospital. The patient who is very ill, however, may feel safer in the hospital than at home and may choose to enter voluntarily. Patients may find the hospital a place in which they can let down their defenses and allow themselves to be "sick." They learn how to ask for the help that they need, and most of the time, they get it, although mental hospitals, like general hospitals, are often understaffed and overpopulated.

Depressive Illness:
The Uniformity Myth

We're going to take a bit of a side trip here and become more technical. We will discuss terminology and some of what we've learned about the various manifestations of depression from reading the psychiatric literature.

The word *depression* is generally used in a loose fashion, to describe a downward turn in mood (*a symptom*), a mood accompanied by certain cognitive and behavioral changes (*clinical signs*), and, more recently, biologically based but clinically variant forms of major affective disorders (*a syndromal illness*). We will consider each of these usages in turn, recognizing, however, that the separation of sign, symptom, syndrome, and illness is somewhat arbitrary and artificial, as these terms obviously overlap.

Depression by Any Other Name . . .

Depression: A Mood State

Sadness, a normal reaction to negative life events, is a mood state that usually remits without undue laboring. Therapeutically, what may be helpful (if any help is needed at all) is kindness, empathy, interpersonal support, normalization and explanation, and a friendly environment in which one has permission to experience and express this normal human emotion.

Grieving, a more prolonged and intense mood typically precipitated by a major loss, is assisted by a more extended period of support, encouragement, and tenderness. In grief, the focus of the patient is on the loss rather than on the self and self-blame. Freud described it well in 1917: "Now the melancholic displays something else which is lacking in grief—an extraordinary fall in his self-esteem, an impoverishment of his ego on a grand scale. In grief the world becomes poor and empty; in melancholia it is the ego itself" (Jones, 1950).

The mood of sadness, even when prolonged, is neither a necessary nor a sufficient clue to reach the diagnosis of depressive illness. Although 89% of depressed patients complain of sadness (Schuyler, 1984), the remainder do not, perhaps because they do not recognize it, do not feel it, or are more aware of irritability than sadness. One of our consultants pointed out that any symptom gets its meaning from the company it keeps: a cough can mean a cold, heart failure, pneumonia, cancer, nervousness, or an attempt to get someone's attention. A sad mood can be a part of a clinical depression, uremia, hypothyroidism, grief, disappointment, the blues, and even "anger turned inward." Mood, therefore, is merely one clue in diagnosis.

Depression: A Syndrome

More than a blue mood, the syndrome* of depression is a cluster of symptoms that may include an overreaction to a negative activating event, as well as other cognitive, emotive, behavioral, and physical symptoms. Accompanying the dysphoria are appetite, sleep, and sexual cycle changes; energy level changes; and persistent attitudes of helplessness and hopelessness. Beck (1976) described one cognitive cluster as having three "faces": a negative view of the self, a negative view of the world, and a negative view of the future. Cognitively, the distortions may be in the realm of perception (Beck, 1976), process (Burns, 1980), or expectations and evaluations (Ellis & Whiteley, 1979). The full depressive syndrome is typically more debilitating or pernicious than mere sadness and usually results in a referral for psychotherapy of some sort.

A variety of active and directive psychotherapies have been shown to be effective in the treatment of the depressive syndrome (Rush, 1982), but as cognitive symptoms are a central element in the syndrome, it is no surprise that cognitive therapies, especially, have been shown to be a treatment of choice. In those instances in which the individual still maintains the *ability* to exert some control over his or her affective state and continues to have rational thought processes despite some irrational thinking, RET and CBT are useful.

Depression: An Illness

Actually, this heading would more accurately be "Depressions: A Spectrum of Illnesses." There is lack of clarity about the exact nature of the illness of depression, as witness the plethora of descriptive terms for various symptom constellations. Consider this (partial) list: endogenous, exogenous, reactive, neurotic, melancholic, unipolar, bipolar (depressed), dysthymia, bipolar II, bipolar III, pseudounipolar, major depression, psychotic depression, delusional depression, retarded depression, agitated depression, double depression, atypical (nonendogenous), primary, and secondary depression. To complicate matters, many of these terms have different meanings to different clinicians. In addition, the same patient may present different symptom clusters across different episodes of the illness (Gold, Goodwin, & Chrousos, 1988).

The more research we did in the biological psychiatry sections of the library, the more it seemed that there were many mechanisms that could

*We use the word *syndrome* merely to describe the cluster of signs and symptoms, not in the context of a disease model, in which one seeks to explain syndromes in terms of pathologies and, ultimately, etiologies.

trigger similar affective, cognitive, and behavioral end products. Patients with what may turn out to be different forms of the illness or different illnesses may exhibit common symptoms (Gold et al., 1988; Norman, Miller, & Dow, 1988). In individuals with the "same" disorder, different etiologies may be operating, so that different treatments may be required for the same phenotypic expression of a disorder (Mash, 1989). Even the common distinction between "endogenous" and "exogenous" depression has not been shown to be reliable and is far too dichotomous to be useful (Free & Oei, 1989).

Depressive illnesses are recurrent. The majority (estimates range up to 80%–100%) of patients with major depression will have at least one other episode (Goodwin, 1988). The duration of each episode of depression tends to be relatively consistent for the individual, and the typical cycle length, averaged over a large population, is approximately one year (Goodwin, 1988). There are some patients who have been diagnosed with a "personality disorder" because their depressions are so prolonged; they may describe themselves as "always being depressed" or "depressed for as long as I can remember." Among this group are those studied by Akiskal (1985), who were, in fact, shown to be drug-responsive.

A Brief Review of Some Varieties of the Illness

Strong evidence is accumulating for a genetic predisposition to psychiatric disorders, and to affective disorders in particular (Blehar, Weissman, Gershon, & Hirschfeld, 1988; DePaulo, 1989; Johnstone, 1988). We are close to being able to identify genetic markers, and in an affected family, over 30% of a proband's siblings and offspring may have some type of affective disorder (DePaulo, 1989). Although symptomatic affective disorders resembling genetically transmitted depressions may occur after stroke, the administration of certain chemicals, and so on, we will discuss only the heritable illnesses.

Bipolarity and Unipolarity

The patient with *recurrent unipolar depression* experiences bouts of depressions interspersed with periods of euthymia, in the absence of mania. Older texts taught that unipolar depression was the most prevalent form of the illness. Current diagnostic research, however, indicates that the *bipolar spectrum* of disorders, many of which are "soft" or more subtle in form, may constitute the largest population by far. *Bipolar I* disorders, often florid, are those formerly referred to as *manic-depressive*. The more recently described *bipolar II* syndrome is characterized by major depressions, interspersed with mild depression and brief, mild hypomanic periods. In the third edition of the American Psychiatric Association's *Diagnostic and Statis-*

tical Manual (DSM-III; APA, 1980), the soft bipolar spectrum was labeled the "atypical bipolar" condition. Akiskal and Mallya (1987) suggested that the descriptor *atypical* is statistically incorrect. According to DePaulo (1989), the prevalence statistics for the major subtypes of depression are atypical depression (76%), bipolar I (17%), and unipolar (7%).

Bipolar II illness is often unrecognized and, consequently, therapeutically mismanaged. This condition is typically of mild to moderate severity and rarely leads to hospitalization, and the psychopathologic manifestations appear to be more in the "personality" sphere than in classic symptoms of mood disorder. The patient is often self-described as "moody," and his or her problems are usually assumed to be caused by problems in living (DePaulo, 1989). Many of these patients function so well that they may not be considered ill, and the bipolar nature of the illness may thus go unrecognized.

Hypomania, which is critical in identifying the bipolar II patient, is often overlooked by the clinician as well as the patient because it may be quite adaptive. The patient feels more functional than usual, more productive, more clearheaded, and more energetic. He or she can stay up later than usual, solve more problems, accomplish more tasks, and not feel tired the next day. People around her or him may shake their heads and say, "How do you get so much accomplished in a day?" but they most likely will not identify the state as pathological.

The cycle length may vary greatly, from rapid cycling to extended mood periods. These patients may report internal "racing" sensations and typically have high BDI scores during the acute phase of the depression, plunging rapidly into this depressed phase. This affective lability, in which they seem to become extraordinarily and disproportionaly depressed in response to an environmental event, has led some clinicians to describe these patients as showing *borderline features.*

Recent studies point to the reactivity of the bipolar II patient to many different stimuli:

1. Hormonal (e.g., pregnancy, parturition, PMS).
2. Seasons of the year (see SADS, below).
3. Exercise or engrossing "projects" (which may lead to obsessive involvements).
4. Drugs and alcohol (which may lead to secondary substance-abuse problems).
5. Eating, sleeping, and sex (which may be associated with abuses as well).

From such a list, it would be easy to imagine how this reactive individual would make many false attributions and come to many incorrect conclusions, would develop many faulty habits, would become very self-doubting, and would reinforce the clinical impression of an Axis II or personality diagnosis. Small wonder that he or she would develop into what Bowlby (1977) described as either a "compulsively self-reliant" or "anxiously attached" person.

Bipolar II patients also seem to be hypersensitive to abandonment, perhaps because they feel themselves to be biologically more vulnerable and more emotional, and the idea of being alone may be more frightening. Many have had separation anxiety or phobic or panic symptoms, which may have set the stage for their vulnerability. Thus, they may have a hard time in interpersonal relationships, being particularly reluctant to give up relationships that are not very functional. In this example, we may be observing the interaction between the biology, the environment, and the cognitive schemata of dependence laid down in early life.

Bipolar II patients are more likely to have relatives exhibiting bipolar II disorder than bipolar I disorder, and thus, the illness seems to breed true. The diagnosis of bipolar II is stable over time and does not progress to bipolar I disorder. Similarly, the illness has no greater kinship with non-bipolar disorders than it does with bipolar I disorders.

Seasonal Affective Disorder Syndrome

Since the time of Hippocrates, it has been proposed that there is a relationship between depression and the seasons. Statistically, there is a higher incidence of endogenous depression in the spring, but some patients have regularly occurring winter depressions. Rosenthal and Wehr (1987) suggested that the syndrome was first reported by Esquirol in 1845 and was later described by Kraepelin in 1928. Rosenthal and his colleagues at NIMH (Rosenthal, Sack, Gillin, Lewy, Goodwin, Davenport, Mueller, Newsome, & Wehr, 1984) suggested the following diagnostic criteria for seasonal affective disorder syndrome, or SADS:

- A history of major affective disorder (Research Diagnostic Criteria).
- The development of depressive episodes in fall or winter and remission by the following spring or summer, a pattern observed for two consecutive years.
- The absence of other psychiatric disorder.
- No psychosocial variables accounting for these regular, cyclical changes in mood.

The trigger for the individual with SADS is shortening daylight periods, so that in the Northern Hemisphere, as autumn fades into winter, the person sinks into a depression, characterized by weight gain and increased appetite, often accompanied by carbohydrate cravings, decreased physical activity, and hypersomnia. The patient shows a depressed, anxious, or irritable mood and experiences work and interpersonal difficulties. The most outstanding symptom of SADS, however, is the reactivity of the individual to changes in environmental lighting and climate. Day length, not the cold temperature, seems to be the relevant factor. It has been suggested that this version of the syndromal depression may have to do with melatonin suppression, a substance ordinarily released by the tiny pineal gland (Rosenthal & Wehr, 1987).

SADS is estimated to affect about 450,000 people, the majority of whom are women. Over half of these women report PMS mood changes, often worse in winter. The onset of the illness is typically in the third decade, although the syndrome has been identified in school-aged children, many of whom had been misdiagnosed as school-avoidant or -phobic.

A primary treatment for this syndrome is phototherapy, or exposure to panels of daylight-spectrum lights for one or more hours a day. Bright light (2500 Lux) seems to have a therapeutic effect within three days, whereas ordinary room light or dim light has no mood effect (Rosenthal et al., 1984). The condition does not invariably respond to lights, but it may respond to medication.

There is also a subset of patients who have a "reverse SADS" syndrome, in which too much light seems to trigger depressions. Some individuals seem to be heat-sensitive, and others, cold-sensitive; temperature regulation is healing for them. It seems that there are a number of elemental environmental triggers for what may be many different patterns of recurrent, cyclical affective episodes. The primitive nature of these syndromes surprised and fascinated us, but systematic work on them is far from complete.

An Incomplete Etiological Model

Interaction of Biology, Development, and Stressors

Figure 1 depicts three circles that help one to conceptualize three etiological factors that may be operative in depressive illness. These circles should be thought of as variable in size and degree of overlap.

Circle 1 represents *biology*—the genetic contribution made by all the birds who sit up in our family tree. Circle 2 represents our *developmental environment*—the experiences we had while growing up, largely in our families of origin. The third circle represents *current circumstances*—stress, loss, illness, and any number or combination of events in the environment, including "microstressors," the daily minor unpleasant events (Lewinsohn, Hoberman, & Rosenbaum, 1988). The impact of any one factor—genetics, early environment, or current stress level—may vary from individual to individual, and from time to time in any one individual. Similarly, the interaction between these factors can change.

It is possible to imagine a patient who may have come from a healthy primary family (neither mother nor father had depressive illness ex-

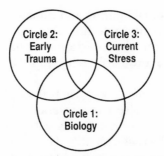

FIG. 1. Some factors influencing depression.

pressed), but who nevertheless has a genetic predisposition to depression. The healthy messages imbibed from a healthy family may serve a protective function when depressive illness is activated. Conversely, a child may have grown up in a home with a depressed parent but may have been bypassed genetically for the illness. Or an individual may have been spared the biological factors and may have come from a healthful home yet may have some overwhelming stressors in current life that result in cognitions of despair and helplessness.

Things are rarely simple, however, because these factors interact. For example, Circles 1 and 2 may intersect: if one or both parents have contributed genetically to a patient's biological diathesis to depression (that is, if there is affective illness in the family), it is typical that they have also contributed to making "home" a stressful place, and the family, a dysfunctional unit. Similarly, if a child has a "sensitive nervous system" (the genetic diathesis), he or she may be more reactive to these (home) environmental stressors than a child who was spared the diathesis.

It is in this interface between circles that we may see the development of core cognitive schemata or underlying assumptions about the world that may come to color the individual's thinking so deeply as to be represented as her or his "personality." Growing up in a dysfunctional family may predispose the patient to behaviors and thought patterns that mimic aspects of a personality disorder and may complicate management of the depression and require further aggressive treatment after recovery from the depressive episode (Pilkonis & Frank, 1988). In turn, a severe biological depression with strong genetic diatheses may intensify the features of a disordered personality and may thus complicate its treatment (Klein, Taylor, Harding, & Dickstein, 1988b).

The cognitive distortions and underlying assumptions of the truly personality-disordered individual generally are not responsive to short-term cognitive therapy (Young, 1989). There is some possibility that long-term therapy may eventually correct the basic dysfunctional ways of relating, and that RET may be useful in ameliorating "symptom stress" (Walen, DiGiuseppe, & Wessler, 1980).

Putting the Model to Work

Our etiological model suggests that an individual may experience varying sorts of negative affective responses, which may be more or less engulfing. When the current stress circle is enlarged, the emotive experience may be one of normal *sadness*, the kind of reaction that virtually everyone has had in response to a loss or a deprivation or a hassle. This is a nonpathological, although clearly unhappy, state. When the loss is more severe or prolonged (e.g., the death of a beloved spouse), the reaction is more intense and prolonged, and we speak of *grief*, another normative, time-limited response. When the reaction is intense and out of proportion to the negative stimulus, we may speak of *reactive depression*. The individual not only mourns a loss but has significantly distorted thinking about it, tending to personalize, overgeneralize, and awfulize, thereby making a bad situation worse, which may feed into the negativity of the reaction. At this point, we can suspect that Circle 2, developmental experience, is involved in the heightening of the intensity of the depressive response. If this overreaction continues long enough, and if the family history is positive for depressive illness, we may suspect that a biological diathesis (Circle 1) is operating, and chemotherapy may be required.

Mary: I had a large "dose" of all three circles. The biological diathesis (Circle 1) became evident from an exploration of my family tree. In addition, I've realized in the course of psychotherapy that my family of origin was highly dysfunctional. I had learned early never to show feelings—and later, not to feel them. To ask for help or comfort automatically brought punishment. In fact, anger and punishment—physical or verbal—were the standard response to questions, the expression of wants or needs, illness, injury, and even fear. I internalized this response, and as an adult, I punished myself. My Circle 2 was loaded! Environmental stressors (Circle 3) in the year preceding my first hospitalization included the deaths of four significant persons, including a grandmother with whom I identified. There was also my completion of a second master's degree in a field about which I was ambivalent. Our daughter, to whom I was probably overly close, left for college. Physically, I was struggling with several chronic conditions that contributed to lack of energy and weight loss. So the biological diathesis to depression, plus deeply entrenched schemata, in concert with considerable environmental stress, united to really zap me. My greatest disappointment after the depressive symptoms were ameliorated with medication was the discovery that many dysfunctional thought patterns were still there. My early family relationships and the resultant cognitive distortions were successfully addressed by insight-oriented and cognitive therapies.

CLINICAL AND TREATMENT IMPLICATIONS

Diagnosis

Our main point thus far is that more precise diagnosis may assist in more helpful treatment. *We must learn to do finely detailed evaluations of the symptom picture, the personal and family history, and the current life story,* in order to make our best guess about what kind of depression is operative, so that we can more prescriptively suggest what kind of psychotherapy we will do and what kind of biological therapy we may need to institute as a prerequisite or adjunct to therapy.

Eliciting the Phenomenological Report

The signs we need to focus on particularly are the vegetative symptoms of depression. The diagnostic issue is whether there is a *change* from the individual's normal state. One of the characteristics of the illness is that "you don't feel like yourself." Maintaining this "change" focus may help patients sift through their phenomenological experience for us.

A BDI is not enough—especially with a new patient or one in whom the depression is being newly observed. The specificity of instruments like the BDI and the MMPI-Depression scale is low. High scores are often false positives. For example, more than half of the patients with high scores on such pencil-and-paper measures did not meet the criteria for a diagnosis of depression. On the other hand, the false-negative rate is very low, as almost no one with a very low BDI score meets the diagnostic criteria for a depressive episode (Lewinsohn, Hoberman, & Rosenbaum, 1988). Tools like the BDI, therefore, may be advantageous, but they are not sufficient to make a diagnosis of depressive illness.

A cognitive analysis of automatic negative thoughts is also not going to give a differential diagnosis. Although the intensity and pervasiveness of negative thinking varies systematically with the depth of the depression (Beck, 1964), the various subtypes of depression are indistinguishable on the basis of the cognitive symptomatology (Eaves & Rush, 1984).

Hypomania

It is particularly important for the therapist to elicit detailed descriptions of the mood periods—especially the easy-to-miss hypomania—in order to differentially diagnose unipolar from bipolar disorders. Making the diagnosis may be treatment-relevant because some researchers suggest that patients with bipolar II disorders may have an elevated risk of developing rapid cycling when they are treated with tricyclic antidepressants (Wehr, Sack, Rosenthal, & Cowdry, 1988), the typical first-line treatment for unipolar depressions. In fact, a trial of a tricyclic may be given as a "challenge" to see if it induces a manic or hypomanic state.*

Hypomania is crucial to the definition of the soft bipolar spectrum, but patients enjoy it and rarely spontaneously label it as pathological. How is the clinician to discriminate it from "happiness" or "joy"? Akiskal (1983) suggested some criteria:

- There is no obvious cause for the emotion, or the response seems disproportionate to a pleasant event that occurred.
- It is labile. It may have a "drivenness" that joy does not contain and may thus be accompanied by a dysphoric agitation.
- It may be associated with substance abuse or impaired social judgment.
- It may be recognized because it is "surrounded" by periods of retarded depression, so that the contrast may make it obvious.
- "And, most importantly, hypomania is a recurrent condition. (Happiness is not!)" (p. 134)

Akiskal proposed that "tricyclics must be used with great caution in individuals with any history of bipolarity" (p. 130) and suggested that, if the patient is not too ill, it would be better to avoid medication if possible. Otherwise, he claimed, the patient may be at high risk of rapid cycling, especially women and those with borderline thyroid indices. Instead, the clinician may want to consider the use of MAOIs, lithium, phototherapy, or, in severe cases, electroconvulsive therapy (ECT), although clearly none of these alternates is risk-free for rapid cycling.

Obtaining Accurate Phenomenological Reports May Be Tricky

Depressed patients have state-dependent memories. For example, if we ask deeply depressed patients how long they've felt the way they feel, they frequently tell us that they've "always felt this way." In other words, when they are depressed, they are selectively retrieving depressed, state-dependent memories. Now, patients who have a depressive illness have probably had recurrent episodes of it, so that based on this selective memory, it may well seem as if they have spent a lifetime being depressed. Even when we try to do a careful life review and invite these patients to tell us times when they were happy, they may not be able to recall those periods. Depressed patients don't see the good, don't have spontaneous access to it, and thus

---

*Other medications, such as the MAOIs, may have a lower probability of inducing a manic rebound, as do mood-stabilizing drugs such as lithium (Wehr, Sack, Rosenthal, & Cowdry, 1988). Recently, there seems to have been an increased use of the MAOIs, particularly with panic disorders, atypical depressions, SADS, and bipolar II disorders (Regier *et al.*, 1988). Some literature suggests that the MAOIs provide more consistent relief from affective lability (Joyce & Paykel, 1989).

passively remember only the bad. Thus, at the time, the individual is not able to be a good historian, as the entire past looks bleak.

Our diagnostic prescription is to educate the patient about state dependence in memory retrieval. Although depression renders the positive memories passive, they can be retrieved with reminders and prompts. Don't settle for "I've always been depressed." Instead, gently but persistently assist patients to do a detailed life review. Insist that they go through their life story bit by bit to figure out spells when things were going along differently. Outside informants—family or friends—may be important in getting more accurate data. Bringing in these assistants may also serve the purpose of allowing the therapist to educate family members about depressive illness and to help them understand the kind of support required of them.

Some depressed patients make inappropriate use of stoicism. A somewhat peculiar aspect of our depression seemed to have to do with a denial mechanism that may result from an inappropriate stoicism—almost a perversion or distortion of RET. Even when we were feeling very ill, we would assure others, including our therapists, that we were all right, that we could do without medication, could probably drop out of treatment, and so forth.

> *Mary:* When I was hospitalized, I was trying to be very, very stoic. The hospital staff picked up on that immediately, and I was confronted about trying to be in control and not letting out my feelings as I "needed" to do. In truth, my overcontrol was inappropriate. Assurance that my feelings were acceptable and that I would be kept safe as they emerged facilitated my laying aside the stoic posture I'd taken.

It is important to reach around the patient's bland or facile facade and, with an understanding of the phenomenological experience of the illness, to help the patient continue the fight against it.

> *Sue:* When I felt a little bit better, I told my psychologist that I thought I could stop coming for treatment, assuring him I was at least 80% recovered and could certainly stand this much discomfort without whining. He confronted me on this assertion, however, and suggested strongly that it really wasn't necessary to struggle as much as I was struggling. He shared many stories of other patients and their various responses to medication and how, with continued experimentation on dose and type, they could get finer and finer control of the symptoms while balancing the therapeutic effects against the side effects of medication. His stories provided hope of change to me when I had prematurely decided that coping was all that I had left.

There is a strong tendency to put on a mask and act bravely for many different reasons, which may change at different times. Sometimes, the reasons are cognitive (e.g., not wanting to appear "weak" or to be a "burden"), or emotive (feeling numbed or inured to the symptoms), or behavioral (e.g., patients may not want to "tip their hand" if they are hanging on to the promise of relief afforded by the option of suicide).

> *Sue:* I determined that the present state was as good as the depression was going to get, and that I was simply going to have to live my life in the void and accept that that was how it was. Then, after I had done the next several years of necessary parenting and had organized my estate, I could opt out. I calculated how long I needed to tolerate my life and laid long-range suicide plans. That idea sustained me for some time, but the date for my intended suicide moved about, in tandem with the intensity of my despair.

This is the most dangerous source of "stoicism"—hopelessness and despair that anything will ever change. It's a very small step from here to suicide.

The antistoicism prescription recommended is a mixture of loving confrontation, education, support, encouragement, and prodding by the sharing of the hopeful stories of others. As recovery proceeds, suggest that it's not necessary to feel merely "80%"; the patient can aim for 100%. Let the patient know that there are many medication options, singly and in combination, and that new medications are being tested every year. Encourage the patient to be persistent; push the patient to believe that he or she *can* truly feel *good*.

Other patients have little access to stoicism. These individuals may be somewhat more impulsive in style, and either have low tolerance for pain or have developed fast-acting coping strategies for reducing discomfort. They may, for example, overeat, oversleep, abuse drugs or alcohol, and even cut themselves as a distraction from their internal pain. It is useful to see these behaviors as coping strategies, although not cognitive or intellectual ones. However, as with the overly stoic patient, we need to use RET to replace these coping styles, as, of themselves, they may be self-destructive as well as frightening to the patient's family.

Depressed patients may overestimate how well they are. A related aspect of the denial of, the dissociation from, or the blindness to the severity of the illness is seen in an "overestimation of wellness."

> *Sue:* When I was announcing that I was 80% better and could stand it if I showed no further improvement, I see now I was overestimating. When I was encouraged to push for still finer affective recovery and arrived at 95%–100%, I could look back and realize that what I thought of as 80% better was no more than 40%–50% better. I was much sicker than the depression would allow me to know.

Again, our prescription is to educate and encourage patients to be persistent in working to feel as good as they possibly can, not to "settle for less," and to be assertive in dealing with the medical establishment.

Sue: I was on 30 mg of Parnate and feeling better, but my psychologist kept urging me on. He'd say, "You know, if you ever get the feeling that, if you could just get a hair better, you could talk to your doctor about taking 40 mg instead of 30. You know, lots of patients here at our hospital use 40–50 mg of Parnate a day." I appreciated his pushing me to push on the system to feel as good as I possibly could.

Each of the factors above—including difficulties in the recognition, evaluation, and reporting of symptoms—singly and in combination, suggests a multipronged approach to the differential diagnosis. Another important clue can come from an evaluation of the patient's family history.

Getting the Family History

Depressive illnesses of the sort we describe above have a genetic diathesis, run in families, and, to a certain extent, "breed true." When one accepts the conception of biological depressions and accepts the hypothesis that one may have inherited the tendency to such depressions, a paradigmatic shift in the perceptions of family stories may take place.

Sue: Before I got to see my psychiatrist, but knowing that I was sick, I decided to do a biological interview and "pedigree" study of my family by interviewing my parents. A detailed examination of my father's side indicated no affective illness. On my mother's side, however, the old family stories suddenly took on a new cast. They were stories of symptoms and tales of bouts of depression and fits of anxiety. Probands were found in three of my mother's siblings and her own mother. To summarize an afternoon's worth of listening, I found her childhood affective state unclear, but my mother seems to have suffered major depressions in her teens, her early 30s, and her mid-40s and had a partial symptom picture in her mid-60s. Although I had never applied the label of depression to myself, looking back over my own life I can now identify periods of childhood dysphoria, a teenaged anorexic depression, a postpartum depression in my mid-30s, and a symptom cluster almost identical to my mother's in my 40s. It is as if I am walking in my mother's biological footprints. The family interview also yielded an alcoholic uncle and a chronically depressed grandmother, facts of which I had never been aware. So there is a biological diathesis or predisposition or pedigree for depression that seems to have passed down through the maternal gene pool.

Mary: I just found out about two years ago that my father's mother had had periods of depression. My father has been severely depressed intermittently for the past seven or eight years and probably would have been diagnosed as dysthymic before that. I can look back at my own development and identify depressive symptoms in the fourth grade, and possibly even earlier. I had a brief but intense major depression in college and postpartum depressions after the births of each of my children. At age 45, I had the most serious episode so far and the first for which I sought treatment. Major depression and other affective disorders, as well as substance abuse, appear in various other family members. There were also dysthymic indicators in several members of my mother's family.

What we learned from this experience of reexamining our lives and looking up into the family trees was that *things look quite different when we use a different frame of reference:* the concept of a biological affective illness, rather than a purely psychological one (Klein, Clark, Dansky, & Margolis, 1988a).

The use of multiple criteria, including the dexamethazone suppression test (DST) and sleep EEG studies, may help to establish the key diagnostic discrimination: between endogenous and nonendogenous depressions. In one study, for example, Rush (1983) found that *zero* out of five patients with endogenous diagnoses, abnormal DSTs, and abnormal sleep EEGs responded to cognitive-behavioral therapy (CBT), whereas eight out of nine patients with an opposite clinical picture responded well to CBT.

Looking for Precipitants

Don't be fooled by tricky As. Look for the precipitants of depression, and pay attention to the subtle ones.

> *Mary:* We can make an analogy to blood sugar levels. Mild variations in my diet over a long period of time can lead to symptoms such as moodiness, shortness of breath, fuzziness in concentration just creeping up. After a sugar binge, I'll have a clear high, followed by a crashing low.

How does this relate to depression? When we interview our depressed clients about the precipitants of their depression, what we tend to look for are binges—some sort of psychiatric binge or a crisis or a major loss—some sort of trauma. We may not find any because the depression may have just crept up on the person.

> *Sue:* I think I had been gradually sliding into depression over the past several years. The onset was long, slow, and subtle.

Alternatively, merely because the person has experienced a negative life event, it may be foolhardy to assume that the depression is simply reactive. Who doesn't have negative life events, day in and day out? One may make an erroneous—or at least, oversimplified—diagnostic attribution: we may fool ourselves into thinking that we have a clear case of reactive or neurotic depression, eminently suitable for our most elegant RET or CBT, only to discover much later that we missed the boat at the diagnostic port of entry.

A similar misattribution, relating depression to reinforcement contingencies in the environment, was suggested by a client's story. This young woman had come from a large family and, as one of the middle kids, had endured a certain amount of predictable, if benign, neglect. During her high school years, she slid into what we later recognized as the first of her major depressive episodes, and as a result, she got a lot of attention at home and at school. Her first reaction to the suggestion that she might have a cyclical illness was met with staunch disbelief. She had quite convinced herself that she had done so poorly in school, suffered so much social isolation, and felt so badly *because* of the attention she'd received. It took a good deal of detailed historical life review to disabuse her of this self-abnegating belief.

In order not to be fooled by the coincidental or merely contributory presence of a negative trigger or activating event, don't be trigger happy. Ask the patient if he has ever had such a negative event occur at other times. Has he always reacted so strongly? If not, why *now* is he overreacting? Has he ever *over*reacted before? When? Is there any *pattern* to this overreactivity? Does it have any periodicity or any sense of a cycle to it? Diagnostically, think in terms of cycles of varying lengths: daily, weekly, monthly, yearly, and so on. The difficult assessment at which we're trying to arrive is whether the triggering event caused a flood of negative thinking and consequent emotional turmoil, or whether a biological state has been activated, in the throes of which the patient merely *seems* to be overreacting.*

Importance of Doing Formal Assessment

Sometimes, it is very difficult to recognize a biological depression in a relatively high-functioning patient. Many of the patients whom we have recognized as suffering a depression had been in previous therapies, often for long periods of time, and (blush), in a few instances, with the authors before our own consciousness about biological depression was raised. In these cases, none of the patients had been interviewed systematically about the symptoms of affective disorders. None had received formal mental status examinations. None had been considered as candidates for medication. Misdiagnoses in this high-functioning population may be similar to that in other clinical populations; that is, an "epiphenomenon of the fact

---

*A life review of the cycles of the illness may be prepared graphically (Post, Roy-Byrne, & Uhde, 1988). One can superimpose on a longitudinal plot of episodes of mood disorder the patient's treatment record, hospitalization frequency, and course of major life events. This graphic depiction can help one to assess (1) the pattern of the episodes; (2) their relationship to environmental, endocrine, and seasonal factors; and (3) their response to treatment, especially when the response is subtle. A graphic representation of the illness may help the patient to understand the disorder and may help the therapist in case management.

that many patients who initially present as intact, 'good neurotics' do not receive a comprehensive assessment" (Kluft, 1986, p. 724).

In summary, we need to do very detailed reviews of symptoms, and we need particularly to learn to focus on the physiological, phenomenological, and family history details, learning to listen with what the analysts call our "third ear." We have a very tricky job to do, because our clients' distorted perceptions and derailed memories often make them poor historians.

> *Sue:* I was a reasonably seasoned clinician, but I didn't recognize that I was depressed until I was so sick that it was staring me in the face. I also lived in a family riddled with depression and never labeled their problems either.

We may need to help clients to elucidate their feelings and explore their family history, as they may be relatively unable to recognize or label their own or the family's pathology.

Beginning Treatment

If the Patient Has an Acute Affective Illness

When we enter the domain of depressive illness, self-control of feeling and thought is often not possible. The best role for the counselor may be the one appropriate for dealing with any illness: kindness, nurturance, education, and a reaching out to the patient so that she knows that she is dealing with someone who understands her sensations and frightening experiences, that her condition has a name, that it will improve, and that the doctor's office is a safe place, in which she can allow herself to feel the symptoms and will receive the doctor's support until she gets the medical help that works for her. In other words, the help needed is that of a loving nurse, keeping hope alive while trials of medication are being conducted.

Other experienced clinicians and students of depression have suggested the same concepts:

> [In affective illness,] the depression is a state imposed on the patient out of impaired biology. . . . Affective disorder is a biological condition, best construed as a disease. The patient did not bring it on himself in any real way. It wasn't learned, it wasn't the result of the way he thinks, or the way he was raised, it isn't the result of the way he relates to others, or the way he strives. (Kaminsky, 1986)

> In true endogenous depression, any attempt at systematic psychotherapy is contraindicated as it often leads to a deepening of the patient's sense of worthlessness. But it is essential to penetrate the barrier created by the patient's self torment and despair and to establish a warm rapport with him—a difficult task which requires much patience and skill. (Slater & Roth, 1969, p. 229)

> Look upon your distressed friends as under one of the worst distempers to which this miserable life is exposed. Melancholy incapacitates them for thought

or action: it confounds and disturbs all their thoughts and fills them with vexa-
tion and anguish. I verily believe, that when this malign state of mind is deeply
fixed and has spread its deleterious influence over every part, it is as vain to
attempt to resist it by reasoning and rational motives, as to oppose a fever or the
gout or pleurisy. . . . Do not urge your melancholy friends to do what is out of
their power . . . if you can innocently divert them, you would do them a great
kindness; but do not urge them to do anything which requires close and intent
thinking; this will only increase the disease. (Timothy Rogers, 1658–1728, Pref-
ace to *A Discourse on Trouble of Mind and the Disease of Melancholy*)

Beck and his colleagues, who did the seminal work on cognitive therapy in the treatment of depression, recognized that cognitive therapy, in
and of itself, is not always sufficient, and that antidepressants are "of
significant value in the treatment of various kinds of depressions" (Beck *et
al.*, 1979, p. 354). He suggested the use of cognitive therapy for patients
who have incomplete remission with chemotherapy, to increase compliance with the medication regimen, and to counter premature termination.

The Iatrogenic Message of CBT and RET

Unfortunately, an oversimplification of a core principle of RET and
CBT may send an erroneous message to the patient: Your emotional distress is a product of your dysfunctional thinking. If you tidy up your
thinking, you'll feel better, and if you can change your thinking, you'll get
better. We have seen this message over and again in the self-help literature:

The negative thoughts that flood your mind are the actual cause of your self-
defeating emotions. These thoughts are what keep you lethargic and make you
feel inadequate. (patient handout used in one clinic)

In other words, cognitive therapy has been associated with a theory on the
etiology of depression, which is that the *proximate* etiological factor is cognitive. Although this model may very well be partially correct and not
harmful to the patient with milder dysthymia or reactive depression, it
may be a pernicious idea to apply to a patient who is seriously ill with
depressive illness. The implication to the ill patient is that she or he is
causing the illness by faulty thinking. Personal and clinical experience as
well as more recent research suggests the need for a modification of this
idea (Barnett & Gotlib, 1988; Bedrosian, 1989; Bradley & Power, 1988).
Although the relationship between negative cognitions and depressive illness has been observed (Seligman, Castellon, Cacciola, Schulman, Luborsky, Ollove, & Downing, 1988), cause and effect have *not* been demonstrated (Barnett & Gotlib, 1988; Klein *et al.*, 1988a; Lewinsohn *et al.*, 1988).

The message is this: Inappropriate yet persistent reliance on a cognitive therapy with a patient who is in the throes of an affective illness may
have dire iatrogenic consequences. It is likely to fail and may seem like the
"final blow" to a patient who has already accumulated a list of perceived

failures. Parenthetically, we might point out that the patient and the therapist may spuriously congratulate each other on a successful course of therapy, when the depression was lifting spontaneously. This comment is not meant to disparage the humanity of the therapeutic effort or its importance, but to remind us that correlation is not the same as causation.

As a function of personally experiencing this illness, our consciousness and sensitivity to its biological nature and intractibility in response to psychotherapy are enormously heightened. *There is something phenomenologically distinct about the thinking that goes on during severe affective illness.* The thinking is, indeed, negative, but the quality of the thinking is beyond what we see in reactive depression. It is not merely self-downing or filled with catastrophic prophesies. It is highly obsessional, highly ruminative, quasi-delusional in quality, and impervious, we assure you, to logic. It is as if the thinking has moved to a different dimension and is more like a thought disorder. It is *determined* by the illness.

> *From Sue's journal:* I worked my fool head off to try to do something about my thinking when I was sick. So did the friends who cared for me. I tried out all of my RET and CBT tools. And although I could wrestle the negative thoughts down for perhaps a minute, very quickly it was clear to me that the Real Truth was embodied in my negative thoughts.

There is a fixed, rigid, delusional quality to the thinking that seems to *be* the illness. The brain seems to be processing information in a vastly different way. The process, more than the content, is what is salient. Stated another way, we suggest that *there is a palpable difference between* irrational thoughts *(the content) and* irrational thought processes. It is the latter that are so pressing in acute affective illness, and that seem to be relatively impervious to rational-emotive therapy. One can dispute an irrational thought, but not an irrational process. The patient's belief in the thought that is produced by the ruminative process seems impermeable. For example, one female patient who had made a successful and stable adjustment to her newly single status commented repeatedly on her ability to be productive, social, active, and "in charge of her life" after her disengagement from her male partner. Some time later, after she entered an acute phase of her depression, her core belief was that there was no reason for her even to stay alive if she did not have a male partner, a thought that preoccupied her during the day and marred her sleep at night. Once her medication took hold, she not only reverted to her former belief system about relationships, but she barely even gave them much thought and looked back on her ruminations with disbelief!

The fruitlessness of dealing with thought content when the "biology circle" is enlarged may be further illustrated by a clinical vignette.

Sue: The patient was a 17-year-old female diagnosed with SADS on the basis of a careful historical review of her life with depressions. She quickly responded to light therapy, but, as is often the case with teenage clients, precise compliance with the treatment regimen was somewhat of a problem.

One day, she came in for her appointment looking not well. When I asked how things were going, she began a recitation of how terrible the various aspects of her life were, especially in school. She moaned, "School is really awful. I'm flunking out, I just know it. I just flunked a chemistry test today, and that's going to bring my average down so low that there's no way I can salvage the semester. I just can't do science," and so on. I dutifully wrote each of the negative statements on my chalkboard, and when she stopped for a deep sigh, I asked if she had any further negative thoughts about school, and she continued to spew them forth until my board was completely full. At that point, I turned to the client and suggested that we start at the top and do a little cognitive therapy work on these thoughts. But when we tried to examine the first negative statement, the result was a cascade of further negative statements. It felt as if we'd tried to put a rock in front of a torrent of rushing black water, and all that happened was that the stream bounced over and around the tiny barricade. No matter which thought we tried to challenge, the same result occurred.

I must have struggled for 10 or 20 minutes with her until the lightbulb went on over *my* head: "Stop. No more cognitive therapy. Tell me about your lights." Indeed, she had been managing her phototherapy rather haphazardly, so we shifted treatment gears. "OK, let's add an extra hour's light per day. I'll call you tonight, I'll call you tomorrow, and I'd like to see you in three days to see how you are." Three days later, she was fine and totally euthymic. When I showed her the notes I'd taken of her negative thoughts from previous days, she smiled and looked at me quizzically: "That's easy to see, now. Those aren't true. They're full of distortions." I suggested that we go through the exercise of challenging the negative thoughts anyway, which we did as a rehearsal, but it was clear that she no longer thought that way. She was on a different mental track.

Another way to think of it is that the patient's negative cognitions were state-dependent (Klein *et al.*, 1988b).

This patient was, at the earlier appointment, ill and unable to think her way out of it. Her thought *process* was illogical and was impervious to logical argument. Trying harder would have produced more failure experiences and would have added reality to her beliefs about failing. At that point, it was more useful for her simply to "take her medicine" and try "not to think," which isn't as easy as it sounds.

The point is that all depressions are not the same. Some seem more clearly to be illnesses of the limbic system and other structures in the brain, affecting the physiological economy of the body in the most profound and painful ways—disrupting energy, sleep, feeding, sexual appetite, and the "vital sense" of oneself. These depressions feel like raging fevers, whose bodily and mental symptoms are only marginally under conscious control. Styron (1988) said it succinctly: "It is the brain as well as the mind that becomes ill."

The differential diagnosis for *melancholic* depression in the revised third edition of the American Psychiatric Association's *Diagnostic and Statistical Manual* (DSM-III-R; APA, 1987) suggests the unique experience of the patient who is "ill." In addition to loss of reactivity and loss of the ability to sense pleasure, the mood is said to have a "distinct quality—i.e., the depressed mood is perceived as distinctly different from the kind of feeling experienced following the death of a loved one." Some data (Belsher & Costello, 1988) suggest that a patient with melancholic depression, even if treated with an aggressive psychotherapy such as RET or CBT, has a very high probability of relapsing into depression within a two-year period. *Four out of five patients with melancholia, treated with cognitive therapy, will relapse (if they do not suicide).* Among despondent patients who do *not* have melancholia, four out of five will *not* relapse within two years.

Therefore, we suggest that the *primary* therapeutic tool for the management of acute depressive illness is *not* cognitive therapy. This sort of depression is a reality of dysfunction within the patient's nervous system. For these illnesses, treatment must include medication and a modification of cognitive approaches (which we discuss later) during the patient's critically ill period.

But Isn't CBT the Treatment of Choice for Depression?

In the history-making research literature on the treatment of depression with cognitive therapy (e.g., Rush, Beck, Kovacs, & Hollon, 1977), it was indeed shown to be significantly more effective and longer lasting than a standardized dose of imipramine. Unfortunately, the depressed patients were not well described, nor had they been followed for a long enough period of time to allow for the relapse potential of the illness to be expressed. In addition, we cannot tell which of the more current diagnostic categories would be most descriptive of the patients studied.

Then How Can We Use RET?

Our suggestion would be that RET and CBT therapists be cautious about introducing the ABC model, because, as we have shown, when the patient is in an acute phase of a depressive illness, his or her ability to wrestle with negative thoughts may be quite minimal because of the thought *processes* by which the brain is operating. It may be more useful (as well as a kinder and gentler message) to say to such a patient, "Of course, you're thinking this way. That's part of your illness. People who have your illness tend to think this way. We don't need to challenge this thinking right now; in fact, that may be a fruitless venture for a while. For right now, I want you to *try not to think too much*, and just try to get help in taking good nursing care of yourself." *Learning not to be frightened or depressed about the illness may be the most important function of cognitive-behavioral treatments.* This is where RET can be efficaciously applied—to "symptom stress," which we discuss in more detail further on.

In addition, CBT or RET can serve a *diagnostic* function. The first few meetings with the patient are assessment sessions. During this period of data collection, one kind of assessment can be a "pretest" of the patient's receptivity to cognitive interventions. The therapist may determine what some of the negative cognitions are and gently test the patient's responsiveness to disputation of that thinking. This process may be undertaken collaboratively as an empirical test of the appropriateness and/or timeliness of cognitive therapy. Hollon (1984) stated that 90% of the eventual reduction in symptomatology is evident by six weeks of treatment. Clinically, informal observation suggests that one or two good illustrative disputations can provide useful feedback about the viability of the use of a cognitive intervention. If the patient feels no relief from an adequate disputation or rapidly returns to the emotional low point, the *sufficiency* of RET or CBT at that time should be questioned.

There is some empirical data to suggest that cognitive therapy can reduce the risk of relapse, even in apparently endogenous or biological depressions (Hollon, 1988). Research patients who were given CBT in addition to a mere 12 weeks of tricyclic antidepressants had the same relapse rate at the end of a year as the patients who remained on medication for the full year but did not receive CBT.

We must not be too cavalier or overconfident about this prophylactic effect, however. Recent studies of long-term follow-up (20 years) suggest that the prognosis of depressive illness is much more serious than is commonly realized, for both endogenous and neurotic depression (Kiloh, Andrews, & Neilson, 1988). Although these two variations have different courses, "over the years there was no difference in overall severity, and both varieties of depression appear to produce the same amount of despair and disability" (p. 756). Lewinsohn *et al.* (1988) concluded that general pessimistic outlooks may predispose one to depressed *moods*, but cognitive style is *not* related to the probability of developing a diagnosable episode of depressive disorder.

Other Less Elegant Strategies

Distractions can be very useful. Mary took up art:

> I began doing pointillism (an art form which uses tiny dots) because it made me concentrate very carefully. I could not think about anything except

the characteristics of what I was trying to capture, and I chose this discipline for that reason. I also worked with sculpture to take my mind off myself and my feelings.

Sue, at her nadir, took nursing notes every 10–15 minutes:

> I had taken up Nautilus exercising and spent a lot of time fussing with record keeping on that, until I got too ill to leave the house because the symptoms were too pressing. So I logged them in a journal, which gave me a little distance from the symptoms, as I was observing them with a bit of scientific detachment. I didn't try to challenge my thinking at that point; I merely logged it in, along with frequent medical bulletins on my blood pressure and other symptoms. My psychiatrist supported this position. He said, "I don't want you to think about your life now. You're too sick. I don't want you to think now." I thought that was a strange assignment to give to an intellectualizing cognitive therapist, but it was relieving to hear it.

Thus, Mary distracted herself with an "outward" focus, and Sue focused inward.

It may seem counterproductive to have the depressed patient keeping careful note of symptoms and thoughts. The patient's attention already seems to be overly self-absorbed. Nonetheless, keeping detailed logs may help because the patient begins to pull a part of the self outside the self in order to observe and thereby achieves a small measure of objectivity. We both found that *the process of shifting from introspection to self-observation was helpful*. It ameliorated the sense of being caught in something beyond ourselves and gave us at least a small sense of control.

Avoid "Deep" Cognitive Therapy—Till Later

Confrontational psychotherapy, directive therapy, or affectively charged therapy such as the kind that focuses on deeply rooted schemata may be not only unprofitable during depressive illness, but actually harmful. Digging up painful childhood memories—the traumata that may be connected to the negative schemata—is difficult work in the best of times, by its very nature.

> *Sue:* When my depression was coming on but had not yet reached its nadir, I had begun a course of schema-focused cognitive therapy with a therapist in another city. As my symptoms became worse, I called to cancel further sessions until I could be seen by a biological psychiatrist. The next time I went for a therapy session, I was medicated, but not yet effectively. Although I put on what I thought of as a very good 'face,' I was frightened of the emotion that might be stirred up in the session. At the end of the meeting, I commented on the relief I felt that we hadn't delved back into our schema-focused work. "No," replied my therapist, "I can see that you're too

sick for that now. You don't have a floor under you emotionally. I wouldn't do that to you now!" I burst into grateful tears at his empathy and kindness.

Mary: I knew that I needed to work on some extremely dysfunctional emotional and cognitive characteristics from both psychodynamic and cognitive perspectives, but I also knew that the lowering of defenses necessary to do the former work was dangerous, leaving me too vulnerable to self-destructive urges. In addition, my thought processes at that point were extremely irrational. Attempts to counter my thoughts simply reinforced my view of myself as the cause of the depression. Later, when I was able to return to exploratory work, cognitive techniques not only facilitated the uncovering process (the "downward arrow" is simply a structure that facilitates free association) but were very useful in dealing with all the ghosts and garbage that floated to the surface.

Symptom Stress: An Important Role for RET in Affective Illness

The cognition we need to impart to patients is that they are suffering from an *illness*. The negative cognitions, self-blaming, dire predicting, and lack of energy are all part of the same syndrome. *Patients need help to reframe their experience as indicative of the "disease" of depression, not a characterological flaw.* Even when we've sold them that idea, however, they may still put themselves down for being so "weak" as to have an illness in the first place. This is what RET therapists know as *symptom stress* (Walen *et al.*, 1980), or a secondary reaction to their problem (Ellis, 1973).

Below are some other examples of negative thoughts about the illness or the symptoms of the illness that we typically hear from patients:

Shame. "I should be able to handle this myself. If I can't handle it myself, then I'm weak. It's shameful to be weak."

"I can't let new people who don't know me learn about my psychiatric history. They'll be turned off and not want to have anything to do with me."

Guilt. "I'm not taking care of my family. They need me. I can't be sick."

"All I think about is myself."

Anxiety. "I'll never feel better."

"I'll never be able to work again."

"My diagnosis says 'recurrent depression.' It's going to come back. And I can't stand to feel like this again, ever."

Secondary Depression. "I can't stand the way I feel. I feel totally overwhelmed. I feel terrible."

"If I were as smart as everybody says I am, I wouldn't be depressed."

An Interpretive Hypothesis

One of the things Sue concluded about the physiological or vegetative symptoms of the depression is that they may have some homeostatic value that she, as a clinician, had not appreciated:

For example, when my appetite shut down and I could not eat, it seems to have been appropriate not to do so. My attempts to nurture myself with soup merely led to bowel distress. It was as if my guts were saying to me, "We're too sick, so don't feed us now; we're busy doing other things and don't have a good blood supply for the stomach and its digestive work. . . .

The sleep disorder may also have a corrective homeostatic function. In fact, some research suggests that a sleep-deprivation period may serve to elevate mood, potentiate drug effects, and reset the disturbed sleep cycle (Goodwin, 1989). A sleepless night can be used to advantage if the patient can be encouraged to be sure to stay fully awake through the night and the next day, returning to bed at the normal time the following night.

The homeostasis of appetite loss and sleeplessness seem akin to Mother Nature's use of "paradoxical intention" (prescribing the symptom) and can be used to advantage by the therapist if cognitively reframed for the patient so that he or she will come to welcome these symptoms rather than be frightened by them. The reconceptualization is that the body is "taking a break" and trying in some way to heal itself and recover physiologically. Even suicidal thinking can be viewed as a comforting option; as depression can be such an extraordinarily painful experience, the thought that one will not have to struggle unremittingly and eternally can paradoxically provide a sense of hope. The contemplation of suicide may be an effective way of keeping oneself from committing suicide out of total hopelessness and despair. As one wounded healer said, "It's always my ace-in-the-hole."

A Note on Anxiety

Much of what we have said about depressive illness parallels what has evolved in the diagnostic and treatment literature on panic as discriminated from other anxiety disorders. The older conceptualization of anxiety was that it was elicited by an external threat (the phobic stimulus), and therapies had been devised to help the sufferer to approach the feared stimuli. In more contemporary formulations, panic disorders are thought to have a genetic diathesis. When in a panic attack, the patient often reports that cognitions are relatively unavailable for observation, let alone disputation. In the midst of a panic attack, the patient is not able to do cognitive therapy or elegant RET. Instead, the therapeutic focus lies in (1) breaking the panic cycle; (2) learning not to be frightened of the panic state; and (3) learning not to make incorrect associations with an outside "threat." In addition, the patient may need help to understand that the inability to "talk herself or himself out of a panic attack" is not a matter of weakness or ineptitude. It is a reality of the integration of the nervous system (Beck & Emery, 1985).

Some Additional Clinical Tips

Empathy and Understanding

What can you say to your sick patient? The most salient elements in rapport during the critical parts of the illness seem to us to involve (1) a sense of true understanding of the patient's experience; (2) a sense of loving acceptance; and (3) a realistic sense of hope.

> *Sue:* During the worst part of the illness, it felt like a lifeline when my doctor would roll his chair close to me and lean in toward me as he listened to me tell of the symptoms. The words that were most comforting to me were when he'd simply say, "Yes, I know" or "Listen, I understand." Or he would remind me "You know, the illness runs in my family, too. I really understand this." Then, as the medicine began to take hold and I began to recover, he didn't roll up as closely to me. It was, in a funny way, a measure of my recovery that he felt I could tolerate the distance between us.

Respect for the Patient

The patient not only views himself as worthless, he invites others— including the therapist—to share his opinion. It is vital that the therapist avoid falling into pitfalls dug by the patient. Helping the patient to participate in the treatment process by exploring his history and observing his symptoms, asking the patient to collect data about the effects of medication, reassuring without patronizing, expecting and reinforcing "victories," however small—all communicate the therapist's respect for the patient's efforts. Respect from the therapist can be treasured and clung to until the patient recovers enough to begin to respect himself again.

Assertively Reaching Out

Although some patients may be able to reach out for help, many are not. Remember that part of the depressive aspect is the poignant sense of isolation, existential aloneness, and worthlessness. This is what Sylvia Plath described so vividly in her metaphor of the bell jar.*

Reach out clearly, lovingly, and frequently to the patient who is ill.

---

*Plath, author of *The Bell Jar* (1971), suffered major depressions, and was treated with ECT and hospitalization before her ultimate suicide. She described her illness as "A time of darkness, despair, disillusion—so black only as the inferno of the human mind can be—symbolic death, and numb shock—then the painful agony of slow rebirth and psychic regeneration." She tried to show "how isolated a person feels when he is suffering a breakdown . . . I've tried to picture my world and people in it as seen through the distorting lens of a bell jar." And in her last pages, "How did I know that someday . . . the bell jar, with its stifling distortions, wouldn't descend again?"

Sue: My doctor asked me to call him. He'd say, "Call if there's any change at all. Call if there are any questions you have. Just stay in touch with me." But, of course, I didn't. I was trapped in my black hole, and I certainly didn't want to burden him with my worthless self. So he called me frequently and kept finding little excuses to do so, just to touch base with me. He'd say, "I just thought I'd check and see whether I have the time right for our next visit. . . . That was just an excuse to call you and see how you're doing. How are you feeling today? . . . Yes, I know. . . . Listen, I know." And that was so wonderful for me.

Mary: I was very suicidal, even after I was on the medication that ultimately turned the illness around. My doctor would have felt more comfortable if I had been in a hospital, but I explained to him that my suicide plans had taken hospital life into account and that the hospital could not provide a safe place. I needed just to go ahead and handle the suicidality. So he agreed and said, "OK, what's a good time of the day for me to call you?" I offered to be the one to make the call, but he said, "No, I will call you"—and he did, faithfully, every day that week. Once I got through that rough period, he let me take over more responsibility. But his being available provided the strength I needed to keep myself safe.

These patients may need us but probably won't be able to tell us that. One important lesson we learned, therefore, is how important it is for professional helpers, family, and friends to *be assertively and stubbornly loving and supportive.*

Impact on the Family: The Need for Prophylaxis

Until we lived through it, we did not realize how dastardly this illness can be on family members. One of the clinical hints we would like to pass on is the need to bring the immediate family into therapy. When a parent is ill with depression, it is particularly hard on the children. It is important to intervene prophylactically rather than waiting for the patient to discover that the children are upset. The patient, in fact, may be so negatively self-absorbed that the children's pain is missed.

Sue: Before I was adequately medicated, my son spent a very unhappy season, complaining bitterly about his school. I had decided to enroll him in a private school, but the day before his admission interview (several months into my treatment), he said to me, "Mom, you know, I don't think we really have to go through with this. Now that you're better, I feel fine. I really like my old school. I'm going to be on the swim team. I think I was just feeling bad because you were feeling so bad and I felt like I lost my mom and kind of lost my home, and everything sort of fell apart." I hadn't realized that. I had no idea I had had so much impact on my teenaged son's life! And I thought I'd been successfully hiding my pain from him!

One little 8-year-old, whose mom was very deeply depressed, worked with a colleague of ours, Barbara Mandell, who runs groups for children of divorce. The boy told his therapist, "I just got bored trying to help my mom." But then he stopped himself, and said, "No, bored isn't the right word. I just got so tired of it that I had to put it away. It's like when you take something apart and then you try to put it back together again, but you're missing a piece and you keep trying and you keep trying, and then, after a while, you get so tired of it that you just give up." That's how it felt to him, being around his mother, watching her cry night after night and not being able to do anything about it. He needed supportive counseling himself and a chance to take a break from worrying about his mom by himself.

The family also needs help to encourage the patient to engage in activity—while understanding that even the smallest effort is incredibly difficult for the patient.

> *Mary:* I remember standing in the shower, staring at a shampoo bottle, feeling as if I did not have the energy to pick it up and take off the cap!

Redistributing family chores to alleviate pressure while still helping the patient to maintain some activity is challenging but necessary. Gently encouraging the patient's participation in activities with family and friends is also important. Be mindful, however, that family patience wears thin at times. Frequent support and occasional respite for all family members involved can be highly recommended.

Commonly Asked Questions

Will I Get It Again?

> *Mary:* The first time I received the diagnosis of "recurrent" depression, I was devastated. I still had the idea that the illness was my fault, and "recurrent" simply meant that the psychiatrist thought I was so screwed up that I wouldn't be able to keep myself well. As information about the biological nature of the illness began to trickle out, "recurrent" came to mean I would probably experience additional episodes but hopefully would recognize the symptoms and begin medication before the episode became too severe.

At this time, recurrence is likely, especially for those patients who have already had more than one episode of the illness (Belsher & Costello, 1988). The situation is becoming more hopeful, however. Research is being done that may identify means of preventing further episodes. Lithium, for example, may serve this very important function in unipolar depression (Regier *et al.*, 1988).

Will My Children Get It?

Children and adolescents do indeed get depressed, and often the first episode of recurrent depressive illness is seen during these young years.

> *Sue:* After I had recovered enough to travel to visit with my daughter, who was studying overseas, we spent some time discussing the details of the episode. When I shared the stories of my symptoms, she came to my arms, hugged me tightly and said, "Mom, I know about that. That's what was happening to me between the fifth and seventh grade." What I had seen as pubescent crankiness and the slimming of her body into that of a more stylish teen, I had attributed to the difficult period of adjusting to adolescent peer pressures. I had no idea that she had struggled—alone—with anorexia, insomnia, suicidal ideation, self-loathing, and the "bell jar" of existential isolation! Now that we have identified her first episode, we are all on the lookout for early identification of a subsequent attack. My other two children seem to be free of the illness—at least so far.

Educate family members about the illness; education may provide important prophylaxis.

How Long Do I Have to Take This Medicine?

What a difficult question, and yet it is often at the top of the list in terms of frequency.

> *Sue:* I view weaning from my medication as an experiment to be done, perhaps. Right now, I have no interest in doing the experiment because I am feeling so good and it is such a relief. When I decide to do it, I plan to line up my support systems and get friends to help keep watch on me. Part of me is curious to know if the disease process is quiescent, as it is a cycling and recurrent illness.

How Can I Tell if I'm Getting Sick or Merely Overreacting?

Encourage your patients to keep an account of their affective state and daily functioning, even—perhaps especially—after "recovery." A simple plus or minus recorded morning and evening on a calendar will do. More information is provided by an analogue scale; the patient can draw a 10-centimeter line on an index card each day and put a cross-hatch along the line to indicate the amount of disorder felt that day. A still more helpful strategy is keeping brief journal notes on events and the patient's responses to them, which may help to identify trends, particularly in the vegetative signs. Over a period of time (and in true depressive illness, we may be talking about *years*), patterns may emerge indicating cycles, hypo-manias, SADS, and so on. Just as a diabetic learns to watch for blood sugar cycles, persons with depressive illnesses must learn to watch for affective symptom patterns. As cognitive therapists, we must help them to become good observers and researchers of themselves.

We have found that every day we learn something new about our illnesses. There is a constant series of puzzles to be solved. Sue realized that she was not simply overreacting with anger to a series of social stressors but was experiencing breakthrough depression, which required an increase in medication dosage. Mary found that a chronic fatigue was due to being overmedicated; cutting back on her medicine made her feel much better.

CONCLUSION

We've Come a Long Way, Baby

Mary: When I began the slide into the most recent depressive episode late in 1981 and early 1982, the predominant assumption of my mental health colleagues and myself was that depression was primarily a product of negative early life experiences and the resultant dysfunctional thinking of the patient. Medication was prescribed but was generally viewed as a crutch to be used by those who weren't able to use psychotherapy effectively. Requests for medication indicated resistance to psychotherapy. As the evidence of actual chemical imbalance accumulated, the use of medication became somewhat less suspect but still tended to be viewed as a booster for "real" therapy. My own perspective was similar when medication was prescribed for me. I hoped that there might be a true biological basis primarily to remove some of my self-blame and to give hope for control of the illness. But my suspicion was still that it was "all my fault" or my rotten parents or . . .

By the time I discussed my experiences with Sue in 1984 and 1985, as the initial lifting of my illness began in response to imipramine, I had recognized that some of what had happened truly felt physiological, but my suspicion remained that this was wishful thinking on my part. Sue made the conceptual breakthrough first with her own experience of depression a couple of years later. She convinced me that this was indeed a physical illness, itself the source of many irrational beliefs, complicated by dysfunctional thinking, but not a shameful product that I had manufactured myself.

As we've shared and worked with our experience the last two to three years, and scoured the literature as well as talking to our colleagues and our own therapists, it's been gratifying to be able both to confirm and to be confirmed by the evidence of chemical changes in the brain and the discovery of genetic markers for the illness. We are in an exciting time. The promise of control, prevention of recurrence, and perhaps eventually of onset brings huge hope for us and for the estimated 13.7 million people in the United States who suffer, generally untreated, from the illness. We're grateful to families and friends who stuck by us, to those who have treated us and kept us safe, to the theoreticians who sought and found some ways to relieve the symptoms with psychotherapy, and to the researchers who are discovering more efficacious medication for this often fatal disease.

Each of us has found the experience of a major depressive episode shocking and miserable, yet also the pivotal point for a great deal of new learning about diagnoses and treatment issues, and about the biological revolution in psychiatry. We became far more appreciative of the art of empathically recognizing, reaching out to, and knowing how to be helpful to our own affectively ill patients. Our learning took place in libraries, consultation rooms, and therapists' offices, and through critical examination of our own experiences. Our use of RET in the clinical work that we do has been significantly altered by this experience, and we have wanted to share our learning with our colleagues. In "coming out of the closet" as "wounded healers," we have discovered many others similarly afflicted— and isolated. To battle that isolation, we have formed a support group for affectively ill mental health workers, which has been a particular source of strength and growth for each of us. It also provides a safety net as we confront one another about blind spots where we may be fooling ourselves—and our therapists—about our thinking and our functioning.

In some ways, writing this chapter seems premature. Every time we discuss the illness, each day that we live with it, each patient we help to wrestle with it, we learn something else about it. In some ways, it has caused us to question our most fundamental assumptions about psychology, but unarguably, it has helped us to become much better clinicians. The experience of depression has been the greatest teacher of all.

SOME RECOMMENDED BOOKS ON DEPRESSION FOR PATIENTS

DePaulo, J. R., Jr., & Ablow, K. R. (1989). *How to cope with depression.* New York: McGraw-Hill.
Klein, D. F., & Wender, P. H. (1988). *Do you have a depressive illness?* New York: New American Library.
Papolos, D. F., & Papolos, J. (1987). *Overcoming depression.* New York: Harper & Row.
Rosenthal, N. E. (1989). *Seasons of the mind.* New York: Bantam Books.

REFERENCES

Akiskal, H. S. (1983). Diagnosis and classification of affective disorders: New insights from clinical and laboratory approaches. *Psychiatric Developments, 1,* 123–160.
Akiskal, H. S. (1985). A proposed clinical approach to chronic and "resistant" depressions: Evaluation and treatment. *Journal of Clinical Psychiatry, 46,* 32–36.

Akiskal, H. S., & Mallya, G. (1987). Criteria for the "soft" bipolar spectrum: Treatment implications. *Psychopharmacology Bulletin, 23,* 68–72.

American Psychiatric Association. (1980). *Diagnostic and statistical manual of mental disorders.* Washington, DC: Author.

American Psychiatric Association. (1987). *Diagnostic and Statistical Manual of Mental Disorders* (3rd ed., rev.). Washington, DC: Author.

Barnett, P. A., & Gotlib, I. H. (1988). Psychosocial functioning and depression: Distinguishing among antecedents, concomitants, and consequences. *Psychological Bulletin, 104,* 97–126.

Beck, A. T. (1964). Thinking and depression: 2. Theory and therapy. *Archives of General Psychiatry, 10,* 561–571.

Beck, A. T. (1976). *Cognitive therapy and the emotional disorders.* Philadelphia: University of Pennsylvania Press.

Beck, A. T., & Emery, G. (1985). *Anxiety disorders and phobias: A cognitive perspective.* New York: Basic Books.

Beck, A. T., Rush, A. J., Shaw, B. F., & Emery, G. (1979). *Cognitive therapy of depression.* New York: Guilford Press.

Bedrosian, R. C. (1989). Treating depression and suicidal wishes within a family context. In N. Epstein, S. E. Schlesinger, & W. Dryden (Eds.), *Cognitive-behavioral therapy with families.* New York: Brunner/Mazel.

Belsher, G., & Costello, C. G. (1988). Relapse after recovery from unipolar depression: A critical review. *Psychological Bulletin, 104,* 34–96.

Blehar, M. C., Weissman, M. M., Gershon, E. S., & Hirschfeld, R. M. A. (1988). Family and genetic studies of affective disorders. *Archives of General Psychiatry, 45,* 289–292.

Bowlby, J. (1977). The making and breaking of affectional bonds: 1. Etiology and psychopathology in the light of attachment theory. *British Journal of Psychiatry, 130,* 201–210.

Bradley, V. A., & Power, R. (1988). Aspects of the relationship between cognitive theories and therapies of depression. *British Journal of Medical Psychology, 61,* 329–338.

Burns, D. (1980). *Feeling good: The new mood therapy.* New York: Morrow.

DePaulo, R. (1989). DRADA: Lecture on depression. Depression and Related Affective Disorders Association, annual meeting, Johns Hopkins Hospital, Baltimore.

Dryden, W., & Golden, W. L. (1986). *Cognitive-behavioral approaches to psychotherapy.* London: Harper & Row.

Eaves, G., & Rush, A. J. (1984). Cognitive patterns in symptomatic and remitted unipolar major depression. *Journal of Abnormal Psychology, 33,* 31–40.

Ellis, A. (1973). *Humanistic psychotherapy.* New York: Crown and McGraw-Hill Paperbacks.

Ellis, A., & Whiteley, J. M. (Eds.). (1979). *Theoretical and empirical foundations of rational-emotive therapy.* Monterey, CA: Brooks/Cole.

Endler, N. S. (1982). *Holiday of darkness: A psychologist's personal journey out of his depression.* New York: Wiley-Interscience Press.

Free, M. L., & Oei, T. P. S. (1989). Biological and psychological processes in the treatment and maintenance of depression. *Clinical Psychology Review, 9,* 653–688.

Goethe, J. W., Szarek, B. L., & Cook, W. L. (1988). A comparison of adequately vs. inadequately treated depressed patients. *Journal of Nervous and Mental Disorders, 176,* 465–470.

Gold, P. W., Goodwin, F. K., & Chrousos, G. P. (1988). Clinical and biochemical manifestations of depression: Relation to the neurobiology of stress. *New England Journal of Medicine, 319,* 348–353.

Goodwin, F. K. (1988). Talk presented at the Depression and Related Affective Disorders Conference, Johns Hopkins Medical Center, Baltimore.

Goodwin, F. K. (1989). *Mood disorders: Diagnosis and treatment.* Presented at the Mood Disorders Symposium, Spring Grove Hospital Center, Catonsville, Maryland.

Hollon, S. D. (1984). Cognitive therapy for depression: Translating research into practice. *The Behavior Therapist, 7,* 125–127.

Hollon, S. D. (1988). Presentation at the Cognitive Behavior Therapy Meeting, Washington, D.C.

Johnstone, E. C. (1988). *Depression: An integrative approach.* Report of a Joint Conference of the Royal College of Physicians and the Mental Health Foundation. *Journal Royal College of Physicians, 22,* 185–187.

Jones, E. (Ed.). (1950). Mourning and melancholia. In *Collected Papers.* London: Hogarth Press and Institute of Psycho-Analysis, 4, 152–170.

Joyce, P. R., & Paykel, E. S. (1989). Predictors of drug response in depression. *Archives of General Psychiatry, 46,* 89–99.

Kaminsky, M. J. (1986). *Psychotherapy with patients with endogenous depression.* Grand Rounds, Department of Psychiatry, Johns Hopkins University Hospital, Baltimore.

Kiloh, L. G., Andrews, G., & Neilson, M. (1988). The long-term outcome of depressive illness. *British Journal of Psychiatry, 153,* 752–757.

Klein, D. N., Clark, D. C., Dansky, L., & Margolis, E. T. (1988a). Dysthymia in the offspring of parents with unipolar affective disorder. *Journal of Abnormal Psychology, 97,* 265–274.

Klein, D. N., Taylor, E. B., Harding, K., & Dickstein, S. (1988b). Double depression and episodic major depression: Demographic, clinical, familial, personality and socioenvironmental characteristics and short-term outcomes. *American Journal of Psychiatry, 145,* 1226–1231.

Kluft, R. P. (1986). High-functioning multiple personality patients. *Journal of Nervous and Mental Disease, 174,* 722–726.

Lewinsohn, P., Hoberman, H., & Rosenbaum, M. (1988). Risk factors for unipolar depression. *Journal of Abnormal Psychology, 97,* 251–264.

MacKensie, A. (1985). Personal view. *British Journal of Psychiatry, 291,* 1044.

Mash, E. J. (1989). Treatment of child and family disturbance: A behavioral-systems perspective. In E. J. Mash & R. A. Barkley (Eds.), *Treatment of Childhood Disorders.* New York: Guilford Press.

Norman, W. H., Miller, I. W., & Dow, M. G. (1988). Characteristics of depressed patients with elevated levels of dysfunctional cognitions. *Cognitive Therapy and Research, 12,* 39–52.

Pilkonis, P. A., & Frank, E. (1988). Personality pathology in recurrent depression: Nature, prevalence, and relationship to therapeutic response. *American Journal of Psychiatry, 145,* 435–441.

Plath, S. (1971). *The bell jar.* New York: Bantam.

Post, R. M., Roy-Byrne, P. P., & Uhde, T. W. (1988). Graphic representation of the life course of illness in patients with affective disorder. *American Journal of Psychiatry, 145,* 844–848.

Regier, D. A., Hirschfeld, R. M. A., Goodwin, F. K., Burke, J. D., Jr., Lazar, J. B., & Judd, L. L. (1988). The NIMH Depression Awareness, Recognition, and Treatment program: Structure, aims, and scientific basis. *American Journal of Psychiatry, 145,* 1351–1357.

Rippere, V., & Williams, R. (Eds.). (1985). *Wounded healers: Mental health workers' experiences of depression.* Chichester, England: Wiley.

Rosenthal, N. E., & Wehr, T. A. (1987). Seasonal affective disorder. *Psychiatric Annals, 17,* 670–674.

Rosenthal, N. E., Sack, D. A., Gillin, J. C., Lewy, A. J., Goodwin, F. K., Davenport, Y., Mueller, P. S., Newsome, D. A., & Wehr, T. A. (1984). Seasonal affective disorder: A description of the syndrome and preliminary findings with light therapy. *Archives of General Psychiatry, 41,* 72–80.

Rush, A. J. (Ed.). (1982). *Short-term psychotherapies for depression.* New York: Guilford Press.

Rush, A. J. (1983). Cognitive therapy of depression. *Psychiatric Clinics of North America, 6,* 105–127.

Rush, A. J., Beck, A. T., Kovacs, M., & Hollon, S. (1977). comparative efficacy of cognitive therapy and imipramine in the treatment of depressed outpatients. *Cognitive Therapy and Research, 1,* 17–37.

Schuyler, D. (1984). Cognitive therapy of depression. Presentation at the first Post-Doctoral Institute Symposium, Taylor Manor Hospital, Ellicott City, Maryland.

Seligman, M., Castellon, C., Cacciola, J., Schulman, P., Luborsky, L., Ollove, M., & Downing, R. (1988). Explanatory style change during cognitive therapy for unipolar depression. *Journal of Abnormal Psychology, 97*, 13–18.

Slater, E., & Roth, M. (1969). *Clinical psychiatry* (3rd ed.). Baltimore: Williams & Wilkins.

Styron, W. (1988). Why Primo Levi need not have died. Editorial, *New York Times*, December 19.

Styron, W. (1989). Darkness visible. *Vanity Fair*, December.

Walen, S. R., DiGiuseppe, R., & Wessler, R. (1980). *A practitioner's guide to rational emotive therapy*. New York: Oxford University Press.

Wehr, T. A., Sack, D. A., Rosenthal, N. E., & Cowdry, R. W. (1988). Rapid cycling affective disorder: Contributing factors and treatment responses in 51 patients. *American Journal of Psychiatry, 145*, 179–184.

Young, J. (1989). Schema-focused cognitive therapy for personality disorders. In A. T. Beck & A. Freeman (Eds.), *Cognitive therapy of personality disorders*. New York: Guilford Press.

Psychological Messages and Social Context

Strategies for Increasing RET's Effectiveness with Women

JANET L. WOLFE AND HEDWIN NAIMARK

> There will be some fundamental assumptions which adherents of all the various systems within the epoch unconsciously presuppose. Such assumptions appear so obvious that people do not know what they are assuming because no other way of putting things has ever occurred to them.
>
> Alfred North Whitehead
>
> If you just bought the culture, the average person will never get around to the answers because he or she hasn't begun to ask the right questions.
>
> Bonnie Strickland

Effective RET involves helping clients to help themselves by questioning the should's, the awfulizing, and the self-downing that lead to emotional disturbance and that limit one's options in living a happy, productive, and fulfilled life.

The question that prompted us to write this chapter is: Are the working principles of RET equally effective in treating women and men? As RET practitioners, we would like to think they are. But to date, we have virtually no outcome or process research to answer this question definitively. What we do have, instead, is knowledge of our own lives and an awareness of the differences in the way men and women are perceived in

JANET L. WOLFE AND HEDWIN NAIMARK • Institute for Rational-Emotive Therapy, 45 East 65th Street, New York, New York 10021.

contemporary Western society (Block, 1973; Chesler, 1972; Spence, Deaux, & Helmreich, 1985), despite strides made recently in redressing imbalances in the workplace and the home (Milwid, 1983; Naimark et al., 1987).

Most likely, then, there are important differences between the experiences and perspectives of men and women that had better be explicitly addressed in doing RET with women, if this therapeutic modality is to be optimally effective.

For example, many women who present for therapy have grown up in a culture that frequently places them in a double bind. By following traditional feminine models, women are more likely to receive social acceptance and relationship maintenance. Yet, the traditional feminine role also incorporates behavioral deficits, lower self-esteem, and more characteristics labeled unhealthy or neurotic (Davis & Padesky, 1990; Resick, 1985).

If women's sex-role socialization produces possible skill deficits that militate against their achieving power and autonomy, as well as rules for living that sabotage their pursuit of self-actualization while they involve themselves in giving to others, then therapy had better overtly question and challenge these messages about sex-role stereotypes. But many mental health professionals believe that they should help clients make their own choices in an atmosphere that is "value-free" (Lerner, 1978). Thus, considerable controversy exists about whether bringing into the therapy sessions a discussion of often unexamined and unconsciously held assumptions about the "feminine" role undermines therapy's value neutrality. Despite the therapist's best intentions, his or her own values and attitudes *will* influence the goals, process, and outcome of treatment and may affect both the interventions that are made and those that are *not* made in the course of therapy (Denmark, 1980; Frank, 1973; Lerner, 1988). Therefore, the issue is not so much whether there are values in therapy. Clearly, there are. One is to help the client function better in the environment in which he or she wishes to live. This is an essentially conservative value; that is, it is good to adapt to the situation in which one finds oneself. The fundamental problem with values in therapy is not that they exist, but that they are frequently not made explicit; instead, they are unspoken assumptions about the nature of truth and reality.

The thesis of this chapter, then, is that most people in this so-called liberated age are, to some extent, still unaware of how sex-role values or stereotypes impinge on people in general, and specifically on both clients and therapists involved in the therapeutic process. We present a model and outline the ways in which these subtle attitudes about sex roles become part of our automatic repertoire of cognitions, and how they influence our behavior. In the second part of the chapter, we describe methodologies and provide sample materials that can help both therapists and clients to become more aware of, to challenge, and perhaps to opt to change these values in the interest of improving people's mental health, productivity, and satisfaction. These methodologies are divided into three sections: (1) the case study; (2) exercises for challenging stereotypes; and (3) exercises designed primarily to encourage women's self-empowerment.

It should be noted that this chapter focuses on the problems of female clients. However, women do not live in a vacuum. Most interact with men in the workplace, in the family, and in their social lives. Therefore, men's perceptions and experience will be addressed as they relate to the lives of women. But more important, the principles presented here can easily be applied to men's lives in a way that may enhance their psychological growth and well-being. Although engaging men in the questioning process (and noting the possible benefits to men of becoming involved in challenging sex-role values) is not the focus of this chapter, the reader is invited to make the necessary analogies and to consult the appropriate literature in order to apply the principles to men (Lamb, 1976; O'Neil, 1981; Pleck, 1981, 1985).

THE VICIOUS CYCLE OF SEX-ROLE STEREOTYPES

The psychological literature is replete with theoretical positions and concrete examples of sex-role stereotyping and the detrimental and sometimes debilitating effects of this process on women (Bem & Lenney, 1976; Brehoney, 1983; Broverman, Broverman, Clarkson, Rosenkrantz, & Vogel, 1970; Kelly, Kern, Kirkley, Patterson, & Keane, 1980; Rothblum, 1983). Below, we suggest a model for the way in which this process may operate (see Figure 1). Although our focus is on the woman as the target, keep in mind while reading that the process of sex-role stereotyping also occurs in the lives of men. Although it can be shown historically that women, as a group, have been deprived more than men because of stereotyping (Baruch & Barnett, 1983; Norton, 1981; Reskin, 1984), this is not to say that the process is not detrimental to men.

The process of sex-role stereotyping begins with messages that infants, toddlers, children, and adolescents receive as they grow up in their social context (Step 1 in the cycle). These messages begin early (Block, 1973) and start to affect children's behavior and ideation even before language capacity evolves (e.g., the way adults physically handle boy and girl infants, the toys and clothing that are provided, and the activities that are offered). The messages come from many sources: parents, siblings, teachers, other members of the social milieu, and the media (Fodor, 1990; Heriot, 1983).

By the time children are grown, these messages have been internalized and have developed into belief systems within the individual (Step 2). Many of these beliefs are irrational in that they represent demandlike proscriptions, or should's in RET parlance. In the case of women, beliefs are

FIG. 1. The "vicious" cycle of sex-role stereotypes (its effects on women).[1]

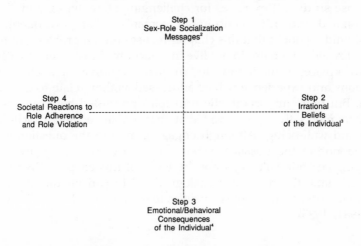

[1]The cycle is not unidirectional. Note the various directions in which influence occurs.
[2]For example, little girls should wear pink. Girl babies need lots of gentle handling and soft toys. Girls shouldn't play rough games. Girls are good at English and bad at math. Women must be thin and keep their mouths shut.
[3]For example, I *must* be thin to attract men (and I *must* attract men).
[4]For example, I'm anxious because of my diet. Or: I'm depressed because I can't get a man, so I eat to comfort myself. I don't let him see how smart I am because I'm nervous that he'll think I'm "too much" for him.

common that they "should" or even "must" talk, behave, feel, look, and think in certain ways if they are to be accepted, valued, and appreciated by men.

Such demanding thoughts or beliefs in the individual's head create both affect, often dysfunctional, and motivation to behave in specific ways (Step 3). Feelings of diminished self-worth, anxiety about the consequences of sex-role-inappropriate behavior, and depression over lack of control are not uncommon in the "normal" female population and are frequently found in women seeking therapy. Self-defeating behaviors, including procrastination, lack of assertiveness, failure to follow through on self-generated goals, pleading and nagging with significant others, and hesitation or inability in reaching and implementing decisions are often present in women. Moreover, these behavioral and affective outcomes have attitudinal correlates. The individual woman may herself have biases and may behave in discriminatory ways toward other women and toward men. In the least benign case, the woman may not be simply emotionally distressed and biased but may experience severe psychopathology.

The cycle is completed as society reacts to women (Step 4). Institutional principles and programs (e.g., school curricula, media messages, political policy, health care services, business practices, and financial relations) are designed to serve as reminders of the existence and value of sex-role stereotypes. Society notices whether a woman is adhering to implicitly agreed-upon norms, and it reacts negatively to breaches of those norms (Heriot, 1983; Kelly et al., 1980). Furthermore, society is constantly reacting not only to the actual behavior and affective display of women, but to sex-role messages that abound. These messages, even when expressed in stereotypical but not irrational terms (i.e., women "are" loving creatures rather than women "must be" loving creatures), directly affect societal patterns.

Clearly, links between the steps in the cycle are not unidirectional. Women's irrational beliefs, many of which were learned in childhood, are passed on through the socialization messages that women provide to their own children. Moreover, people often react negatively to the behaviors and feelings of women. These reactions then fuel the fires of socialization efforts. At the same time, socialization efforts feed into societal reactions to women. Societal reactions also affect women's behavior and feelings. Finally, societal reactions both affect and are affected by women's irrational beliefs (e.g., a woman believes that she must diet until she dies or she believes she must eat to comfort herself for the societal problems she faces). Society reacts negatively to the fat woman but has mixed reactions to the dieter. Whereas the "thinness" is admired, the "dieting" is a sign of demeaned status and value.

The Content of the Steps in the Cycle

The model of the vicious circle can be applied to many topic areas and distinctive types of messages. Some of these have already been suggested above. Some may vary across subcultures, social classes, or even geographical regions, and certainly many vary across historical periods. But currently, four major content areas seem prevalent in Western society: sex and love relationships, physical image and sexuality, work and career, and victimization and self-sacrifice. The material presented in Tables 1–4 reflects these four content areas and describes the four steps of the vicious circle in each area. The first step is presented in the far left column and summarizes typical sex-role socialization messages. The second column of each table contains examples of Step 2: individuals' irrational beliefs that emanate primarily from these sex-role socialization messages. The third column describes Step 3: the emotional and behavioral consequences for individual women who espouse irrational beliefs about their sex roles. The last column presents some examples of Step 4: societal reactions to women, especially to their adherence to or violation of female sex-role stereotypes.

Sex–love relationship messages to women (Table 1) seem to center on the notion that women are born to be loved and loving. Motherhood comes naturally; so does caregiving and gentility. Women without men are to be

TABLE 1. Sex–Love Relationships

Sex-role socialization messages	Irrational beliefs[a]	Women's emotional and behavioral consequences[b]	Societal reactions (to role adherence and role violation)
1. A woman without a man is unfulfilled.	1. I must be loved and approved by significant others to be worthwhile. I am nothing without a man. I need someone stronger on whom to rely.	Guilt Anxiety, phobias Low self-acceptance Boredom Depression Lack of assertiveness Trying to stay in a relationship at all costs (even if battered) Not focusing on career advancement Searching desperately for a mate Failing to self-actualize Psychosomatic illnesses	If passive/submissive: accepted but not valued. If assertive: called "castrating," "nag," "shrew." If married: homemaker role trivialized ("She's just a housewife"). If in dual-career marriage: is expected to do majority of housework. If a mother: accepted but not valued. Expected to be primary caretaker. If single: stigmatized as "old maid." If divorced: stigmatized; income goes down (while mate's goes up). If a lesbian: considered perverted, a loser, a manhater.
2. Nice, sweet girls get husbands.	2. I must not act assertively in front of men. I must not put my desires first.		
3. For women, work is nice, but love is better.	3. I must not take my work too seriously.		
4. A woman without children is like a tree without leaves.	4. I am nothing without a child.		
5. Women without men are weird or pitiable.	5. I must find a man, or people won't accept me, and I couldn't stand that.		
6. Women's main job is to catch a man.	6. As above.		
7. Bad kids come from bad mothers.	7. If my children are screwed up (or my marriage falls apart) I'm no good, a failure.		

[a]The irrational beliefs column derives directly from the sex-role socialization column.
[b]Any of the emotional and behavioral consequences and/or societal reactions can result from the sex-role messages and the irrational beliefs in the first two columns.

pitied and viewed as aberrant. Work never takes the place of love for women; if it does, there's something wrong with the woman.

Still more confusing are the messages about women's sexuality and physical appearance (Table 2). The paradoxes are numerous and the resultant double bind is stultifying. Women who are young, beautiful, and thin are valued. Although men want women to be sexy, the messages say, they do not want them to show it in the "wrong" way. There is the marrying kind of woman and the "other" kind, that is, the kind you take home to meet the family and the kind you take home to bed. And if a woman has won a man by displaying her sexuality, she is not to define or request the ways in which the sexuality will be expressed.

At work, women are described as being interested in and facile at "affiliation" but not at "tasks" (Table 3). It is common to hear such comments as "Women are to be trusted only with menial work" (everyone knows that they might have PMS and mess up the deal!); "Women can't add two and two"; and "They're really better off at home." Although the fabric of the business and professional world often subtly denies women access to the highest levels of authority (Kanter, 1977; Milwid, 1983), those in power usually assess women's failure to advance as a sign of their inherent incompetence (Naimark et al., 1987). The message: One really can't bring women into the boardroom (or the operating room) and expect anything to get done. On the other hand, women who do succeed are frequently described as "bitchy," or as conniving users who've probably "slept their way to the top."

Finally, women are implicitly, though rarely explicitly, envisioned as willing victims in their own situation (Table 4). They are seen as born to be self-sacrificing; the role they love is to serve others. Many people believe that there's really nothing wrong with pushing women around sexually (Colao, 1983; O'Hare & Taylor, 1983), professionally, or personally: it's what they want and expect. Should women happen to resist or shed the role of victim, they are to be feared and detested not only by men, but by other women as well.

Although some dramatic license has been taken in the examples of stereotypical messages included in the tables, and although there are many men and women who would not subscribe to any or all of them, it is our contention that none of us has fully escaped their impact.

The Direction of Influence

These tables do not imply a unidirectional relationship between one column and another, and it is important to note that RET does suggest a definite direction in the relationship between Steps 2 and 3. Irrational beliefs, it is hypothesized, are the cause rather than the effect of behaviors or emotions (Ellis, 1962; Ellis & Becker, 1982). In other words, each person

TABLE 2. Physical Image and Sexuality

Sex-role socialization messages	Irrational beliefs[a]	Women's emotional and behavioral consequences[b]	Societal reactions (to role adherence and role violation)
1. Thin, young, beautiful women are valuable; others are not.	1. If I'm not thin (young, beautiful), I'm disgusting. If I'm middle-aged, my life is essentially over. I must do everything to look beautiful (wear makeup, enlarge my breasts, decrease my thighs, shorten my hair, lengthen my legs!).	Anxiety and self-downing for even slight weight gain or other physical imperfections. Preoccupation with food. Eating disorders (85% of anorexics). Support billion-dollar cosmetic and weight reduction industry. Rage (at self or others). Terror of aging.	Deification of thin, young, beautiful women. Older women at parties: invisible. Double standard for overweight women and men (women ridiculed). Sexually unresponsive women: considered "frigid"; "uptight."
2. Nice women don't tell men what they want sexually.	2. I should look sexy but not act sexy, lest I make him feel inadequate.	Lack of sexual fulfillment; fear of rejection or "hurting" partner if assertive sexually.	Sexually assertive women considered "castrating"; "loose."
3. There are two kinds of women: sexy and motherly; the two don't go together.	3. I should be sexy but not look sexy, lest he not marry me.		Industries designed to sell women endless beauty products, diet pills, cosmetic surgery, books, etc.; appeal to their fears of aging and spreading. Media, religious, educational, medical, etc., messages often designed to maintain status quo.

[a]The irrational beliefs column derives directly from the sex-role socialization column.
[b]Any of the emotional and behavioral consequences and/or societal reactions can result from sex-role messages and the irrational beliefs in the first two columns.

TABLE 3. Work and Career

Sex-role socialization messages	Irrational beliefs[a]	Women's emotional and behavioral consequences[b]	Societal reactions (to role adherence and role violation)
1. Women are emotional.	1. I really don't belong in a position of power (I'm an impostor).	Lower aspirations; less risk-taking and assertiveness. Fear of failure *and* success.	Discrimination in promotions, salaries. Women concentrated in lowest occupational groups, so aspiring women have few role models or access to people in power.
2. Women are not good at mechanics, math, and management (the 3 "M's").	2. I'll never learn to do math, so I mustn't even try.	Avoidance of tasks leading to job advancement (public speaking, generating new ideas).	Salary differentials for men and women of equal training, experience, and rank (least $ to single mothers).
3. Women are responsible for making relationships work.	3. I have to spend my time at work helping people to get along.	Nonassertiveness in seeking promotions, salary increases.	Assertive women in management positions considered "castrating," "dykes," "not real women," or have "slept their way to the top."
4. Be nice, be sweet; don't be too assertive.	4. I shouldn't rock the boat or be too pushy.	Trying to fit existing structure.	Working mothers especially discriminated against on the job, then blamed for being "bad mothers" or "bad workers."
5. Men need higher pay more than women.	5. I don't deserve more money.	Developmental lags in agentic functioning (autonomy; skill mastery).	Sexual harassment.
6. A woman's "real work" and sources of happiness is in taking care of her home and family.	6. I must have a sex–love relationship to be happy; work is only temporary; I must not be too involved.	If successful: anxiety about lesser chance of mating; sense of being an "impostor."	Gender isolation. Little institutional support (day care, help at home from spouse).
7. Successful women are "ball-breakers" or "sluts."	7. I have to be careful not to disturb anyone as I try to move ahead. I can't really show them what I know.	If mated, fear of (and guilt about) losing partner's love. If a parent, guilt over "abandoning" children.	

[a]The irrational beliefs column derives directly from the sex-role socialization column.
[b]Any of the emotional and behavioral consequences and/or societal reactions can result from sex-role messages and the irrational beliefs in the first two columns.

TABLE 4. Victimization and Self-Sacrifice

Sex-role socialization messages	Irrational beliefs[a]	Women's emotional and behavioral consequences[b]	Societal reactions (to role adherence and role violation)
1. Women's role is to please men sexually.	1. I must give him what he wants sexually.	Anxiety about being alone, resulting in bad mating choices.	Rape, incest, sexual molestation, and harassment.
2. Nice women take care of men.	2. I must satisfy his wishes.	Staying in abusive relationships.	Blaming women for messy house, noisy children, bad sex.
3. It's a woman's fault if the man is unhappy or the relationship fails.	3. If he's displeased, I'm bad, a failure.	Saying yes to unwanted sex.	Physical and psychological battering (one woman battered every 15 seconds).
4. A woman without a man is worthless.	4. I'm nothing without a man (i.e., incapable of coping, being fulfilled, or being happy).	Enduring abusive treatment in workplace and/or home.	37%–50% of women have experienced sexual or physical abuse before age 21.
5. Women's needs come last.	5. I must not take care of myself until everyone else is taken care of.	Depression about helplessness.	71% of women have had a significant instance of sexual harassment on the job.
6. Men lead; women follow.	6. I must accept the man's decisions.	Shame about not taking risks.	Portrayal of women as willing victims in media.
7. Women put up or shut up.	7. I must not argue or dispute the man's wishes or commands.	Fear of asserting desires.	Portrayal of women who do not accept victimization as dangerous "troublemakers."
8. Women expect to be pushed around.	8. It's my job to bear the burdens of womanhood in silence.	Harboring unresolved anger.	Lack of avenues for redress of women's grievances.
9. Women who open their mouths can expect to get them shut.	9. It's too dangerous to take a risk.		

[a]The irrational beliefs column derives directly from the sex-role socialization column.
[b]Any of the emotional and behavioral consequences and/or societal reactions can result from the sex-role messages and the irrational beliefs in the first two columns.

is free not only to accept or reject the early sex-role socialization messages, but to ignore or attend to society's reactions to particular behaviors. Although this line of reasoning makes logical sense, *we are arguing that for an individual to make the decision to reject or accept a value—defy or adhere to a norm—he or she must be aware of its existence, must understand something about its impact on his or her life, must have the opportunity to weigh the consequences of different approaches to it, and, in some cases, must receive some support or reinforcement for an atypical decision.*

Thus, although Steps 2 and 3 are not completely bidirectional, they are each more or less powerfully influenced by the presence of Steps 1 and 4.

THE VICIOUS CYCLE AND THE RET PROCESS

Consider the following cases, taken from supervisory presentations at the Institute for Rational-Emotive Therapy in New York.

A female therapist treating an obese female client focuses on the low frustration tolerance that prevents the client from sticking to her diet. She fails to address adequately the client's fundamental irrational belief, self-downing (influenced by the societal message that "Thin is beautiful"). The self-downing prevents the client from accepting herself though overweight. No serious challenge is raised to her belief that she must be thin to be acceptable and happy.

A male therapist learns of a female client's decision to accept a pickup offer from a male cab driver and her embarrassment about her decision, commenting to the supervisor that he thinks it was a "bizarre" thing for her to have done. In session, the therapist encourages the client not to engage in this behavior. He fails to make explicit the sex-role stereotype (women mustn't pick up men) and does not adequately reinforce the client for assertiveness. He thus subtly supports the client's belief that there is "something wrong with me if I pick up a cab driver."

A female therapist counseling a European woman about her marriage (to a European man) assumes, as does the client, that the stereotypical roles of the client's culture will prohibit change in her partner. The therapist concentrates on showing the woman that she can accept her husband as he is or leave him. She does not adequately explore the client's own stereotype (e.g., "He must take care of me even though I want to take care of myself"). In conjoint sessions, the therapist does not question the male partner about his sex-role stereotypes or explore whether he would be willing to challenge some of his stereotypes for the sake of keeping his partner.

A male therapist tells his female client to "kiss the ass" of her male boss who acts condescendingly because that behavior will help her keep her job. He does this without exploring other alternatives (e.g., talking to someone in the personnel department, investigating the possibilities of getting another boss, attempting to discuss the issue with the boss in a professional manner, or weighing the consequences of losing or giving up the job). Most important, the therapist does not corroborate the client's appropriate perception that there is sexism in the workplace.

These vignettes suggest that even therapists well trained in RET can be trapped by the processes of the vicious circle of sex-role stereotypes. The therapists' reactions do not appear to be purposeful attempts to harm the clients; yet, the omissions and commissions are, at best, thwarting the therapeutic process or, at worst, influencing the client to think rigidly and not to consider new options. By leaving sex-role stereotypes unexamined, the therapists in these vignettes have fallen prey to the vicious circle.

How could this have happened? RET certainly provides an effective and well-defined self-help system for facilitating personal growth and emotional well-being in men and women (Ellis, 1974; Ellis & Becker, 1982; Wolfe, 1975, 1985). It offers also a humanistic, presumably nonsexist vehicle for helping women work through their emotional and practical problems via a realistic, logical examination of their beliefs and philosophies (Ellis, 1974; Zachary, 1980). RET presumably teaches a woman how to define her problems, identify the variables that influence her present feelings and actions, and alter both her environment and her behavior in positive ways.

More than any other school of therapy, RET (and some other cognitive-behavioral therapies) appears to meet the criteria for effective, nonsexist therapy (Brodsky & Hare-Mustin, 1980; Robbins & Siegel, 1983). RET is designed (1) to deal with the should's, must's, self-rating, and love-slobbism inherent in sex-role messages, and to provide a concrete method for disputing them; (2) to help women to stop condemning themselves for their emotional disturbances and ineffective behavior; (3) to encourage autonomy, through disputing irrational beliefs, offering client involvement in goal setting and self-therapy, and including a behavioral component meant to teach more effective behaviors and skills; (4) to show women how to stop depressing themselves or making themselves dysfunctionally angry about their frustrations with unfair behavior (including sexism); and (5) to help them to reduce their anxiety about the consequences of changing (Wolfe, 1980).

Returning to the vignettes cited above, we must acknowledge that all the profound theoretical statements on RET (Oliver, 1977; Wolfe, 1985; Zachary, 1980), all the appropriate guidelines in the practical manuals (Ellis, 1985; Walen, DiGiuseppe, & Wessler, 1980; Wessler & Wessler, 1980), and all the good intentions of trainees and RET supervisors are not sufficient to guarantee that therapists will recognize their own or their clients' sex-role stereotypes or will intervene to question these stereotypes at salient moments.

In order to make possible the kind of vigilant awareness and readiness to question that are required if therapists are to interrupt or challenge the vicious circle, much work still needs to be done with RET and other therapies. The subtle force of long-held, and now implicit, assumptions about women's roles is as great and invisible as the air we breathe. Uncovering the layers of prejudice and, not infrequently, attacks against challenges to these assumptions will require courage, practice, and patience.

BUILDING AWARENESS OF AND CHALLENGING SEX-ROLE STEREOTYPES

Many strategies exist in the literature for enhancing awareness of sex-role stereotypes (Naimark et al., 1987; Sargent, 1977). How effective they are depends on many factors. For one, the atmosphere or setting in which an awareness-building exercise is generated needs to be a safe one. By *safe*, we mean free from anger, hostile responses to others, or danger of recrimination beyond the setting. Several tactics may help create this atmosphere.

First, if working in one-on-one sessions (i.e., a therapist and a client, or two therapists), acknowledgment of the participants' gender differences or similarities can be helpful. If, for example, a male therapist simply acknowledges that, as a man, he cannot know with any certainty what the female client or therapist has experienced (or vice versa), the atmosphere is made safer.

Second, when working with either mixed-sex or single-sex groups of clients or therapists, it is desirable to have both male and female leaders. The presence of both a male and a female leader makes it easier for a sense of equality to be established and maintained within the group. Moreover, the group has the opportunity to consider both the male and the female point of view, and to evaluate any discrepancies that arise. Finally, the male and female leaders, if adequately trained and aware of their own particular tendencies to think in sex-role-stereotypical ways, can provide behavioral models for the group.

Third, when training professionals, ground rules need to be clearly defined. A firm commitment to confidentiality, acceptance of everyone's admission of stereotypical thinking (including the leader's or therapist's), permission to disagree about any aspect of the training, and a forthright guarantee that all verbal responses, as long as they are not abusive, will be tolerated and not punished in any way are some of the rules that can sufficiently free the trainees so that participation will be open and honest. It should be noted that most of the procedures in dyadic situations may be applied to working with groups as well.

Strategies for Increasing RET's Effectiveness with Women

Each of the strategies described in the sections below can be used in different settings. Where counterindications are present (e.g., where a strategy is not appropriate for clients), they will be mentioned. In one sense, what one does may be less important than how one does it. The best exercise in the world will have little impact if, for example, the presenter is seen to be coercing change in the participants. Thus, in using any of the materials that follow, the reader is advised to work *first* on his or her own level of anxiety or anger, as well as on any existing stereotypes that may impede the processes described.

Case Studies

The use of case studies is highly recommended. They are vivid. The comments of the participants are generally easier to elicit when case studies are presented than in any other format. People report that it feels like giving one's opinion about some event that occurred rather than being tested for knowledge or checked for appropriate responses. One way to generate case studies of therapy or "real-life" experiences is to think about an occasion when some element of sex-role behavior or attitude seemed to be involved. Such simple experiences as hearing a parking attendant call a woman "honey" and immediately afterward call a man "sir," noticing that a male colleague seems short-tempered or silent whenever a female offers criticism of performance, or observing that a female therapist often speaks rudely to a female secretary but not to other female therapists can serve as "case studies."

The main questions to ask when a case is presented are:

1. Was sex-role stereotyping probably involved?
2. What was the stereotype?
3. Who expressed it?
4. How was it expressed?
5. What damage might it do to anyone involved?
6. How can it be questioned or challenged?
7. What benefits might accrue if it were given up?
8. Who might benefit if it were given up?
9. Are there any reasons to keep it?
10. What steps might help the person with the stereotype to give it up (e.g., identifying the feelings and irrational beliefs involved, disputing those beliefs, and trying out new behaviors)?

The following therapeutic case study is presented as typical of the issues frequently involved. Errors of omission are pointed out, and strategies for improved intervention are described. In this case, the therapist is a woman, and there are two clients: a male and a female. It is recommended that the reader consult Tables 1–4 after reading the case study to clarify what, if any, of the elements of the tables are present in the case study.

CASE STUDY

The Situation

Lynne, a 33-year-old woman, married for 12 years to Paul and mother of two children, ages 2 and 6, came into therapy to deal with her depression. She described herself as "fat, disgusting, unreasonably jealous, and a lousy household organizer." She indicated that her husband rarely wanted to have sex with her and that he was frequently highly critical of the mess around the house, which he saw no reason for, as she had only a 10-hour-a-week job outside the home in a public relations firm. Lynne's entire week tended to be consumed in caring for others; taking time to nurture herself was not in her repertoire. She was debating, at this point, whether to quit the job, which she enjoyed, to devote more time to house and children. She remarked that her mother and sisters attacked her for neglecting her role as wife and mother. Although the job gave her some income that she felt she could really "call her own," plus a sense of accomplishment, her husband argued that it brought in so little extra money that it was hardly worth sacrificing the well-being of their home life for it.

As Paul expressed willingness to be involved in the therapy, it was agreed that there would be joint sessions alternating with individual ones for Lynne and Paul. As it turned out, Paul came only three times—once individually and twice jointly—asserting that the demands of his job were too time-consuming for him to come more often, and that the problem, in any case, was largely "Lynne."

The Goals

During the early sessions, the goals for therapy were established, as is the practice in RET. Through discussion of the client's wishes and desires for therapy outcome, specific goals were designed for Lynne and Paul as follows:

Lynne

1. Work on her low frustration tolerance to help (a) reduce her "bingeing" (she was approximately 10 pounds overweight) and (b) overcome her avoidance of household tasks.
2. Work on reducing or eliminating anger at her husband's rejection of her.

3. Improve her ability (to act assertively) to express her sexual wants more directly; develop behavioral techniques for being more sexually seductive.
4. Increase capacity for decision making about whether to give up her public relations job.

Paul

1. Work on low frustration tolerance about wife's household organization.
2. Work on irritation about wife's wanting sex when he wasn't interested.
3. Increase assertiveness and decrease aggressiveness when criticizing wife's body and homemaking.
4. Develop relaxation techniques to help him unwind from his stressful work day.

Evaluation

Although basically good cognitive-behavioral therapy, the above treatment plan reveals subtle omissions rather than commissions, that is, blatant forms of sexism that can frequently affect the goals and course of therapy. Although the therapist may have had the best intentions in going along with the goals of the primary client, she failed to recognize the limited (and sex-role-scripted) options provided by the client and did not build into the goals concrete questioning or challenging of these options. She thus became part of the problem, rather than part of the solution. It is not uncommon for an exhausted and fairly isolated woman to begin treatment with the goal: "Make me a better wife and mother to my husband and children" (echoed by her husband, if he is involved). But the therapist, we argue, had better consider the vicious circle's application and at least discuss with the client the possibility of adding new goals or questioning the reasoning that led to the current ones.

Some specific strategies for interrupting the vicious circle are outlined below. They include attention to the stereotypes and irrational beliefs of the clients and a consideration of the links between these feelings and the emotional consequences experienced. Finally, some options are included for intervening in the "societal reactions" step in the cycle by dealing differently with family members and colleagues.

Revised Goals for Lynne

1. Identify and point out the effects of the sex-role messages that have become irrational demands in Lynne's head and that are affecting her self-acceptance. For example:

- I *must* be thin to be worthwhile and sexually attractive to my husband.
- It's *my sole* responsibility to maintain the household and children—especially if my husband works long hours outside the home and is the major breadwinner.
- I am a *bad person* for failing to meet my responsibilities.
- I *must not* think of my job as important.
- I'm being a *lousy mother* by insisting on keeping my job or wanting to have some outside activities and interests unrelated to my family.

2. Suggest support structures to combat Lynne's sense of isolation and to help her recognize her strengths (e.g., a consciousness-raising group and developing female friendships).
3. Legitimize some of Lynne's anger and frustration before jumping in to dispute its cognitive bases; avoid reinforcing the covert message that "Women *should* be nice and sweet and not rock the boat."
4. To combat Lynne's depression, self-downing, and sense of helplessness, encourage the inclusion in her week of several activities designed to increase her own individual pleasure in living, such as taking time to enjoy nature or to giggle with women friends. (It is helpful in combating self-downing to point out that the highest rates of depression are among women with young children who do not work outside the home, and that homemakers, although appearing to have realized "the American dream," are, in fact, in a situation where they get little power, environmental reinforcement, or sense of efficacy.)

Revised Goals for Paul

1. Insist on more therapy participation on the husband's part. (In the case as described, the success of the relationship was made to hinge largely on Lynne's changing her behavior, whereas Paul's "task" was mainly to learn to tolerate her lacks.) Avoid focusing most of the therapy on what is wrong with Lynne, so as not to reinforce Paul's idea that she is "the problem."
2. Encourage Paul to see the benefits he might gain if he were to reconceptualize "the problem" as not just Lynne's but his, the children's, and even society's.
3. Help him to challenge his own sex-role stereotypes and become more involved in the parenting role, pointing out that these new behaviors not only may be enjoyable but may increase Lynne's good feelings toward him.
4. Increase Paul's willingness to support his wife's wage-earner role, thereby perhaps taking some of the financial burden off him.

5. Suggest that Paul engage in more sexual behavior with his wife, not as a reward for her changing but as a desirable behavior in marriage.

6. Help Paul to become more empathic and reinforcing of Lynne's strengths (nurturance, mothering ability, etc.). Challenge Paul to correct his assumption that the stresses of the homemaker role are far less than those of his job.

Revised Goals for the Couple and the Relationship

1. Point out to both partners the depressiogenic effects for the woman of the homemaker role and of being economically dependent on a male provider.

2. Disclose the therapist's own biases, for example, her sense that women really should stay home full time with young children and her tendency to try to control the primary client. (The therapist in this case commented in supervision, "No matter how hard I push her, I just can't get her to be more assertive!")

3. Have statistics and resources available, such as:
   • Rates of depression among homemakers.
   • Weight tables.
   • Lists of resources and support groups for women.
   • Articles about two-career couples.
   • Information (books, articles, and programs at the workplace and in the community) for men.

Conclusions

In revising the goals and strategies for this couple and for each of the individuals, the therapist will intervene in the vicious circle of sex-role stereotypes, irrational beliefs, emotional and behavioral consequences, and even societal reactions, as both Lynne and Paul begin to challenge the status quo in their disturbed marital interactions.

As a result, the emotional climate in the home most likely will be improved, as will the sense of autonomy and the decision-making ability of the wife. Naturally, subtle imbalances in control and authority will be addressed in the process. There may be resistance to this process not only from the husband, who may believe that he is being unfairly asked to relinquish some control, but from the wife, who may hesitate to permit the husband real control over "her turf," in caring for the children and contributing to household management (Naimark *et al.*, 1987).

The therapist can help Lynne and Paul to succeed by repeatedly pointing out their irrational beliefs and their must's and should's about sex roles, and by putting the problems of the couple into a sociopolitical context, letting them know that they are not alone in trying to redefine equitable and satisfying relationships in contemporary society.

STRATEGIES AND EXERCISES THAT CHALLENGE SEX-ROLE STEREOTYPES

The exercises and interventions below are designed to enhance RET's effectiveness in the four content areas presented in Tables 1–4: (1) sex–love relationships; (2) body image and sexuality; (3) work and career; and (4) victimization and self-sacrifice. Each area is divided into two sections. Consciousness-raising exercises designed to clarify the sex-role socialization messages and irrational beliefs basic to women's experiential world are presented first. These exercises can be used either as part of therapist training or directly with clients. Suggestions and caveats for therapists only, including errors of omission and commission, are presented last. Although the organization of these materials is somewhat artificial, as the content areas frequently overlap, it provides an easy reference structure when working with clients or training therapists or, for that matter, other professionals (e.g., guidance counselors, relocation specialists, and corporate managers). As elsewhere in this chapter, the focus is primarily on women. Included, however, are a number of exercises, suggestions, and caveats for working with men. Extrapolating from these exercises to others designed solely to help men challenge stereotypes should not present a problem.

Sex–Love Relationships

To the leader-therapist:

1. Check out your own beliefs about men's and women's roles:
   - Do you believe that a married woman should stay home and take care of the children?
   - Do you believe that the male member of a couple should control and manage finances?
   - Do you believe that working couples should equitably divide housework and child care?
   - How would you define equality within marriage?
   - What do you think are some of the positive (and negative) effects of expanding roles for men? For women?
   - Do you think there are distinct "maternal" and "paternal" qualities that are specific to each sex, and if so, what are they? Do you think these qualities are biologically determined or a product of traditional sex-role socialization?
2. Use the questions and sentence completions below in therapeutic and training sessions with individuals, couples, or groups:
   a. What were some of your early family messages about being male? Female?
   b. Sentence completion (for couples groups):

Males: "In order for me to be a good husband, *you* must . . .";
"In order for me to be a good husband, *I* must . . ."
Females: "In order for me to be a good wife, *you* must . . ."; "In order for me to be a good wife, *I* must . . ."
(Have men and women keep alternating sentences until they've expressed many of their thoughts.)

  c. Do you act differently with men than with women? In what ways?

  d. Do you act differently at work than at home?

  e. Do you do a lot of things because you think it's what a woman (man) "should" do and not because you really want to? Give examples and discuss how you feel about this situation (examples: women afraid of being unfeminine if assertive; men thinking they must make sexual overtures).

  f. What kinds of behavior do you most dislike in a member of the opposite sex?

  g. Imagine you had been born with the genitals of the opposite sex. In what ways do you think your life would have been different?

  h. *For women*: What do you gain by your reliance on having a male in your life? What does it cost you?
    For men: What do you gain by being the major breadwinner and the person in charge? What do you lose?

3. Use these behavioral in- and out-of-session exercises with your clients and trainees:

  a. Go on a date with a member of the opposite sex. Each of you is to take on the sex-typed behaviors of the other gender, continuing the role playing throughout the date (for example: female orders wine, makes menu suggestions, orders, pays, and initiates after-dinner activity, including, if appropriate, sex; male acts submissive and supportive, goes along with female, lets female do most of the talking). Discuss your experiences together afterward.

  b. At a party or in a work situation, observe the behaviors of males and females, paying attention to such factors as nonverbal behavior, the quality and quantity of participation in conversations, male behavior toward older females as opposed to younger and/or more attractive females, and female behavior toward other females as opposed to males.

  c. Observe examples of "egalitarian" relationships—in life and in the media (e.g., Joyce and Frank in the "Hill Street Blues" TV series)—and study the attitudes and behaviors that underlie them. Think about what makes them egalitarian.

  d. Classroom or group workshop exercise: generate "nasty" slang words to describe each of the following four categories:

Sexually active women	Sexually selective women	Sexually active men	Men in general
Slut	Frigid	Don Juan	Fairy
Whore	Uptight	Swinger	Sissy
Tramp	Dyke	Stud	Pussy-whipped
Loose	Prude	Ladies' man	Bastard
Easy lay	Prick tease		Son of a bitch

Discuss the above labels as a reflection of attitudes toward women and men in our culture. Consider what they suggest about how people react to *behavior* as if it defined the person's totality. Reflect on the kinds of criticism involved.

4. Refer clients and trainees to some of these books of readings:
   Sisterhood Is Powerful (Morgan, 1970).
   Women and Psychotherapy: An Assessment of Research and Practice (Brodsky & Hare-Mustin, 1980).
   Women Changing Therapy (Robbins & Siegel, 1983).
   Women in Sexist Society (Gornick & Morgan, 1972).

Suggestions and Caveats in Working with Women

1. Given that much of a woman's self-worth is strongly tied to having a sex–love relationship, finding and keeping a relationship with a man frequently become the woman's major focus in therapy. To avoid tacitly feeding into the idea that a woman's worth and happiness depend on having a man, help the woman to explore other options, such as friendships with females, children, or males who will not become partners; and provide statistics and anecdotes countering the myth of the "lonely spinster." Clinicians have an ethical obligation to correct their own and their clients' prejudices and distortions about "women alone," helping to reframe living alone as a valid life status, rather than a condition to be alleviated (Gigy, 1980; Nadelson & Notman, 1981).

2. In helping the female client focus on her own dysfunctional feelings and behaviors in a relationship, take care not to reinforce the common cultural belief (held by men and women) that if a relationship fails, the woman is to blame. (Witness the titles of recent self-help books: *Women Who Love Too Much; Smart Women, Foolish Choices.*) Challenge women's tendency to blame themselves for bad relationships by validating women's experiences with abusive or exploitive behavior by males. Reinforce the point that men are equally responsible in relationships, and try to put the entire issue of relationship difficulties in the context of a sexist society. This approach is not meant to imply that women are helpless victims and men are

criminals; rather, it is to encourage equitable responsibility for each person in a relationship.

Questions and Caveats for Therapists Working with Couples

- Do you tend to see the more overtly upset partner (usually the woman, as it is expected that women will cry) as more disturbed than the calmer, quieter, and perhaps emotionally constricted partner? Do you view emotional excess as a higher order disturbance than emotional suppression?
- Do you collude with the husband because you are more sympathetic to his views (e.g., wives should do most of the housework), because you may yourself have a "nagging" wife at home (if male), or because you believe that a woman has no choice but to tolerate and accept the man's behavior (if female)?
- Do you use extra energy to engage the male partner in an alliance, perhaps because you sense his reluctance to be in therapy, or because you accept him as the person who holds the power in the relationship, and thus the power to keep the couple in therapy?
- Do you collaborate with the husband to "cure" the wife's passivity, neurosis, lack of assertiveness, and overdependence?
- Do you overemphasize the woman's and overlook the man's anger? (Some male therapists may be reactive to female "bitchiness" in that they see the active female as inappropriately angry and the active male as appropriately reacting to his partner's anger; Haan & Livson, 1973.)

Caveats for Nonsexist Therapists Sensitive to Feminist Positions

- Do you collude too much with the wife, perhaps sensing her passivity and wanting to help support her, thereby reinforcing her passivity and dependency?
- Do you get angry with males and lose touch with your ability to be a sensitive reflector of what's happening when men become evasive and deny feelings?
- Do you fail to notice the male's legitimate complaints about the relationship or the female?

Work

1. Check out your own beliefs about women in the workplace:
   a. Do you ask married women, "Do you work?" (as opposed to "Do you work outside the home?").
   b. Imagine yourself as a boss or policymaker in an organization. Do

you think that it would be your responsibility to provide paternity leaves? If a woman wished to stay on a career path but take
some time off to spend with her young child, would you be
willing to advocate for flextime? Would you hold her job open? If
so, for how long? Do you see it as part of your responsibility to
push for day care centers or day care referrals in your organization?

   c. Do you view the job of a full-time homemaker as less stressful or
      less important than that of the major breadwinner?
   d. Do you view it as more important, when push comes to shove,
      to give the male's career advancement priority over the female's?
   e. Can you imagine counseling a couple to relocate to benefit the
      female's career?

2. Group discussion questions:
   a. Do you act differently with men than you do with women in
      work situations? If so, in what ways?
   b. *For males*: Have you ever blamed your working wife for neglect-
      ing household work or child care?
      For females: Have you faulted yourself more than your mate for
      having an unclean house? For having problem kids?
   c. *For males*: Would you take a paternity leave if your company
      offered one and your spouse's career was at stake?
      For females: If your spouse wanted to take full responsibility (not
      just "help out") for major child care chores (e.g., making and
      keeping a doctor's appointment or planning a meal), would you
      let him?

3. Exercises outside the session:
   a. *For males and for women without children*: Spend a full week (pref-
      erably) or weekend in full charge of one or more young children.
   b. *To sensitize yourself to the situation of a lower-income single parent*:
      Keep on a tape of a baby crying and no air-conditioner.
   c. Spend a minimum of two days observing the behavior of men
      and women in your work environment, paying attention to gen-
      der-related differences in nonverbal behavior; touching; the
      quality and quantity of participation in discussions; interrup-
      tions; and special verbal styles such as prefacing sentences with
      "I think" or "I feel."

4. Educate yourself on some facts:
   • Women still earn an average of 66¢ to a man's $1.
   • Women are concentrated in the lowest paid occupations.
   • Companies are beginning to provide programs and information
     to help two-career couples.

5. Encourage women in your professional or work environment or
   among your friends to explore jobs with higher pay and status,

recognizing that it may be difficult for them to begin the process on their own because of guilt and low self-acceptance.

Suggestions and Caveats

1. Encourage women to:
   a. Look for good role models; possibly join a union or professional organization.
   b. Concentrate on the excitement (and not just the difficulties) of "pioneering."
   c. Develop a support network.
2. Advise women in two-career relationships to:
   a. Adopt different standards (e.g., less neat house and kids and less perfectionism in playing the "spouse" role).
   b. View their working as a valuable experience for their children's learning.
3. Have available a list of resources for helping women combat some of the inequities in the work world, for example, Title VII of the Equal Employment Act of 1972, names of agencies dealing with sex discrimination, lists of nonstereotypical educational and vocational options, and lists of professional women's organizations.
4. Be alert to the reduced expectations that women have of themselves, and brainstorm options other than their stated goal (e.g., getting a $15-a-week raise on their secretarial job); ask if they have thought of applying for managerial-level positions.
5. Do repeated assertiveness training to help change habits (e.g., failing to respond effectively to sex-role-biased criticisms or sexual innuendos, and avoiding competition). It is not uncommon for a $50,000-a-year female executive to break down in tears when her boss criticizes something that she has done, to act cute and seductive when her plan is rejected, or to sulk because she has been given a poor assignment.
6. Encourage covert and overt confidence building. Have clients log global self-criticisms (e.g., "I am a fool") and replace them with comments such as "I did that really well" or "I handled that criticism much better than I did last time." To boost confidence and help increase their self-marketing skills, ask clients to write a letter of recommendation about themselves.
7. Encourage women to develop skills that they may have told themselves they "can't do" (e.g., suggest that they take a course in financial management, computer programming, or auto repair).
8. Ask women to do life planning up to age 90, instructing them to do so independently of current constraints (financial, family, etc.).

Body Image and Sexuality

1. Check out your own beliefs about women's weight:
   - Do you believe that thin women are generally more attractive than women who are moderately fleshy? Do you "feel" a negative reaction to "fat" women?
   - When a woman client presents weight reduction as a goal but is in the range appropriate for her age and frame, do you consider helping her to set an alternate goal of self-acceptance of her weight as is (and to skip the weight reduction)?
   - Observe media representations of and your own reactions to a man and a woman who are moderately overweight. Are there any differences?
   - Do you think that sexy women *look* sexy?
   - Can you imagine a *very* sexy-looking woman as a competent mother?
2. Body-image exercises (in and outside the session):
   - Observe representations of "attractive" females in magazines, films, or TV. Record and then discuss in a group (accompanied by illustrations) the body images that are considered attractive for men and women. (Note: You will frequently see a somewhat portly male "success object," but rarely a plump female "sex object.")
   - Group exercise: Draw a picture of how you see your body. Pass the finished drawings around the room. Then, have the participants discuss how they feel about their body: the parts they like and dislike, the feelings they have when the parts they dislike are seen by persons of the same sex as opposed to the opposite sex, and so on.
3. Sexuality exercises:
   Think back to your most recent sexual experience. Who initiated it? Who set the pace? Changed positions? How satisfied were you and your partner with the experience? Did you ask your partner for what you wanted?
   For women: Have you ever faked orgasm? What are the things your partner can do to create the most sexual arousal? Emotional satisfaction?
   For men: How do you feel and act when you have problems getting or keeping an erection? When you ejaculate quickly? When your partner has not had an orgasm? When your partner rejects your sexual overtures?
4. Reading lists
   Body image:
   Fat Is a Feminist Issue (Orbach, 1978).
   Our Bodies, Ourselves (Boston Women's Health Collective, 1976).

Sexuality:
   The Hite Report on Female Sexuality (Hite, 1976).
   The Great Orgasm Robbery (Tepper, 1977).
   For Yourself (Barbach, 1975).
   How to Be Sexually Assertive (Wolfe, 1976).

Suggestions and Caveats

1. If a moderately overweight woman client (or one within the appropriate weight range for her height and build) proposes a goal of weight loss, do not try immediately to set the behavioral and cognitive programs designed to shape women into the thin mold defined by our culture. Establish as her first goal accepting herself with her weight as is, and learning to increase her satisfaction and pleasure in it.
2. Give reading assignments to help sensitize clients to how they've internalized the culture's "fat" attitudes (e.g., *Fat Is a Feminist Issue,* Orbach, 1978).
3. Work on sensuality enhancement: Have the woman learn to experience her body as a source of pleasure and aliveness, rather than disgust. This can include rolling in the grass in the sun; taking warm perfumed, bubble baths; massaging herself with lotion; and so on.
4. Help the woman redefine sexuality as including a wide range of behaviors, and not only penile-vaginal intercourse.
5. If a female client presents sexual issues such as sexual aversion or orgasmic and other arousal difficulties, refer her to a female therapist trained in sex therapy and, if available, to a women's sexuality group.
6. Be sure to validate the woman's own views of sex before you encourage her to consider other views. Remember that sexual pleasure is a personal experience. Your preferences may not be your client's.
7. Be careful not to infer that a female client who takes nontraditional approaches to sexual expression (with same- or opposite-sex partners) is somehow deviant.

Victimization

1. Check out your own beliefs about the following:
   Incest
   • It is usually a child's fantasy.
   • It happens mainly in lower socioeconomic groups or in the psychiatrically disturbed.

- A bad mother is responsible for the abuse.
- It may be OK because the child is at least getting sex education at home and receiving affection.

Rape

- Women provoke or incite attack by being in the wrong place or by wearing sexy clothes.
- Women rarely get raped by men they know.
- Women invent stories of rape to get men into trouble.
- Women frequently say "no" when they mean "yes."

2. Exercise:

In the workplace:

- Observe who puts an arm around, or a hand on the back or shoulder, when a male boss is talking to a male or female worker.

In the home:

- Who touches whom and how? Between parents and children? Between siblings? Between parents?

Touching another person is frequently a sign of power. Many men are apt to put their hand on a woman's back or an arm around her, or to chuck her under the chin or pat her on the head even during intellectual discussions. Many men feel free to put their arm around a woman, but not a man, and a woman rarely puts her arm around a man with whom she's not sexually involved. A potential conclusion: A woman's body is anyone's property (Henley, 1977).

3. Learn some facts (and share them, when appropriate, with clients):

- A woman is battered every 15 seconds in the United States.
- There are more shelters for abused animals than for abused women.
- Studies suggest that 25%–50% of women experience physical abuse or coercion in relationships; as many as 71% are sexually harassed; and 14%–20% report marital rape (Turkington, 1989).

4. Suggestions and caveats for dealing with victims of sexual, physical, or psychological abuse:

- In disputing a female client's "anger" cognitions, do not move too quickly to squelch her anger; first, empathize with her upset feelings. If you dispute her irrational beliefs about her experience too quickly, the client may continue to blame herself for her experience or leave therapy!
- Do not reinforce in any way the idea that the victim did something to provoke the abuse.
- If you experience frustration in dealing with a battered woman who is reluctant to leave her spouse, be wary of doing your own psychological battering by pushing her too hard when she resists. It is better to use a more evocative or option-planning approach, such as asking her, "How would you advise a high school student

on how to deal with this issue?" or "Let's look at some of the pros
and cons of staying with and leaving your partner."

- Help restore a sense of autonomy in the victim by a graduated set
  of behavioral tasks designed to help her get some control over her
  environment and awareness of her potential personal effectiveness.
- Keep an updated list of resources for incest, rape, and abuse
  victims. These can include shelters and self-help groups in your
  community; 24-hour hotlines; sources for low-cost career training;
  medical and legal assistance; women's career, assertiveness, sexuality, and other groups; women's martial arts training centers;
  women's centers; and women's resource directories.
- Be careful not to ignore reports of psychological abuse, such as
  yelling and screaming, swearing, threatening, and criticizing
  harshly. Such experiences need to be addressed and strategies
  developed to alter not only the beliefs about such experiences, but
  the behavioral responses to them.
- Refer clients, where appropriate, to a female therapist.

Special Considerations in Helping Women Become Self-Empowered

So profoundly are many women lacking in a sense of their own worth
and power that they may need even more help than has been provided so
far in this chapter. Thus, the final section is devoted to what amounts to a
basic retraining program in self-efficacy. Two areas will be discussed: (1) in-
session and at-home exercises for developing autonomy and self-acceptance (a basic emotional "muscle-building" workout) and (2) characteristics
of therapeutic settings and structures that maximize the possibilities for
women's self-efficacy.

The rationale for this basic training is the extraordinarily high incidence among women of chronic self-downing, low self-esteem, and feelings of helplessness, as well as the fact that at least 25% of women will be
affected by depression at some time in their lives. Many of these dysfunctional states are a result of their training to be submissive, dependent, and
passive, as well as their guilt over acting in their own interest. Thus, even
when they have the opportunity to be "captains of their own ship," they
perceive themselves as having little ability to decide what may be good for
them and even less capacity to act in ways that make these things happen.
Having failed to attempt the things that may help them achieve a sense of
success and mastery over their environment, they then give themselves
still more messages about their helplessness and worthlessness, thus per-
petuating the vicious circle of stereotypical feelings described above. These
themes get expressed repeatedly in women's ruminative beliefs that they
are stupid, helpless, inadequate, and incompetent, and in their concentra-

tion on what they cannot do and lack of attention to what they can do. In therapy sessions, the theme may prevail in terms of a female's reluctance to question the therapist out of fear of losing his or her approval. In life, even when women have the power to make decisions and influence their personal relationships or work environments, they frequently avoid using it out of a sense of basic self-distrust.

The following exercises (which can be tailored for use in individual or group therapy, or in workshop settings) provide an "enriched psychic workout" to help individual women combat their hopeless–helpless–worthless cognitions and enable them to be better equipped to go out and deal with their external world.

In-Session Exercises

The following five exercises can be used in ongoing therapy groups, one-day workshops, or time-limited groups such as a six-session women's weight or assertiveness group. They are presented in evocative language (sometimes in the second person) that the leader or therapist may find helpful in introducing the exercise:

1. *Goal setting.* Imagine yourself three years in the future, with your life being at its most ideal. Visualize the details of where and with whom you are living. What kind of work are you doing? How do you spend your leisure time? Now, change the picture to the worst possible one on the same future date, painting in the most unpleasant details. Finally, imagine your life as you realistically expect it to be in six months. (Share experiences and discuss.)

2. *Strongest hour.* Recall a time when you relied on yourself to deal with a difficult situation, a time when your inner strength pulled you through. Bring the situation into clear focus by remembering the details (the setting, the persons who were involved with you, the time and place, the things you and others said and did, your physical sensations, your emotions, and your reactions to others). Get a clear sense of yourself in the situation. Now enjoy your sense of satisfaction and pride about your successful handling of yourself in that situation. Experience the inner power that you used then, and that you're nurturing in yourself now. (Share experiences and discuss.)

3. *Autonomy.* Do exactly what you want to do now for the next two minutes. Keep checking to make sure this is really what you want to be doing. (Share experiences.)

4. *Resistance.* Relax. Begin to contemplate a change that you want to make in your life within the next year (examples: a career change; going on a trip alone; going back to school; changing your relationship with your partner, children, or parents; making new friends; adding fun to your life). Imagine as clearly as possible the effects in your life that your new change

may produce. Imagine a "tiny" figure of a person in your support network, either yourself or someone else who supports your growth and development. Let this support figure enumerate the reasons why you *can* make this change (how competent you are, how you can achieve what you set out to do, and so on). Then, imagine a "tiny" figure of a resistor. Have this resistor enumerate the reasons why you *can't* make this change ("You can't do this; there's no way"; "Who do you think you are?"). Now have the supporter and the resistor argue with each other, and listen to them. The time for decision has come. You must rip one of them out of your being, and that person will determine whether or not you make the contemplated change. Look the figure you yanked out in the face. Who is it? Look at the person you left in your body. Who is it? (Share experiences.)

5. *Running the session* (recommended for individual sessions). Tell your female clients that they can begin each session (without waiting for the therapist to do so), reporting on homework and establishing goals for the session. Let them know that they can be assertive when they feel their goals are not being addressed or if they disagree with a therapeutic intervention.

Homework Exercises for Clients and Participants

Self-Acceptance

1. Each day and evening, stand in front of the mirror and *enthusiastically* tell yourself three positive things about yourself—without any minimization or qualification. Do this every day for a month.
2. Keep a log of each time you put yourself down (overtly or covertly).
3. "Brag" at least three times a week about some strength or accomplishment to another person (e.g., boss, friend, or mate).
4. Write a "love letter" to yourself.
5. Interview a woman you know well (or even slightly) who appears to have a high level of self-confidence. Ask her the following questions: (1) How do you feel about yourself? (2) Did you always feel this way? (3) What were the big turning points in your life? (4) What risks did you take? (5) What was helpful to you in taking these risks? (Report on the interview to the group, or to your individual therapist.)

Self-Nurturance

These exercises are designed to combat cognitively and behaviorally women's internal messages about putting others first and not being selfish:

1. Be your own "prince" for one day a week. Do not take care of others; take care of *you*. Go for a walk in the park. Prepare (or

purchase) your favorite foods. If you can afford it, buy yourself flowers. Take a perfumed bubble bath or a leisurely shower. Treat yourself to caviar and cognac—in your own home or a country inn.

2. Consolidate a friendship with a new woman, child, or older person, as a means of getting loving, caring, sharing, intimacy, nurturance, and giggling into your life.

Assertiveness

1. Construct a hierarchy of assertiveness situations, from low-anxiety-provoking to high-anxiety-provoking ones. Do a minimum of one item a week on the list (e.g., make one comment each week in class; volunteer at work to do an important presentation or take a union responsibility; say "no" to an unreasonable request; or initiate a request for a kind of sexual stimulation you like).

2. Make an audio- or videotape of yourself in a simulated assertiveness situation. Note (without self-downing) both content and nonverbal areas for improvement. Pay special attention to things women frequently do to reduce their impact, including oversmiling, using a low voice tone, ending sentences with question marks, and qualifying ("This probably sounds stupid, but . . .").

3. Contact an organization that can provide resources to help you with a problem area (e.g., a city agency dealing with sexual harassment, a women's professional organization, a battered women's support group, a women's health organization, a financial management course, an organization providing assistance in dealing with chronically ill parents, or a list of corporations offering the best opportunities for women).

Physical Survival Skills

1. Take an Outward Bound wilderness survival course, or join a hiking club.
2. Enroll in a martial arts course.
3. Walk two or three miles alone in parts of the city or countryside that you do not know.

Therapeutic Structures and Settings for Maximizing Client Self-Efficacy

Considerable attention has been given, especially by feminist therapists, to the best structure for therapy with women. The following is offered to help the clinician assess such issues as individual versus group therapy, male versus female therapists, the recruitment of male partners into therapy, and participation by therapists and clients in consciousness raising and social-system change.

1. *All-women's therapy groups*. Dependence on others' approval and poor self-acceptance make it particularly difficult for women to accept themselves and persist in new behaviors in the face of heavy environmental "flak" for departures from feminine behaviors. In a women's group, validation and positive reinforcement for change can be an excellent facilitator of growth (Brody, 1987; Krumboltz & Shapiro, 1979). A second major benefit of women's groups is that, in viewing other women struggling with the same issues, the members tend to move from self-blame into viewing their deficits as due in large part to social forces. In addition, women are likely to participate more actively when in same-sex rather than in mixed-sex groups (Walker, 1987), to experience multiple models of women at various stages of change, and to have more opportunities for assertiveness training and resource sharing. Finally, women's groups provide a powerful message that women can support each other, feel good about themselves, and grow, without the presence of men.

2. *Female therapists*. Recent research has suggested that female clients may benefit from female therapists more than from male therapists (Howard & Orlinsky, 1979; Mogul, 1982). The quality of the relational bond between females, the female therapist's sensitivity to inherent power differences, same-sex role modeling, and the willingness of women to use themselves as vehicles for reaching empathic understanding may account for these effects (Maracek, Kravetz, & Finn, 1979; Walker, 1987). Others have asserted that it may not be as important to see a woman therapist as to see a male or female therapist with a nonsexist or feminist orientation, one who supports and understands desires for female equality and has made a special effort to work on sex-role issues (Freud, 1985). When Chambers and Wenk (1982) interviewed women who had experienced both nonsexist-feminist and traditional therapies, the women said that their traditional therapist had attempted to force them into a traditional mode, and that they had had more freedom of choice with their nonsexist/feminist therapists.

The potential disadvantages of male therapists for female clients include the following:

  a. It may be so gratifying for women to get support and empathy from a warm, nurturant male authority that the therapeutic relationship itself fosters dependency without facilitating autonomous problem-solving.
  b. Cultural pressures for women to please men are so profound that a woman's desire to be attractive and admired by her therapist may override a more honest process of self-definition and self-determination (Lerner, 1988).

c. Even the male therapist who is highly informed about sex-role issues may unconsciously persist in certain sexist behaviors. The research of Krulewitz (1981) and Krulewitz and Nash (1979), for example, has shown that some men find it difficult to identify with female victims, especially those victims of rape who have not offered resistance. As a result, these men deal more harshly with such women. There is evidence that males are more likely than females to react negatively to women's expression of anger. Men are also more likely than women to overlook subtle aspects of female compliance, dependency, and other factors, as these are the expectable and familiar ways that women relate to men in close dyadic relationships (Lerner, 1988).

3. *Female supervisors.* For many of the same reasons that female therapists may better facilitate the growth of women clients, so may female clinical supervisors help enhance the growth of female (and male) therapists. Female supervisors may be more likely to be sensitive to the subtle shifts by which female clients adapt to biases or empathic failures on the part of the therapist (Mendell, 1984). For example, female therapists may more easily notice a therapist's use of male gender pronouns when talking about doctors or the therapist's too quickly jumping into disputing a client's anger cognitions without first reinforcing her ability to feel and express her "unfeminine" feelings of anger. There is also some evidence that same-sex role models are more likely to facilitate career advancement in clinicians. Goldstein (1979) found the academic productivity of female scholars was positively associated with having had a same-sex dissertation adviser. In addition to increasing the percentage of female supervisors in training programs, formally incorporating the relationship between sex-role socialization and pathology into curricula is also advised.

4. *Participation by therapists in consciousness-raising groups.* An American Psychological Association Task Force (1978), in its recommendations for therapy with women, cited "awareness of all forms of oppression and how these interact with sexism" as an important principle. Participation in same-sex consciousness-raising groups provides the best vehicle for getting in touch with the subtle attitudes, behaviors, and sanctions that result from growing up male or female (Heppner, 1981; Kravetz, 1978). A portion of the group's time may be allocated to a discussion of how some of their beliefs about women may be influencing the therapy process with their own clients. Following participation in same-sex consciousness-raising groups, being in a mixed group may help to further elucidate male–female power differentials in action, as well as to provide opportunities for practicing underdeveloped skills (e.g., empathy training and listening skills for men, assertiveness training for women).

5. *"Recruiting" male partners into therapy.* Because a high proportion of

therapy clients are female, and a large percentage of these clients focus on relationship issues, a good deal of "couples" counseling is done with only the woman. It is recommended that strong efforts be made to bring the reluctant spouse into therapy. When this is not done, the therapist may be reinforcing the idea that the woman is the disturbed person who must be "fixed," as well as creating a further gap between the woman, who is changing in therapy, and her nonevolving spouse. Relationships are likely to continue to be dysfunctional and to suffer from major power imbalances until there is an active challenge to fundamental assumptions, such as male entitlement to unconditional and unilateral nurturance from females. One approach that has been successful in recruiting reluctant male partners is to have the female client relay to her mate that the therapist is concerned that she or he is only getting a biased, one-sided view from the female partner and needs more information. In many cases, the therapist's "calling in" the spouse has resulted in the beginning of a therapy process that actively involves both partners. Other means for inducing male involvement in therapy include establishing couples' groups and men's consciousness-raising and/or therapy groups.

6. *Attention to ethnic and other variables and stereotypes.* It is important to be aware of the subtle biases that influence *subgroups* of women. Examples include a black woman's belief that her husband will never amount to anything; a therapist's assumption that all Hispanic women are somewhat "hysterical," or that menopausal women are no longer interested in sex; or an assumption that in every lesbian relationship, one partner is "butch."

CONCLUSION

Conservative RET involves helping our female clients maneuver their way with less pain through the society as it is. In nonsexist or feminist-oriented RET, an attempt is made to awaken clients' interest in going beyond the status quo; for the status quo for women means fitting themselves into a role that binds, that keeps them from fully experiencing their humanness.

Effective RET with women means that, as therapists, we (1) repeatedly and conscientiously address sex-role issues with our clients (both female and male); (2) challenge our own stereotypes as regularly as we can; (3) seek to enhance our training wherever possible through consciousness raising and familiarization with special techniques for working with women; (4) strive to promote therapist–client relationship egalitarianism; (5) model nonsexist beliefs and behaviors for our clients; (6) actively involve ourselves in the bigger societal issues and, when appropriate, share that involvement with our clients; and (7) encourage our clients to seek (and offer) support for challenging sex-role stereotypes in the wider environ-ment (through familial, political, social, and community activity).

Failure to do all this—to address the social and cultural context of the client's problems as legitimate and important foci of treatment—is as inap-propriate as attempts to treat black persons while denying that racism is an ugly reality that affects us all (Bernardez-Bonesatti, 1976), or to draw con-clusions about females' reality from research based only on male samples.

REFERENCES

American Psychological Association Task Force. (1978). Report of the Task Force on Sex Bias and Sex Role Stereotyping in Psychotherapeutic Practice: Guidelines for therapy with women. *American Psychologist, 33,* 1122–1133.

Barbach, L. (1975). *For yourself: The fulfillment of female sexuality.* New York: Doubleday.

Baruch, G., & Barnett, R. (1983). *Correlates of fathers' participation in family work: A technical report.* Wellesley, MA: Wellesley College Center for Research on Women.

Bem, S. L., & Lenney, E. (1976). Sex-typing and the avoidance of cross-sex behavior. *Journal of Personality and Social Psychology, 33,* 48–54.

Bernardez-Bonesatti, T. (1976). Unconscious beliefs about women affecting psychotherapy. *North Carolina Journal of Mental Health, 7*(5), 63–66.

Block, J. (1973). Conceptions of sex role: Some cross-cultural and longitudinal perspectives. *American Psychologist, 28*(6), 512–526.

Boston Women's Health Collective. (1976). *Our bodies, ourselves.* New York: Simon & Schuster.

Brehoney, K. (1983). Women and agoraphobia: A case for the etiological significance of the feminine sex-role stereotype. In V. Franks & E. Rothblum (Eds.), *Sex role stereotypes and women's mental health* (pp. 112–128). New York: Springer.

Brodsky, A. M., & Hare-Mustin, R. T. (Eds.). (1980). *Women and psychotherapy: An assessment of research and practice.* New York: Guilford Press.

Brody, C. (Ed.). (1987). *Women's therapy groups: Paradigms of feminist treatment.* New York: Springer.

Broverman, C., Broverman, D., Clarkson, F., Rosenkrantz, P., & Vogel, S. (1970). Sex role stereotypes and clinical judgments of mental health. *Journal of Consulting and Clinical Psychology, 34,* 1–7.

Chambers, D. L., & Wenk, N. M. (1982). Feminist versus nonfeminist therapy: The client's perspective. *Women and Therapy, 1*(2), 57–65.

Chesler, P. (1972). *Women and madness.* Garden City, NY: Doubleday.

Colao, F. (1983). Therapists coping with sexual assault. In J. Robbins & R. Siegel (Eds.), *Women changing therapy* (pp. 205–214). New York: Haworth Press.

Davis, D., & Padesky, C. (1990). Enhancing cognitive therapy with women. In A. Freeman, K. Simon, L. Buetler, & H. Arkowitz (Eds.), *Comprehensive handbook of cognitive therapy* (pp. 535–557). New York: Plenum Press.

Denmark, F. (1980). From rocking the cradle to rocking the boat. *American Psychologist, 35*(12), 1057–1065.

Ellis, A. (1962). *Reason and emotion in psychotherapy.* Secaucus, NJ: Citadel Press.

Ellis, A. (1974). Treatment of sex and love problems in women. In V. Franks & V. Burtle (Eds.), *Women in therapy* (pp. 284–306). New York: Brunner/Mazel.

Ellis, A. (1985). *Overcoming resistance.* New York: Springer.

Ellis, A., & Becker, I. (1982). *A guide to personal happiness.* North Hollywood, CA: Wilshire Books.

Fodor, I. (1990). On turning 50: No longer young—not yet old. *The Behavior Therapist, 13*(20), 39–44.

Frank, J. (1973). *Persuasion and healing.* New York: Schocken Books.

Franks, V. (1982). *Psychotherapy and women: Letter No. 79.* Belle Mead, NJ: Carrier Foundation.

Freud, S(ophie). (1985, December). *Women.* Workshop presented at The Evolution of Psychotherapy Conference, Phoenix, Arizona.

Gigy, L. L. (1980). Self-concept of single women. *Psychology of Women Quarterly, 5*(2), 321–340.

Gornick, V., & Morgan, R. (Eds.). (1972). *Woman in sexist society.* New York: Signet.

Haan, N., & Livson, N. (1973). Sex differences in the eyes of expert personality assessors: Blind spots? *Journal of Personality Assessment, 37,* 486–492.

Henley, N. M. (1977). *Body politics: Power, sex and nonverbal communication.* Englewood Cliffs, NJ: Prentice-Hall.

Heppner, P. P. (1981). Counseling men in groups. *Personnel and Guidance Journal, 60,* 249–252.

Heriot, J. (1983). The double bind: Healing the split. In J. Robbins & R. Siegel (Eds.), *Women changing therapy* (pp. 11–28). New York: Haworth Press.

Hite, S. (1976). *The Hite report.* New York: Macmillan.

Howard, K. I., & Orlinsky, P. E. (1979). *What effect does therapist gender have on outcome for women in psychotherapy?* Paper presented at the American Psychological Association, New York.

Kanter, R. M. (1977). *Men and women of the corporation.* New York: Basic Books.

Kelly, J. A., Kern, J. M., Kirkley, B. G., Patterson, N. N., & Keane, F. M. (1980). Reactions to assertive versus nonassertive behavior: Differential effects for males and females, and implications for assertive training. *Behavior Therapy, 11,* 670–682.

Kravetz, D. (1978). Consciousness-raising groups in the 1970's. *Psychology of Women Quarterly, 3*(3), 168–186.

Krulewitz, J. E. (1981). Sex differences in evaluations of female and male victims' responses to assault. *Journal of Applied Social Psychology, 11*(5), 460–474.

Krulewitz, J. E., & Nash, J. (1979). Effects of rape victim resistance, assault outcome, and sex of observer on attributions about rape. *Journal of Personality, 47*(4), 557–574.

Krumboltz, H. B., & Shapiro, J. (1979). Counseling women in behavioral self-direction. *Personnel and Guidance Journal, 4,* 415–418.

Lamb, M. E. (Ed.). (1976). *The role of the father in child development.* New York: Wiley.

Lerner, H. E. (1978). On the comfort of patriarchal solutions: Some reflections on Brown's paper. *Journal of Personality and Social Systems, 1*(3), 47–50.

Lerner, H. E. (1988). *Women in therapy.* New York: Harper & Row.

Maracek, J., Kravetz, D., & Finn, S. (1979). Comparison of women who enter feminist therapy and women who enter traditional therapy. *Journal of Consulting and Clinical Psychology, 47*(4), 734–742.

Mendell, D. (1984). *Cross-gender supervision of cross-gender therapy.* New York: Postgraduate Center for Mental health.

Milwid, B. (1983). Breaking in: Experiences in male-dominated professions. In J. Robbins & R. Siegel (Eds.), *Women changing therapy* (pp. 67–79). New York: Haworth Press.

Mogul, K. M. (1982). Overview: The sex of the therapist. *American Journal of Psychiatry, 139,* 1–11.

Morgan, R. (Ed.). (1970). *Sisterhood is powerful: An anthology of writings from the women's liberation movement.* New York: Vintage Books.

Nadelson, C. C., & Notman, M. T. (1981). To marry or not to marry: A choice. *American Journal of Psychiatry, 138*(10), 1352–1356.

Naimark, H., & the staff of Catalyst. (1987). *New roles for men and women: A report on an educational intervention with college students.* New York: Catalyst.

Norton, E. (1981). Remarks at First Annual Women in Crisis Conference. In P. Russianiff (Ed.), *Women in crisis* (pp. 24–31). New York: Human Sciences Press.

O'Hare, J., & Taylor, K. (1983). The reality of incest. In J. Robbins & R. Siegel (Eds.), *Women changing therapy* (pp. 215–230). New York: Haworth Press.

Oliver, R. (1977). The "empty nest syndrome" as a focus of depression: A cognitive treatment model, based on rational-emotive therapy. *Psychotherapy: Theory, Research and Practice, 14*(1), 87–94.

O'Neil, J. M. (1981). Male sex role conflicts, sexism, and masculinity: Psychological implications for men, women, and the counseling psychologist. *Counseling Psychologist, 9*, 61–80.

Orbach, S. (1978). *Fat is a feminist issue*. New York: Paddington Press.

Pleck, J. H. (1981). *The myth of masculinity*. Cambridge: MIT Press.

Pleck, J. H. (1985). *Working wives, working husbands*. Beverly Hills, CA: Sage.

Resick, P. (1985). Sex role considerations for the behavior therapist. In M. Hersen & A. Bellack (Eds.), *Handbook of clinical behavior therapy with adults*. New York: Plenum Press.

Reskin, B. (1984). Sex segregation in the work place. In *Gender at work: Perspectives on occupational segregation in comparable worth*. Washington, DC: Women's Research and Education Institute of the Congressional Caucus for Women's Issues.

Robbins, J., & Siegel, R. (Eds.). (1983). *Women changing therapy*. New York: Haworth Press.

Rothblum, E. (1983). Sex role stereotypes and depression in women. In V. Franks & E. Rothblum (Eds.), *Sex role stereotypes and women's mental health* (pp. 83–111). New York: Springer.

Sargent, A. (1977). *Beyond sex roles*. St. Paul, MN: West Publishing.

Spence, J. T., Deaux, K., & Helmreich, R. L. (1985). Sex roles in contemporary American society. In G. Lindzey & E. Aronson (Eds.), *Handbook of social psychology* (3rd ed., Vol. 2, pp. 149–178). New York: Random House.

Tepper, S. (1977). *The great orgasm robbery*. Lakewood, CO: RAJ Publications.

Turkington, C. (1989). Body image in girls pushes rate of depression up. *APA Monitor*.

Walen, S., DiGiuseppe, R., & Wessler, R. L. (1980). *A practitioner's guide to rational-emotive therapy*. New York: Oxford University Press.

Walker, L. J. (1987). Women's groups are different. In C. Brody (Ed.), *Women's therapy groups: Paradigms of feminist treatment* (pp. 3–12). New York: Springer.

Wessler, R. A., & Wessler, R. L. (1980). *The principles and practice of rational-emotive therapy*. San Francisco: Jossey-Bass.

Wolfe, J. L. (1975, September). *Rational-emotive therapy as an effective feminist therapy*. Paper presented at the American Psychological Association Convention, Chicago.

Wolfe, J. L. (1976). *How to be sexually assertive*. New York: Institute for Rational-Emotive Therapy.

Wolfe, J. L. (1980, September). *Rational-emotive therapy women's groups: New model for an effective feminist therapy*. Paper presented at the American Psychological Association Convention, Montreal, Canada.

Wolfe, J. L. (1985). Women. In A. Ellis & M. Bernard (Eds.), *Clinical applications of rational-emotive therapy* (pp. 101–127). New York: Plenum Press.

Zachary, I. (1980). RET with women: Some special issues. In R. Grieger & J. Boyd (Eds.), *Rational-emotive therapy: A skills based approach* (pp. 249–264). New York: Van Nostrand.

Using RET Effectively in the Workplace

Dominic J. DiMattia

Since the inception of rational-emotive therapy over 35 years ago, many professionals have recognized the application of RET to problems in the workplace. Needless to say, thousands of individuals have been helped by their therapists in dealing with problems relating to work. Helping individuals not to upset themselves with events at work, which they cannot change immediately, has always been a goal of rational-emotive therapists. Ellis in his book on *Executive Leadership* (1972) also proposed that effective managers develop what he labeled "Rational Sensitivity." No doubt, RET can and will continue to help humans deal with problems at work in the confines of their office. However, rational-emotive therapy—or, as we have begun to label it, rational effectiveness training—is making a more direct contribution to the workplace by introducing the concepts of RET into management training, and into the development of "corporate cultures." However, in order for the concept to be accepted, and to be effective in the workplace, it is important to understand that a change in focus is required from the traditional approach used in therapy. In this chapter, I provide several specific applications of RET to the workplace and discuss specific techniques that I have found successful in applying RET to the workplace.

PROBLEMS IN THE WORKPLACE

In order for professionals to be effective in using RET in the workplace, they must first understand the problems facing organizations today and

DOMINIC J. DIMATTIA • Department of Counseling and Human Resources, University of Bridgeport, Bridgeport, Connecticut 06602, and Institute for Rational-Emotive Therapy, 45 East 65th Street, New York, New York 10021.

then clearly conceptualize that RET is one of the best approaches to helping organizations function more effectively.

What are some of these problems facing business and industry? First, most organizations are plagued with *low productivity*. A substantial percentage of the work force is seemingly unable to focus for any length of time on the assigned tasks. Organizations are trying desperately to confront problems of *absenteeism, chronic tardiness,* and *high turnover.* All the traditional behavioral techniques of reinforcement and punishment seem to be failing. Money, power, and recognition seem to maintain behavior only in the short run. Over the long run, organizations around the world are confronted with "burnout" and "low frustration tolerance." One president of a corporation complained to me that, no matter how much he rewarded young, bright, ambitious employees, they were constantly badgering him with their demands for more and more money and recognition. They weren't willing to wait to move up the ladder; they wanted it instantly. It seems to me that organizations are confronted with work forces that have self-defeating attitudes and beliefs about work that the organizations reinforce. It is necessary that these beliefs be confronted directly in corporate training programs and in the propaganda issued to motivate and maintain workers.

A second problem facing organizations today seems to be extensive *low morale,* which, of course, is related to the low productivity mentioned above. Even though work environments have constantly improved over the past 30 years, employees are steadily dissatisfied with their jobs. One only needs to visit the offices of major corporations to discover the country club atmosphere that has been created in executive parks. Even manufacturing facilities often include modern, aesthetically pleasing cafeterias, lounges, and health clubs. As we look out the window, we see beautiful surroundings. Corporations are constantly experimenting with color, light, and temperature as they try to create optimal working conditions for their employees. Yet, these workers never seem to be satisfied. Anyone who has any awareness of human behavior from an RET perspective recognizes that changing As when self-defeating Bs are present is only dealing with the external symptoms and is not focusing on the underlying issues causing the disruptive behavior. Therefore, organizations need to be taught the relationship between beliefs and behavior. They must be reeducated to recognize that humans do not function by Stimulus = response exclusively and that cognition is a significant factor in maintaining high morale.

A third problem facing most employers is a *significant change in the nature of their work force.* Increasingly, women and minorities make up a substantial percentage of the work force, and *they bring to organizations different values and desires.* They are motivated by different goals. The increasingly diverse nature of the work force creates clashes among workers that must be effectively handled rather than ignored in attempts to force all individuals to submit to the preordained procedures that have existed for years. When differing values and beliefs exist in organizations, it is important that the organizations create a climate and a work force that are flexible and adaptive. Obviously, this requires that the individuals within an organization free themselves of the rigid, absolutist attitudes that interfere with cooperation and problem solving. RET can make a definite contribution to organizations by teaching individuals to acknowledge and dispute their rigid attitudes.

Finally, organizations are confronted with *extreme international competition*. No longer can the major powers expect a guaranteed market at home and their share of the market in underdeveloped countries. With increased free trade and the industrialization of Third World countries, organizations must be alert to changes in the marketplace and must be able to respond to them quickly or, even better, anticipate them and plan for them. This requires a work force that is farsighted and does not focus on short-term profits. This presents a balancing act for most companies that are responsible to shareholders, who want immediate and steady profits. The companies must constantly decide between investing time and resources in projects that will result in immediate profits and investing in projects that may in fact result in a temporary reduction in profits. The leadership of such organizations requires a high degree of confidence and must have techniques that are self-reinforcing rather than externally reinforcing. Once again, it requires major changes in the attitudes and beliefs at every level of the organization. RET's clear and didactic approach to teaching humans high frustration tolerance and self-acceptance is a natural approach to be integrated into corporate training programs. RET has always been a preventive educational method for solving problems. It is this aspect of RET that is most acceptable to business and industry. With the exception of its use in employee assistance programs, RET is best introduced to organizations as an approach that will prevent problems and will help organizations meet their goals more efficiently.

Applications of RET in the Workplace

RET has been effectively applied to the following four areas within the workplace: employee assistance programs, training and development, managerial leadership development, and the training of human resource professionals. In the sections that follow, the ways in which RET can be effectively introduced in the workplace are discussed and illustrated.

Employee Assistance Programs

Ellis (1985a) introduced ideas on how RET can most effectively improve employee assistance programs (EAPs). Klarreich, DiGiuseppe, and DiMattia (1987) also demonstrated the effectiveness of RET in EAPs. I discuss here some ideas I have about how to use RET more effectively in this area.

EAPs have traditionally developed from the alcohol rehabilitation goals of corporations. Although many have expanded their roles to a more broad-brush approach and often treat a wide range of problems that interfere with worker efficiency, it is still important in introducing RET to EAP professionals to avoid challenging concepts religiously held by Alcoholics Anonymous (AA) supporters. It is not necessary to capitulate to their concepts totally, but when discussing RET concepts, it is better to draw attention to the similarities to the 12 steps than to challenge them openly. EAP professionals are more amenable to incorporating RET if they see it as complementary rather than competitive. As Ellis (1985b) pointed out, there are several steps in the 12-step program that help individuals significantly (see Table 1).

Because many EAPs insist that counselors make quick diagnoses and effective referral decisions, it is helpful to show these counselors how using the ABC model can help them quickly determine how disturbed an individual is. For example, if an employee is sent to the EAP counselors because his or her work performance has deteriorated, the counselor may begin to teach the employee that his or her own thinking and beliefs keep him or her from producing adequately; an employee who rigidly refuses to accept that he or she is, in part, to blame for the situation may be very rigid and unbending and may need more extensive assistance from trained therapists. However, if the employee quickly grasps the problem and willingly accepts assistance, the EAP counselor can proceed to teach the employee how to manage his or her feelings and behavior by using RET and other cognitive-behavioral techniques in a few sessions, assuming the EAP counselor is trained in RET. Also, it is important to point out to EAP personnel the wide range of self-help materials and educational workshops available to support the RET approach. These adjunctive materials help to reduce the cost of rehabilitation, an issue most organizations and insurance companies are increasingly interested in because of the rising costs of benefits in most companies.

Because most EAPs cannot refer exclusively to one therapist or institution, it is important to avoid overt and challenging criticisms of other approaches. RET will be more readily acceptable if similarities are discussed to other approaches that are action-oriented and have as their goal cost-effective methods of changing disruptive and self-defeating behavior.

I also recommend training EAP counselors in the techniques of RET rather than winning them over as converts to the RET philosophy. If they are at least willing to try the techniques, I believe their experience with its application will result in their wanting to learn more about RET and becoming more proficient. Rather than confronting their current ideology directly, which often requires that they admit that their current mode of

TABLE 1. Comparison of Twelve Steps and RET

AA: The Twelve Steps	RET consistent concepts
1. We admitted we were powerless over alcohol . . . that our lives had become unmanageable.	1. Accept your fallibility as a human.
2. Came to believe that a Power greater than ourselves could restore us to sanity.	4. Discover your irrational beliefs; acknowledge your self-defeating behaviors.
3. Made a decision to turn our will and our lives over to the care of God as we understood Him.	5. Admit to yourself that you have made mistakes but can still accept yourself.
4. Made a searching and fearless moral inventory of ourselves.	8. Be willing to correct your mistakes.
5. Admitted to God, to ourselves, and to another human being the exact nature of our wrongs.	9. Develop new behaviors that will demonstrate you are taking responsibility for your mistakes.
6. Were entirely ready to have God remove all these defects of character.	10. Constantly examine your behavior and change it when it is self-defeating.
7. Humbly asked Him to remove our shortcomings.	12. With your new insight and self-acceptance, help yourself and others to lead more productive lives.
8. Made a list of all persons we had harmed and became willing to make amends to them all.	
9. Made direct amends to such people wherever possible, except when to do so would injure them or others.	
10. Continued to take personal inventory and when we were wrong promptly admitted it.	
11. Sought through prayer and meditation to improve our conscious contact with God as we understood him, praying only for knowledge of His will for us and the power to carry that out.	
12. Having had a spiritual awakening as the result of these steps, we tried to carry this message to alcoholics and to practice these principles in all our affairs.	

operation is ineffective, thus forcing them to come to the conclusion that they have been, in effect, incompetent, it is better to discuss RET techniques as adding to their repertoire and thus making them more effective. For instance, when Arthur Fiedler and the Boston Pops Orchestra added to their repertoire Beatles songs, did the addition make their early performances inadequate? Mostly, EAP counselors see themselves as very skilled and are only looking for more efficient approaches that are consistent with their current philosophy. RET can be introduced and taught, with a few exceptions, to most of these individuals without their rejecting their current philosophy.

For instance, by pointing out to EAP counselors who are trained in behavior therapy that, by focusing on the attitudes and beliefs that clients have, contingency management programs are more efficient. Instead of waiting for clients to change their attitudes after they have engaged in new behavior, counselors can directly confront the self-defeating beliefs by teaching the ABCs of RET at the same time that they use reinforcement techniques when training behavioral counselors to use RET, emphasizing that RET has always been cognitive, emotive, and behavioral. In effect, you are suggesting a more comprehensive approach that includes their current skills.

Many EAP counselors have been trained as social workers, so that usually, their early training is in the medical model and psychoanalytic theory. Many religiously believe that Freudian or neo-Freudian explanations of personality are correct. However, they, also recognize that corporations will not tolerate treatment modalities that take years to yield results. This situation often puts them in a serious bind. They must give up their current beliefs in treatment or face criticism from corporate management. Therefore, they are searching for approaches that are consistent with their current beliefs and yet are more cost-effective. You may be surprised to read that I believe that RET fits the bill, as RET is an insight-oriented therapy in that we are interested in clients' discovering their deeply imbedded philosophical beliefs about themselves, others, and the world in general. We are interested not only in changing behavior but also in having clients understand why they behave the way they do. We are also interested in teaching them a process of challenging these underlying philosophies that has been proved to be more efficient than traditional analysis. In fact, we are interested in the same goals but have developed a different strategy to achieve them. This interpretation is usually more acceptable to EAP counselors and will reduce the resistance to incorporating RET into their approach.

Another example of how we can encourage individuals with a different persuasion to incorporate RET into their approach can be demonstrated with Gestalt therapy. Gestalt therapies focus on teaching an increased awareness of the emotional reactions that clients often deny and then assume that their awareness is therapeutic in and of itself. By encouraging Gestalt therapists to continue with RET's didactic techniques after they have increased the clients' awareness, we are able to blend the approaches, rather than engage in fruitless confrontation over which approach is more beneficial.

The important point in these examples is to reduce resistance to RET by showing similarities rather than differences, and by emphasizing the didactic and efficient aspects of RET rather than engaging in dialogue to win converts during an initial encounter. If we encourage EAP counselors to experiment with RET techniques, the success they experience will convince them to learn more about the RET approach to treatment.

Training and Development

Corporations currently spend over $180 billion a year on short-term training programs (1986). Many of these programs are conducted in-house by human resource professionals who use packaged programs developed by companies specializing in training. Often, they also invite outside consultants to conduct the training directly. How can RET be effectively introduced to companies when so much competition exists? First, it is important to avoid any mention of therapy when integrating RET into training programs. As a trainer you are constantly reinforcing the notion that these techniques will increase productivity by reducing the amount of time that workers spend engaging in self-defeating reactions to frustrating circumstances. Avoid, as often as possible, mentioning emotions or feelings. It is better to use words and phrases such as "your wasteful reactions" or "your impulsive behavior." When teaching the ABC model, constantly use job-related examples. Do not revert to clinical examples. The RET trainer is not increasing job satisfaction but is constantly demonstrating the relationship between job satisfaction and productivity.

For example, if a worker is very frustrated by an organization that does not make decisions quickly or sends mixed messages about the priorities within the organization, he or she may spend an inordinate amount of time ruminating about how unfair this situation is and may be worried about how to accomplish his or her work. Rather than focus on the emotional upset, it would be better to point out that the time he or she spends ruminating is wasted and unproductive. If RET disputing techniques are applied, he or she may be able to focus on his or her work and thus to increase the probability of finding some solution to the problem. *The focus in training is always on the relation of self-defeating beliefs to low productivity*, not on irrationality and emotional consequences. Constantly reinforce the ideas that if each individual in an organization develops flexible, adaptable ideas, the environment becomes less confrontational, and more problem solving can occur.

It is most important to emphasize the preventive nature of RET rather than the treatment aspect. RET incorporated into already-existing training programs will improve the effectiveness of those programs and create a work force that will respond more effectively to changing challenges (DiMattia, Yeager, & Dube, 1989).

What are some of the training programs that RET can improve? There are several: performance appraisals, communication skills, sales effectiveness, conflict management, time management, and a wide range of technical training programs.

Let's start with the application of RET to improving performance appraisals in organizations. As Cayer, DiMattia, and Wingrove (1988) reported in their study of 50 managers, many well-developed performance appraisal systems are not effective because managers have high needs for approval, avoid unpleasant reactions of workers by giving higher-than-earned ratings, and often put themselves down for not more regularly managing their employees. Therefore, at the time of a formal performance appraisal, they again avoid giving accurate feedback to employees, and the result is a perpetuation of the problem of employee ineffectiveness. It is recommended that all supervisors who are expected to give formal appraisal be trained to dispute the self-defeating ideas that interfere with their effectiveness. When it is demonstrated that using RET will strengthen their performance reviews and in the long run may reduce problems, supervisors are more willing to learn the RET techniques. Role playing is an important part of training managers to be effective during performance appraisals. Unfortunately, they are often able to demonstrate effective behaviors when coached in the workshop, but unless a cognitive rehearsal to change their underlying self-defeating beliefs is included in the real situation, they are most likely to revert to old behavior patterns. So, as part of any training program on performance appraisal, RET techniques can be included to help supervisors manage their avoidant behavior and to reduce their ineffective reactions to unpleasant employee reactions.

Another common corporate training program that can be improved by RET is communication skills. Most corporations conduct programs in interpersonal communications as well as public speaking. These programs are often behaviorally oriented and include many role-playing exercises and even video feedback. The skills taught are often important in effective communications. However, these workshops often ignore an important dimension. Individuals who have rigid beliefs, which include "I must always look good in front of colleagues," "I must always receive the approval of my supervisors," and "I should be able to communicate better," experience a high degree of anxiety and tension when applying these new behaviors on the job. If they were also taught RET disputing techniques to manage their anxiety and to increase their frustration tolerance, they would have a better chance of maintaining the new behavior and of improving their ability to communicate. When teaching communication skills, constantly focus on behavioral outcomes and demonstrate the relationship between rigid beliefs and an individual's ability to master the new behavior. Take an existing program and introduce RET concepts periodically throughout the existing program to increase the probability that the new behavior will be maintained and transferred on the job.

Training programs in conflict resolution, negotiating skills, time management, and a wide range of technical training programs can also be improved by integrating RET in the same manner described above in the communication skills example. If RET is to be effective in corporate training and development programs, the focus had better be on changing behavior and not on the reduction of emotional disturbance. If they use a different vocabulary and emphasizing the relationship between self-defeating employee reactions and low productivity, RET trainers will be more readily accepted as consultants in training and development.

Another important training area that can be improved by RET is *sales training*. Corporations spend billions of dollars each year on sales personnel, only to find that their turnover rate is very high. A substantial number of the sales force burns out quickly, and others are often erratic in meeting organizational goals. Most current sales training programs include techniques on how to close the sale. Successful salespeople usually conduct these workshops and share tricks and techniques that they have learned from their experiences. Techniques in time management and how to organize a work day are also taught. Unfortunately, these programs often benefit only a small percentage of salespeople who already have a high frustration tolerance and a low need for approval. It is widely accepted that successful salespeople are very persistent and do not take rejection personally. They are able to continue making new contacts even after a long period of rejection. They attribute their "dry" periods not to their own inadequacies, but to the nature of the business.

RET disputing techniques are very effective in helping individuals change ineffective attitudes that extinguish initiating behavior. Sales training programs that teach salespeople these disputing techniques and provide them with actual material that they can use at the moment of discouragement reduce low frustration tolerance and energy-reducing self-downing thoughts. Effective RET-oriented sales programs focus on the long-term goal of changing two major self-defeating beliefs: (1) "I must be successful immediately," and (2) "I am inadequate when I have been unable to close a sale." Changing these underlying beliefs is a long-term project; therefore, sales training programs had better include short-term coping techniques that salespeople can constantly use at the moment of discouragement. Audiotapes, self-help cards, homework sheets, and coping self-statements are examples of short-term approaches that can be included in sales training programs. Teach salespeople to use these self-help techniques when they are seemingly unwilling to push ahead to the next customer. Once again, you are reinforcing the relationship between applying RET techniques and increasing the probability of greater sales.

Management Leadership Development

The third area in which RET can be effective is in general management or leadership development. Effective managers are individuals who have flexible attitudes and do not let their bias interfere with effective decision making. They respond to change in an adaptive manner rather than sabotage new programs and ideas. Leadership or management development programs can be significantly improved when RET is introduced. By teaching the participants to identify their rigid beliefs and subsequently to dispute and change these beliefs, organizations will develop flexible managers capable of making creative decisions. Using an effective decision-making model that includes brainstorming, consequential thinking, and a realistic evaluation as the foundation of management training and incorporating an RET component that will remove the rigid beliefs that interfere with effective decision making, a leadership management program will be more effective. Managers will not properly use decision-making models if their thinking is limited by preconceived ideas about a solution. If programs include the identification of all beliefs about effective management and a systematic approach of reexamining these beliefs and changing the nonproductive beliefs, decision making will not be limited.

As Lewin's change model (1951) points out, there are three broad steps in the change process: (1) unfreezing, which involves reducing the forces maintaining current behavior; (2) moving, which shifts behavior to a new level; It involves new behaviors, values, and attitudes; and (3) refreezing, which stabilizes the behavior at a new level. It is clear that, at Step 2, RET can effectively assist organizations in identifying those attitudes and values that keep managers from changing—rigid ideas such as "We can not move ahead unless we are sure of success"; "Profits must always go up"; "I must always receive positive feedback from my superiors"; and "My employees should perceive me as a fair manager." The challenging of these beliefs with the RET can move managers to more creative decisions, which in the long run will be productive for the organization. Beginning leadership programs by listing all beliefs that are currently held by the group provides a focus for introducing RET concepts. It is more effective if large groups are divided into small groups of five to eight people, who are allowed to list their ideas and then report to the larger group. Each belief can be examined, and the absolute quality of the belief can be challenged by teaching the group the ABCs of RET.

Training Human Resource Personnel

Training human resource professionals in RET requires a commitment from the participants that understanding the principles of RET and its application to training will enhance their skills and improve their existing programs. Like the employee assistance program professionals, human resource professionals already consider themselves experts in human behavior and are often defensive if one positions RET as the only correct method. It is important to emphasize that RET is an added tool that will make them and their program more effective.

Often, human resource professionals are seeking quick-fix approaches that are well packaged. These individuals are difficult customers because, to use RET effectively, they must make a long-term commitment to training. Start by introducing them to RET in short-term programs similar to those described above. Point out to them that, if they become more knowledgeable and skilled in the RET approach, their work will be more cost-effective, as they will not require outside consultants to conduct training or to redesign the existing curriculum. Also, argue that a consistent view of human behavior by a human resource department will ultimately create a corporate culture of flexible employees able to handle their own frustrations and will thus reduce constant pressure on the organization to change. At the same time, point out that RET is an easily understood approach that can immediately aid employees with daily problems.

It is also important to dispute these professionals' own low frustration tolerance for quick solutions. Emphasize the long-term benefits of becoming an expert in RET in the workplace. RET will allow them to stand apart from the average human resource professional, who follows rather than leads the profession.

When conducting training for human resource professionals, do not lecture extensively. Use job-related examples, and design small-group exercises that will allow them to apply the techniques during the workshops. Systematic curriculum-building exercises are also useful. Start with an existing program, and work as a group to redesign it so that RET principles are included. For instance, if you start with a communication program, step by step design exercises with the group that will strengthen the existing goals of the workshop while introducing RET into the format. Communication workshops include training participants in listening skills, which require them to restate or reflect the content and/or the affect of the individual talking. The techniques taught often include models of effective listening, which are role-played or rehearsed; then, the participant receives feedback and tries again. Unfortunately, most individuals stop listening when they hear information that challenges their existing beliefs, and then they react emotionally, a reaction that interferes with their ability to listen. By having the participants identify the trigger behaviors that result in their emotional reactions and by teaching them that their reactions are a result of their rigid beliefs and not the trigger behavior, you can strengthen their ability to listen and not react.

It is also important to spend time with the individual group members on their own rigid beliefs that interfere with effective functioning. However, never pressure the individual group members to self-disclose. Ask for volunteers to conduct demonstrations, and allow the remainder of the participants to practice disputing techniques individually, using modified homework sheets. Often, the use of triads enhances learning. One member of the triad shares a concern, the second member disputes the rigid beliefs that are interfering with effective problem solving, and the third member observes and gives feedback. This process allows individuals the opportunity to challenge their own self-defeating beliefs and at the same time gives the participants an opportunity to practice disputing techniques.

General Issues When Using RET in the Workplace

It is often difficult to dispute the idea that perfectionist thinking is self-destructive. Many organizations emphasize the need for employees to do an excellent job and often punish employees who make mistakes. Therefore, when the RET concept of accepting yourself as fallible is introduced into a workshop, there is serious resistance because it is misinterpreted as meaning accepting inadequate performances. It is important that you clearly state that using RET will improve performance, as the anxiety and tension created by perfectionist thinking will be reduced, and employees will be focused on the completion of tasks rather than engaging in avoidance behavior to reduce the anxiety. Emphasize that RET helps people to achieve excellence with a minimum of distress; it is not an approach which lowers standards. It focuses on a different strategy to achieve high standards.

Deadlines are another given in organizations. When disputing self-defeating ideas like "I *must* complete all tasks on time," it is again important to emphasize that, by accepting the possibility that one may miss a deadline, one is removing extreme anxiety and tension, which interfere with the accomplishment of the task. Worrying about a task doesn't get it completed more quickly; it only distracts one from focusing on the task. Again, acknowledge that meeting deadlines is important, but point out that obsessing about them is counterproductive. Again, emphasize that RET provides one with strategies for achieving organizational goals that reduce counterproductive behavior.

Case Study

Using RET effectively in the workplace can often be like walking a tightrope. Several potential problem areas have been discussed above. Below, I discuss the process of integrating RET into several programs offered by a major U.S. corporation.

For several years, I had been invited to conduct a one-day seminar on "counseling skills for managers" as part of a five-day training program for newly appointed managers. As I became more committed to RET, I began including the basic concepts of RET in addition to the traditional counseling skills of listening, restating, reflection, and problem solving. The participants soon discovered that their behavioral skills were inhibited if they held rigid or irrational beliefs. The application of RET not only helped their learning but also relieved stress in their high-pressure jobs.

At one of these training programs, the newly appointed director of education expressed considerable interest in RET. He had been a psychology major in college and had heard of Albert Ellis. He was fascinated by the application of RET to the workplace and invited me to call him when the workshop was completed. When we met he expressed concern about his immediate staff, who seemed to be burdened with resistance from trainees to the technical programs they were teaching. His staff also seemed overwhelmed by the amount of work required and often complained. He wondered how RET might help. It is important to note here that, in my experience, it has often been better to have one individual in the organization who is familiar with RET than to try to sell a program to departments that have no knowledge of RET. The corporate structure requires so many individuals to "sign off" on a program that, if there is no one championing the program, it will be lost in the maze of daily tasks. The first suggestion is to connect with a significant supporter in the organization. In this case, it was the director of education. I spent several meetings with him exploring how RET could help his staff. We also decided that I should become familiar with the peculiar problems of their industry, so that when the workshop was conducted, the examples used would be relevant to the participants.

After several meetings, we designed a three-day seminar for the education department that included a basic introduction to RET and its application to management and training. It also included opportunities for participants to apply RET in peer-counseling situations. This served two purposes: (1) it helped them learn how to use RET, and (2) it helped them see how RET could reduce their stress and increase their productivity. The workshop was well received by the group because all of the examples were related to their specific problems and they were given many opportunities to discuss their misgivings, especially those related to making mistakes. Large corporations especially terrorize their employees by dramatizing the need to be excellent, the best. Often, workers are so fearful that they procrastinate completing major projects. This staff was quite typical, as they were being asked to revise the curriculum in all courses. Several were afraid that the new director would find their work inadequate. As soon as the irrational belief that it would be terrible if their director disapproved of their work was disputed, they were freed to begin working. A few weeks after the workshop was completed, several participants phoned me to inform me that they had successfully completed their revised curriculum. The second lesson to be learned from this case study is that workshops should include examples relevant to the organization. Thus, we must spend time acquainting ourselves with each industry. Although time-consuming, such a study will pay off in the long run.

As a result of this workshop, the director of education continued to introduce RET concepts to major officers of the company, and the result was a luncheon attended by the president, three senior vice-presidents, and several other high-ranking officials. The purpose of the meeting was to see if I truly understood their problems and to determine if RET would be effective in their organization. This informal dialogue was very significant because I was invited to conduct a two-day seminar for district sales managers. The seminar was also attended by the president and all the senior vice-presidents.

I began the seminar by eliciting from the participants their most frustrating problems. After these were generated, I had a long list of activating events (A) that were common to the organization. I then proceeded to ask them how they reacted to these situations, thus collecting several emotional and behavioral consequences (C). At this juncture, I introduced the concept that A did not cause C, and that B, or self-defeating beliefs, caused C. This concept was easily demonstrated, as different members of the group had different reactions to the same As. This is an especially effective technique for beginning any workshop. It immediately involves the entire group in activity and verbal interaction. It also allows the participants to express their concerns immediately. Exercises were then introduced in disputing techniques, and the participants were able to practice them in triads, with one person playing the "rational" manager, one person playing the frustrated employee, and one person observing and giving feedback to the manager. All exercises were processed in the large groups, and the frustrations with wanting to be perfect in using RET were also conceptionalized in RET terms, so that the participants were helped to increase their frustration tolerance in the use of newly learned techniques.

It is important in training that high frustration tolerance be reinforced. Participants seem to quickly grasp the concepts and then demand that the implementation be as quickly learned. Behavior change requires practice, and using RET to handle frustrations is not an exception.

SUMMARY

RET can be effectively used in the workplace by changing the emphasis from reducing emotional disturbances to changing the self-defeating behaviors that interfere with the achievement of personal and organizational goals. RET, in effect, provides organizations with a more efficient and lasting method of dealing with motivating workers and establishing a flexible work force able to problem-solve rather than react to daily crises. RET trainers must familiarize themselves with the problems facing business and industry and must tailor their interventions to specific work-related situations. The language of RET, also, must be more consistent with the language of business and industry rather than the language of psychology. And, of course, we must all work on our own low frustration tolerance in working with corporate decision makers who do not readily see the value of RET to their organization.

References

Cayer, M., DiMattia, D., & Wingrove, J. (1988). Conquering evaluation fear. *Personnel Administrator, 33*(6), 97–107.

DiMattia, D., Yeager, R., & Dube, I. (1989). Emotional barriers to learning. *Personnel.*

Ellis, A. (1972). *Executive leadership: A rational approach.* New York: Institute for Rational Living.

Ellis, A. (1985a). Rational-emotive approach to acceptance and its relationship to EAP's. In S. H. Klarreich, J. L. Francek, & C. E. Moore (Eds.), *The human resource management handbook: Principles and practice of employee assistance programs* (pp. 325–330). New York: Praeger.

Ellis, A. (1985b). Why Alcoholics Anonymous is probably doing more harm than good by its insistence on a higher power (3rd ed.). *Employee Assistance Quarterly, 1*(1), 95–97.

Klarreich, S. H., DiGiuseppe, R., & DiMattia, D. (1987). EAP's: Mind over myths. *Personnel Administrator, 32*(2), 119–121.

Lewin, K. (1951). *Field theory in social services.* New York: Harper & Row.

Research Institute Report. (1986). New York–Washington, August 29.

RET with Children and Adolescents

Michael E. Bernard and Marie R. Joyce

RET has a long history of application, with children and adolescents, to the treatment of a variety of childhood problems including conduct disorders (e.g., DiGiuseppe, 1988), low frustration tolerance (e.g., Knaus, 1983), impulsivity (e.g., Kendall & Fischler, 1983), academic underachievement (e.g., Bard & Fisher, 1983), anxieties, fears and phobias (e.g., Grieger & Boyd, 1983), social isolation (e.g., Halford, 1983), obesity (e.g., Foreyt & Kondo, 1983), depression (e.g., DiGiuseppe, 1986), and childhood sexuality (e.g., Walen & Vanderhorst, 1983). This chapter provides an up-to-date conceptualization of how RET can be used effectively with young clients. The foundation of the present material can be found in Bernard and Joyce, *Rational-Emotive Therapy with Children and Adolescents: Theory, Treatment Strategies, Preventative Methods* (1984). We have endeavored to refine the ideas presented in this earlier work, incorporating what we have learned over the years since its publication.

THEORETICAL PERSPECTIVES

A brief overview of the RET model of childhood maladjustment will help to make clearer the rationale for the methods that RET prescribes in treating the social, emotional, behavioral, and learning problems of school-aged children (see Bernard & Joyce, 1984).

MICHAEL E. BERNARD • School of Education, University of Melbourne, Parkville, Victoria, Australia 3052, and Australian Institute for Rational-Emotive Therapy, P.O. Box 1160, Carlton, Victoria, Australia 3053.   MARIE R. JOYCE • Centre for Family Studies, Australian Catholic University, Oakleigh, Victoria, Australia 3168.

RET takes extreme cognizance of the wide individual differences observed in the way students in school (and elsewhere) react to the same event. Whether the event be teasing, performance failure, criticism, parental rejection, unfair treatment, or frustrating and difficult tasks, children and adolescents of the same age experience different degrees of adaptive and maladaptive emotions and behavior. This is especially the case after children have entered the concrete-operational period of thinking as defined by Piaget and begin to actively mediate their environment. As children enter this stage of development, they are less influenced by events in their immediate perceptual environment. They begin to be more independent in their thinking and, in particular, think much more about things that have happened in the past or may happen in the future. From an RET perspective, the belief system and the logical reasoning processes of children determine in a fundamental way the extent to which they react adaptively to particular bad events that they encounter. RET accepts the findings of the cognitive-developmental literature that point to a progressive differentiation and sophistication of perceptual, symbolic-representational, and information-processing abilities. However, RET has a particular theory about why certain children bring with them to their immediate environments irrational belief systems and faulty reasoning processes that are atypical of their cognitive-developmental level.

RET incorporates the findings of Chess and Thomas (1984) and other researchers who have found that children are born with reliable and consistent patterns of behavior that they label *temperament* (activity level, regularity, adaptability, approach or withdrawal, physical sensitivity, intensity of reaction, distractibility, positive or negative mood, and persistence). RET theorists (e.g., DiGiuseppe, 1988) have argued that all children are born with NFT (no frustration tolerance). Additionally, RET theorists (e.g., Ellis, Moseley, & Wolfe, 1966) have for many years described differences in parenting styles and how parenting style, along with parental emotions, influences the development of children. For example, Hauck (1967) identified the "unkind and firm" pattern ("unquestioning obedience to authority combined with a kick in the ego") as contributing in certain children to low self-esteem, insecurity, and guilt, as well as avoidant, overly dependent, and submissive behavior. "Not firm" patterns of parenting, which involve parents' setting few rules and limits, have been linked in the RET literature with children who manifest low frustration tolerance and an inability to delay gratification. Bernard and Joyce (1984) argued that child psychopathology results from an interaction of child temperament with parenting style and, in particular, that adaptive development occurs because of a good match between the parents' child-raising approach and the child's temperament. Clinically, the RET practitioner is "on the lookout" for children who have age-inappropriate low frustration tolerance and who have "ego-related" problems and, in particular, "self-downing" thinking tendencies (e.g., Knaus, 1985). In understanding why these children think, feel, and behave as they do, RET gives attention to their temperament and the way their parents, think, feel, and behave toward them.

RET Treatment Levels

There are a number of levels at which the RET practitioner can involve the parents and the younger client in a RET intervention.

Level 1. Practitioner–Young Client. This is the most traditional form of mental health service delivery and involves the practitioner's seeing the young client and using RET directly without seeing the parents.

Level 2. Practitioner–Young Client–Parent or Teacher. At this level, the RET practitioner works directly with the child or adolescent. The parent (or both parents) or the teacher is present, and the goal at this level is both to help the young person modify his or her problems and to teach the parent or teacher basic RET methods that can be used outside the session (see Waters, in press).

Level 3. Practitioner–Parent or Teacher–Young Client. Just as behavioral approaches are taught to parents and teachers in order for them to manage the specific problems of a child, so, too, do RET practitioners work with parents and teachers in order for them to manage the problems of a child without the direct intervention of the practitioner. Although RET practitioners teach parents a variety of practical problem-solving skills and child management approaches, what differentiates RET from behavioral approaches is that it also assesses and modifies parental emotions that are presumed to be interfering with the effective management of a child's problem (see McInerney, in press).

Level 4. Practitioner–Parent or Teacher. It is sometimes the case that the RET practitioner focuses on improvement of the mental health and reduction of stress as ends in themselves when working with a parent or a teacher (e.g., Bernard, Rosewarne, & Joyce, 1983; Forman, in press; Joyce, in press).

Level 5. Practitioner–Young Client–Family Members. Some RET practitioners prefer to have the total family involved during part or all of the sessions with a child, with the goal of modifying the emotional and behavioral patterns of responding among family members by the use of RET and allied techniques (e.g., Huber & Baruth, 1989; Woulff, 1983).

Level 6. Practitioner–Couple. RET practitioners operate from the belief that a child's problems can be the cause rather than the effect of marriage and relationship problems, it is sometimes the case that the RET practitioner, with the cooperation of the child's parents, will spend some time helping to rid the couple (without the child's being present) of emotional disturbance. An improvement in the marital relationship may bring about a beneficial change in the child and may enable the partners to manage their child's problems more effectively (e.g., DiGiuseppe & Zeeve, 1985).

Level 7. Group Therapy. In recent years, there has been a growing recognition of the importance of working with groups of children and adolescents; RET can be readily modified for such purposes (e.g., Elkin, 1983).

THE RATE MODEL

This section describes a four-stage RET model for working with young clients and their significant others: relationship building, assessment, treatment, and evaluation (RATE).

Relationship Building

Albert Ellis (1962) advocated that rational-emotive practitioners use an active-directive, confrontational style of therapy and that they use humor liberally. In writing about the implementation of RET with children and adolescents, a number of RET theorists (e.g., Bernard & Joyce, 1984; Young, 1983) have placed emphasis on the building of a relationship between the therapist and the young client.

Dryden (1987) used Bordin's concept (1979) of the "therapeutic alliance" to elucidate the issue of the practitioner–client relationship. The three components of the therapeutic alliance are found in (1) the bond between therapist and client; (2) the goals set jointly by them; and (3) the tasks undertaken by each to bring about change. The building and maintaining of a relationship between practitioner and young client require attention to all three areas. Listed here are some strategies for relationship building with children and adolescents:

1. Arrange for the first meeting with a young elementary-school-aged child in an environment familiar to the child (even if just to be introduced there).

2. Use language appropriate to the age of the child.

3. Talk to children about why they are coming. Find out their understanding of why they are there and their expectations of what will happen.

4. Explain the practitioner's role simply (e.g., someone to work together with them to help solve a problem they are having, or someone who can help them learn new ways of getting along with people). If the child is at a concrete-operational stage of thought, this can be done more specifically. Very early in the first session, the therapist can list some common problems that other children have sought help about (e.g., bad feelings, hassles, and worries about the future) and can carefully observe the child's body language. The child will usually react physically when his or her

problem(s) are mentioned, and the practitioner can pick up on this reaction to use in examples of what a therapist does. "Helping boys to feel less worried about school work all the time" and "teaching girls to get along more happily with friends at school and not to have so many fights" would be two examples of explaining the role concretely.

5. Find out the child's special interests and hobbies, and use these in explaining concepts.

6. Deal directly with any anxieties that children may have about coming. The two most common sources of anxiety here are the idea in the child's own thinking that coming for help means there is "something wrong with me" and worry about what peers will think or say. (Helping the child rehearse something that he or she would feel comfortable telling friends by way of explanation often helps.)

7. Arrange appointments with respect for children's preferences, not just those of the teacher or the parent.

8. Listen for idiosyncratic language. Peer groups, especially in adolescence, "define" words in their own special ways. If in doubt, ask!

9. Keep the child informed, if possible, about communications with the parents, at least in general terms, so that the child knows when you are speaking to or meeting her or his parents. In explaining confidentiality to the child, it is also important, especially with adolescents, to discuss how your communication with their parents affects this confidentiality. For example, if there is a "touchy" issue, such as the whereabouts and activities of the adolescent during truanting episodes, the adolescent is unlikely to disclose this to the therapist if he or she thinks that the parents will immediately find out. Before such an issue is dealt with by the practitioner, it can be explained to the young person that this is a good example of something that the practitioner would not disclose to the parents without the adolescent's agreement. "If your parents asked me about that, I would tell them to ask you about that themselves."

10. Maintain open and honest communication. Let children in on your thinking: discuss plans for therapy, involve them in joint goal setting, and get them to participate in the monitoring and evaluation processes.

11. As children and adolescents can rarely formulate by themselves what they want out of therapy, it is useful to spend time integrating goals for therapy with their thinking about themselves. Instead of "Let's work to reduce your anxiety," we would have "Do you want us to work together so that you learn to feel less panicky when you want to ask questions in English class?"

12. For young clients who are difficult to motivate and difficult to hold in therapy, some additional measures can be recommended: visiting them at home, contacting them during their school holidays by phone call or visit, watching them at sport, showing an interest in their current school

work exercises and praising good features, visiting them at school camp, or helping them solve a pressing practical problem (e.g., changing a school subject they strongly dislike).

A variety of possible ways of building and maintaining a relationship with young clients have been described that increase the effectiveness of RET interventions. Although the initial building of a relationship with most young clients is not difficult and a few simple steps are all that is often required early in therapy, it is hypothesized that the implementation of strategies that affect the maintenance of the therapeutic alliance will enhance the effectiveness of the treatment interventions.

Assessment

It is possible to view assessment as having two purposes: *problem identification* and *problem analysis* (see Bernard & Joyce, 1984). Problem identification in work with children and adolescents involves determining the type of problem the young person is experiencing: practical, emotional, manipulative, or vocational. RET problem analysis is geared to considering internal and environmental factors that revolve around the young person's emotional problems. RET is an emotional problem-solving therapy geared to modifying and often reducing the intensity, frequency, and duration of inappropriate negative emotional reactions so that the young person not only feels less miserable and stressed but also can solve practical problems. We concur with DiGiuseppe's comments (1990):

> Emotional disturbance results in behavioral disorders because the disturbed emotions will either interfere with children's acquisition of new skills, interfere with children's ability to problem solve solutions or interfere with children's implementation of old or new skills which could alleviate the practical problem. Therefore, the RET practitioner attempts to assess the presence of emotional and practical problems. Children's problems need not result from emotional disturbance. They may result from skill deficits, maladaptive reinforcement contingencies, unrealistic expectations of adults, or poor instruction. Such cases would not be suitable for RET unless they, in turn, trigger cognitions which mediate reactive emotional disturbance. (p. 288)

Simply put, RET problem analysis is concerned with the detailed examination of a young client's emotional reactions and the cognitions that RET hypothesizes give rise to the nature of the emotional reaction.

Assessing Emotions

Let us summarize the different aspects of the emotional assessment of young clients that can help pave the way for using RET effectively in treatment:

1. *Assess "emotional" and "practical" problems.* It is important that the practitioner clearly separate these two types of problems and explain the

difference to the young client. Most young clients are not accustomed to thinking about emotional problem solving as a means of making themselves less miserable and happier and as providing them with the control and resolve to improve their outside world.

2. *Assess all the possible different emotional reactions.* The major emotional reactions to be on the lookout for are irritation-anger-rage, concern-anxiety-panic, and disappointment-sadness-downness-depression. In assessing anger, separate anger with others, anger with the self, and anger associated with the frustration of the task. Anger with the self is considered a type of self-downing. Frustration is considered healthy and normal; assess the different emotional reactions to frustrating conditions.

3. *Assess "appropriate" and "inappropriate" negative emotional reactions.* Be sure to clearly separate those negative emotional reactions, such as concern, irritation, and frustration, that are appropriate because they do not lead to goal-defeating behavior from those inappropriate negative emotional reactions, such as depression, high anxiety, or rage, that are often associated with goal-defeating behavior.

4. *Assess the intensity, duration, and frequency of different emotional reactions.* Assessing these different dimensions affords the practitioner a clearer picture of the order of severity of the different emotional problems.

5. *Assess emotions in specific situations.* Rather than asking, "How angry are you with your father?" ask "How angry were you when your father entered your room without knocking?"

6. *Assess the behavioral consequences of different emotional reactions.* This information will provide the young client—especially in the case of anger—with additional motivation to try to change her or his emotions.

7. *Assess young clients' understanding of the connection between their emotions and their behavior.* Often gained through Socratic questioning, this information reveals clients' self-awareness of the importance of emotions in modifying their own behavior.

8. *Assess secondary emotional problems.* Especially as children grow older, they can develop emotional problems secondary to their primary emotional reactions much as adults do. For example, depressed adolescents can make themselves further depressed by telling themselves that they *shouldn't* be so depressed for so long and that they really are *hopeless* because of their condition.

9. *Assess young clients' emotional vocabulary.* Listening for the words that a child or an adolescent uses to describe feelings provides an insight into the private language system of the young person and may reveal the type of emotional thinking vocabulary partly responsible for the degree of emotional upset. Helping the young person to refine and elaborate his or her emotional vocabulary will help both the practitioner and the young client distinguish emotional problems. A restricted emotional vocabulary will alert the practitioner to how much prerequisite work will need to be done

in teaching an emotional vocabulary before proceeding with RET interventions.

Assessing Cognitions

RET has a particular interest in certain types of cognitions that it hypothesizes mediate emotional disturbance. In working with young clients, the RET practitioner listens for *errors of inference* (conclusions and predictions) and *errors of evaluation* (irrational beliefs) (see Grieger & Boyd, 1983). While not ignoring other cognitive processes such as selective attention or dichotomous thinking, RET does orient its assessment to specific cognitions that clinical experience and research have shown to underlie childhood emotional problems such as anxiety, depression, and anger (e.g., Bernard, 1984).

Before beginning the specific cognitive assessment, the RET practitioner assesses the young person's stage of cognitive development. Using age and mental maturity as a guide, RET practitioners share the opinion that children need to be in the Piagetian stage of concrete operations, usually reached by the age of 8, before they can effectively engage in the logical processes necessary for disputing (e.g., DiGiuseppe & Bernard, 1983).

Another prerequisite that needs to be assessed is whether the young person knows the difference between a "fact" and an "assumption." If not, it will not be possible for the practitioner to introduce the insight that what the young person may be thinking may or may not be "true." This insight is vital if one chooses to teach disputation as a method of self-examination.

The trickiest part of RET assessment is eliciting a young person's thoughts. It is recommended that the practitioner *not* proceed too quickly and allow young persons to gradually–within and across sessions—become aware of their own thoughts as they concern particular situations and give rise to particular emotional reactions. The question "What are you telling yourself when _____?" often does not yield substantial amounts of cognitive material. Indeed, often young persons reply with negative *rational* thoughts. For example, asking young clients to tell you what they are thinking when they get angry about being teased often produces the response "It's unfair," which may well be true. So, as described elsewhere (e.g., Bernard, 1981), the practitioner attempts to "peel away the layers of the onion" (layers of thought) that are keeping hidden the main emotionally arousing irrational thoughts. DiGiuseppe (1990) pointed out that initial questioning techniques often produce *automatic thoughts* (errors of inference) and fail to get at the major irrational ones. It is therefore important for the RET practitioner to be patient, flexible, and skillful in assessing the cognitive activity of a young client. The practitioner needs to know what he or she is looking for and needs to have a variety of questioning strategies to maximize introspective detail. DiGiuseppe (1990) provided the following four strategies:

Inductive Awareness. In this strategy, the practitioner helps children reveal their errors of inference (automatic thoughts) and then challenges each. As sessions proceed, children are asked to contemplate if there are any similarities in their automatic thoughts. The practitioner waits for the child to see the underlying theme that runs through the automatic thoughts already reported. For example, consider the example of Aaron, who fails to hand in assignments that he finds hard and also lies to his father about his school's requesting that he receive extra tutorial help (a request he was supposed to relay to his father). When asked to consider what he is thinking about in these situations, when he experiences worry, he may report that other people would think he was stupid and he couldn't stand that. This strategy can be effective but is rather inefficient. It can take children a long time to become aware of their irrational beliefs. Although most adolescents will eventually become aware of their irrational beliefs with this strategy, our clinical experience is that preadolescents are less likely to reach these insights themselves.

Inductive Interpretation. In this strategy, the practitioner again encourages young clients to explore and collect lists of thoughts they have when experiencing disturbed emotions. Many of these thoughts are errors of inference (e.g., "I'll never be able to do any work" or "The teacher thinks I'm stupid"), and the practitioner challenges them over several sessions without revealing or suggesting the irrational belief. During this time, the practitioner examines the list of client thoughts that are associated with particular emotions and abstracts the irrational beliefs that run through each. After arriving at a hypothesis, the practitioner shares the hypothesis, which the young client is invited to accept or disconfirm. This inductive interpretation strategy is the one most often recommended by Beck and his colleagues (e.g., Beck & Emery, 1985). Generally speaking, RET advises the practitioner to share the hypothesis with the child more quickly in order to prevent, among other things, the practitioner's failing to accurately recall how often the child actually reported thoughts consistent with the irrational belief.

Inference Chaining. This strategy is the main one suggested for use in uncovering client's irrational beliefs. In this approach, the practitioner does not, as he or she does in inductive interpretation, challenge errors of inference. Rather, when assessing cognitions, the practitioner accepts the client's interpretations as true and probes further to see how the client evaluates the interpretations. For example, consider the following inference-chaining procedure used with the previously mentioned Aaron:

PRACTITIONER: And what do you think would happen if you did hand in your work that was incomplete?

AARON: The teacher would find out.
PRACTITIONER: And?
AARON: He would think I'm stupid.
PRACTITIONER: Well, let's suppose that might happen. What might you think then?
AARON: I guess I'd think I was dumb.
PRACTITIONER: And?
AARON: I could not stand that!
PRACTITIONER: Because . . . ?
AARON: It would be terrible!

This interchange illustrates how thoughts can be chained together (layers of thought peeled away) through the judicious use by the practitioner of conjunctive phrases ("and," "because") that help the young person discover the irrational thoughts that are hidden behind his or her thoughts. Inference chaining is the preferred means of assessing irrational beliefs because it is efficient and allows for self-discovery on the part of the child.

Deductive Interpretation. When young clients are unable to become aware of their thoughts through inference chaining, we recommend that the practitioner not wait longer than 5–10 minutes for the child to locate his or her irrational thoughts. Rather, the practitioner suggests to the young client what he or she may be thinking by using RET theory to suggest likely hypotheses about what the client is thinking.

DiGiuseppe (1990) identified several steps in using deductive interpretation. First, practitioners formulate hypotheses based on their knowledge of psychopathology, clinical experience, and RET theory. Next, they offer their hypotheses using *suppositional language* and directly ask the young client for feedback on the accuracy of the hypothesis. Practitioners are advised to avoid using declarative sentences. Third, practitioners acknowledge to themselves that they may always be wrong and recognize that *interpretations* are only a clinical word for "hypotheses." Fourth, if a young client gives negative feedback, the practitioner starts over, using the child's comments to formulate another hypothesis.

With younger clients and with those with a high need for approval, deductive interpretation assessment has to be used with care to prevent the practitioner's "imposing" the cause. Nevertheless, it has been our experience that this strategy is useful when a roadblock has been reached, yet when the identity of the underlying irrational beliefs is apparent.

Treatment

Treatment Goals: Modifying Negative and Inappropriate Emotions

The goals in the RET treatment of school-aged populations are similar to those in adult treatment, although the means vary, depending on the cognitive-developmental status and the intelligence level of the young client. That is, RET is directed at bringing about a reduction in the intensity of the inappropriate, negative emotions of the client that are seen to be causing misery as well as making it harder for the young person to solve current problems and achieve future goals. RET is designed not to help the young client solve current presenting *practical* problems, but to reduce extreme levels of anger (rage), anxiety, and feeling down (depression), which make it impossible—or much harder—for the young person to figure out how to overcome a specific problem. Extreme emotional upset disrupts the thinking process. The RET practitioner does not ignore practical, manipulative, or behavioral problems. While using RET with a student to solve emotional problems, the RET practitioner will also frequently use different cognitive-behavioral techniques (e.g., interpersonal cognitive problem solving, Spivack & Shure, 1974; self-instructional training, Meichenbaum, 1977; Kendall & Finch, 1979; cognitive social-skills training, Halford, 1983) to help the student acquire skills in order to modify aversive events in the environment and to solve practical problems.

Take the example of Andrew in grade 7, who has been referred because of being very scared and depressed about the amount of teasing he receives. From an RET assessment perspective, Andrew might be assessed as experiencing a high level of depression and anxiety surrounding being teased. (He may also have a deficit in social skills or an inhibition of his social skills because of his anxiety, and he may experience other emotions like extreme anger.) The RET treatment goal for Andrew would be to reduce the intensity of his depression and anxiety so that, not only would he be happier with his friends at school, but he would also, through greater emotional self-control, be more effective behaviorally in decreasing the frequency of teasing. Once Andrew's depression and anxiety are reduced, his high level of anger may also be targeted for change.

In RET, the modification of emotional problems is accomplished primarily through the modification of the young person's assumptions, inferences, evaluations, expectations, and beliefs, which are either *antiempirical* or *irrational*. "Errors" of inference are faulty conclusions (e.g., "*Everyone* is teasing me") and predictions (e.g., "Everyone will *always* tease me") that a student makes about past, present, or future external events, as well as misattributions of cause–effect relationships (e.g., "The reason my classmates tease me is that they hate me"). The term *irrational evaluations* refers to the manner in which the student appraises the significance of the initial interpretation or inference of reality; they are typically manifested in absolutistic statements (e.g., "I need my classmates' approval"), awfulizing statements (e.g., "It's terrible to be teased"), I-can't-stand-it-itis statements (e.g., "I can't put up with teasing any longer"), and global rating statements (e.g., "I'm hopeless").

Said another way, when a young client is assessed as having an emotional problem, according to RET theory, one can anticipate a number of different cognitions that are causing and/or are concurrent with the emotional problems. Erroneous and irrational cognitions are seen as exacerbating bad external circumstances. Andrew's ideas that "No one likes me," "I'll never have any friends," "Everyone is teasing me," "I can't stand being teased," and "I'm hopeless" are seen as leading to inappropriately strong negative emotions. A student with a more rational attitude toward teasing would feel appropriately negative (disappointed, irritated, and concerned) but would not be as upset as Andrew. In order to reduce Andrew's depression and anxiety, RET would use a number of different techniques in order to modify Andrew's way of thinking about being teased.

RET Cognitive Change Methods

Once the RET practitioner has identified specific erroneous inferences and irrational evaluations, he or she then decides which cognitions to attempt to modify and which change methods to use. These decisions are based partly on the cognitions themselves and also on the cognitive maturity of the young client. To begin with, those cognitions that are erroneous and irrational are targeted for potential change—sometimes with the help of the young client. That is, the practitioner is careful not to change negative cognitions that may be true. For example, in the case of severe child abuse on the part of a rejecting parent, you would not target the cognition "My daddy doesn't love me" for change to "Daddy loves me" if the overwhelming amount of evidence points to the conclusion that the parent doesn't love the child. For a more detailed discussion of this idea and how RET differs from Beckian cognitive therapy, see Di-Giuseppe (1989).

The main cognitive change method used in RET is called *disputation*. Disputing is based on the scientific method and involves a close examination of the specific thoughts and beliefs of a student to determine the extent to which they are true (how much factual evidence there is to support them), sensible (logical), and helpful (leading to goal-directed feelings and emotions). Once these thoughts and beliefs are uncovered and identified, the practitioner uses a variety of questioning, didactic, and Socratic techniques so that the student can be provided with the evidence and justification for why some of the ideas that he or she holds are irrational and untrue. The disputing process ends with the practitioner helping the child to reformulate his or her irrational evaluations and beliefs to more rational ones and to acquire a set of rational self-statements that he or she can use in the problem situation. The amount and degree of disputing depend on the client's maturity.

Philosophical Disputation

RET is distinguished by its concern with the philosophical belief system of the client, as this system is seen to contain the basic "trait" attitudes that are responsible for the consistencies in the adaptive or maladaptive functioning of clients. The older the client—especially above the age of 12 or 13—the more the belief system is seen to be at the core of the emotional difficulties of the client.

With certain bright and older students—those who have achieved the capacity for formal operational thought (see Bernard & Joyce, 1984, Chapter 4)—one can use abstract philosophical disputation in an attempt to modify the basic belief system. Termed "preferential/elegant RET" by Ellis (1980), this method engages the client in a consideration of the logical, the empirical basis, and the semantic meanings of irrational beliefs expressed as broad generalities and not tied to specific situations. For example, if Andrew, who was very depressed and anxious about being teased, were older, one could dispute some of his more general beliefs, such as "I need people to approve of me," "People should treat me fairly," and "I'm hopeless when people reject me." Methods for the philosophical and general disputation of beliefs have been described in many texts (e.g., Walen, DiGiuseppe, & Wessler, 1980) and more recently in DiGiuseppe (1990).

Disputation of Irrational Beliefs in Specific Situations

With younger clients, the disputing of irrational beliefs should almost always occur in a specific, concrete context. Disputing at this level involves identifying should-ought-need statements, awfulizing statements, I-can't-stand-it-itis statements, and global rating statements as they are manifested in specific situations (for a discussion of these types of irrational statements, see Walen, DiGiuseppe, & Wessler, 1980).

For example, in the example of Andrew, the RET practitioner would dispute his irrational idea that "I'm hopeless" by examining the belief as it arises with a specific person: "So, when George calls you 'Stupid,' you think you are hopeless. Is that right?" Once Andrew agrees, the practitioner establishes a basis for disputing his irrational self-statement dealing with self-worth by asking Andrew to complete a "self-concept circle" (see Knaus, 1974), which asks students (with practitioner help) to write down the positive and negative characteristics of themselves (e.g., negative: getting teased a lot, not good at math, bad at playing the recorder; positive: fixing my bike, looking after my pet, helping Mom and Dad with chores). The practitioner is then in a position to pose basic disputational questions to dispute self-downing: "Does George calling you 'Stupid' take away all of the positive things about you? Do you lose all your good things? Does it make you totally stupid?" One could also dispute Andrew's idea "I'm hopeless" semantically by defining "I'm hopeless" as meaning hopeless at everything he does. One then asks him, on the basis of his self-concept circle, whether he is hopeless at everything. This disputing results in a rational self-statement: "Although I'm not good at making friends with George, there are other good things about me."

Other irrational evaluations expressed by Andrew in specific situations that could be disputed are "It's awful to be teased by George when I arrive at school" and "I can't stand it when George teases me at recess." Disputing awfulizing irrational self-statements involves helping students to keep "bad" events like teasing in perspective. One very effective way that RET disputes awfulizing is through the use of a "catastrophe scale": a vertical line is drawn, and at various levels on the scale, the following percentages are entered along the vertical line: 100% (at the top), 90%, 50%, 10%, and 0% (at the bottom of the scale). At the beginning of the dispute, Andrew would be asked, "When you get very, very down about being teased, on a scale of 1 to 100, where 100 is the worst thing that could happen to you, 50 is medium bad, and 10 is a little bad, how 'bad' is being teased?" Once having given a rating, which tends almost always to be above 90, Andrew would fill out the catastrophe scale beginning with events in the world that could happen that would be catastrophes (events with a rating between 90 and 100), such as an earthquake, his parents dying, and permanent injury. Andrew would then complete the scale for more moderate "catastrophes" in the 80–90 range, from his house burning down and breaking his leg, to trivial bad things with ratings of 10 or less, such as forgetting his lunch and losing 20 cents. The ratings of specific events will vary a little across students and age. The dispute finishes with Andrew's being asked, "On this (completed) catastrophe scale, how bad is being teased by George when you come to school?" In lowering his initial rating of the badness of being teased from above 90 to somewhere in the more moderate range of bad things that could happen, Andrew will experience a restructuring of his cognition that "teasing is awful" and a reduction in the intensity of his anxiety and discomfort. The rational self-statement that could be substituted now would be something like "Teasing is bad, but it isn't the worst thing that could happen."

The irrational statement "I can't stand George's teasing me" would be disputed with questions such as "You mean it kills you? Where is the evidence that you can't stand it? Have you ever fainted? Have your eyeballs fallen out?" A rational counter-self-statement might be "Although I don't like being teased, I *can* stand it."

Disputing of Inferences

The other main category of cognitions, along with irrational evaluations, that is disputed in RET is "errors of inference." Given their lack of experience and knowledge, school-aged children are even more likely than adults to hold erroneous conclusions and to make faulty predictions about reality. Indeed, one of the prerequisite insights that we teach young clients in RET is the difference between an "assumption" and a "fact" and that just their thinking something does not necessarily make it true. Andrew, for example, may subscribe to a number of errors of inference, including "*Everyone* is teasing me," "Because I'm being teased, *no one* likes me," "I'm teased *all* the time," and "I'll *always* be teased."

The main RET technique for disputing faulty inferences is called *empirical disputation* or *empirical analysis* (e.g., DiGiuseppe, 1981; DiGiuseppe & Bernard, 1983). In empirical disputation, the practitioner teases out with the young person whether there is objective evidence to support her or his conclusions or predictions or whether she or he is distorting reality. For example, to empirically dispute the thought "Everyone is teasing me," a class list could be used, and Andrew could go down the list of names and place a check next to any who do not tease him. This empirical analysis would help him to modify his conclusion to something more accurate, which he would find easier to accept (e.g., "Only four or five kids are teasing me").

An effective empirical disputational method is to design an experiment in which the young person collects data over a short period of time (a week) and compares the results of this data collection with his or her original conclusion or prediction. In Andrew's case, the practitioner could design a chart for collecting the number of times he is actually teased, along with their time of occurrence, to help him dispute some of his distortions of what is happening. (You have to be somewhat careful in anticipating the likely results of empirical data collection, in case the environment is so filled with negative events that the student's inference not only turns out to be true but is strongly reinforced by the results!)

Rational Self-Statements

With children younger than 7, the practitioner provides a list of rational self-statements that they can use in the problem situation (e.g., DiGiuseppe, 1981). Rational self-statements differ somewhat from coping self-statements, positive self-statements, attributional self-statements, and self-efficacy self-statements in that they encapsulate a rational idea. RET practitioners use all varieties of self-statements when working with school-aged children. The point here is that some, but not all, self-statements designed to modify emotions and behavior are rational. Some derive from other therapeutic traditions. When used with children with whom you have done some disputing, rational self-statements are the result of the dispute—a new rational belief that counters the previously disputed irrational belief. With children younger than 7, little if any disputing takes place. Instead, these young children are given extensive practice in "what to think." The RET practitioner models aloud a rational self-statement expressed in very simple language (e.g., "It's not so bad to be teased. I can stand it"). The young child is then given practice in thinking aloud the rational self-statement in a role-playing situation and slowly, over time, practicing saying the rational self-statement silently. If the young clients can read, it is generally a good idea to write the statements down on a card and have the clients practice thinking the statements at home during the week.

In the case of Andrew, the rational self-statements that could be generated to replace his previous irrational beliefs and also to be practiced and used when he is being teased include "Just because I'm being teased doesn't mean *all* kids don't like me," "I can stand being teased," and "There are lots of good things about me."

Evaluation

Evaluation is the process of examining the effectiveness of the interventions; in RET, it can be carried out in two ways:

1. An *overall evaluation* can be done near the end of therapy. The practitioner compares the child's present functioning with some criterion of hoped-for change (e.g., no longer refusing to attend school or no more angry outbursts). This is frequently the main evaluation when there is a single presenting problem; this evaluation is carried out to answer the question "Is it time to terminate therapy?" The child's current functioning is compared with the goals of therapy.

2. A *monitoring process* may occur at different points during therapy. On the basis of this monitoring, the practitioner may decide to alter the treatment or move on to the next problem. This is important when problems change or when there are multiple presenting problems. For example, if an adolescent presents with behavior problems, anxiety, and depression including suicidal thoughts, the practitioner works on the urgent emotional problems or the depression first. An evaluation of the adolescent's improvement enables the practitioner to decide when to move the focus of therapy from one problem to another.

The first type of evaluation is a global one, made against some criterion that is directly related to the main goal established for therapy (e.g., reduction in bed-wetting or elimination of panic attacks). The second type is often a multifaceted evaluation that may combine data from three sources: (1) subjective client reports; (2) objective client indicators; and (3) independent observations.

Subjective Client Reports

Diaries, other written records, and verbal statements provide useful data. Probing questions are advisable in using subjective client reports so that the practitioner's assumptions can be checked. An adolescent who earlier presented with depressed moods may report, "I've felt much happier all this week." The practitioner thinks, "Good; those disputational strategies are working". The practitioner asks, "How did this come about?' The client may reply, "The next-door neighbor asked me to go jogging with her every morning, and it's been great!" Or again, a young client with an anger problem toward a live-in grandparent may say, "I haven't had even one angry outburst this week." The practitioner thinks, "We're really getting somewhere!" The practitioner asks, "What do you think was responsible for the change?" The client replies, "Oh, Grandma moved out."

These examples underline the importance in evaluation of checking out assumptions about *what is changing* and *why*. Changes in the client's emotions and behavior may be related to unexpected changes in the antecedent events rather than in the rational-emotive intervention. In different circumstances, when clients report that change was connected with treatment strategies, they can be asked to report on the relative effectiveness of different components (e.g., rational-emotive imagery, logical disputation, and rational self-statements). Improved practical problem solving may be another indicator that confirms change. For example, tasks that the client has put off may have been completed—an essay written or music practice done.

Objective Client Indicators

Evaluation information can be obtained from the client by the administration of scales such as depression or anxiety inventories, and by using nonstandardised methods such as the feeling thermometer and ABC sheets. Such measures can reflect changes in the intensity and/or the duration of the inappropriate negative emotions troubling the client. Behavioral monitoring can record other types of change, such as the frequency of fights, tantrums, anxious episodes, and bed-wetting.

Independent Observations

Reports by independent observers such as teachers or parents can contribute to evaluation. Standardized scales may be used (e.g., the Eyberg Child Behavior Inventory; Eyberg & Ross, 1978), but frequently these data are gathered in informal ways. Parents may report, for example, on whether the child is doing homework, eating normally, talking sociably, or cooperating with siblings. Teachers may report on the child's academic achievement, sporting activities, or social interaction. Although each of these reports may be associated with validity problems, the practitioner would look for congruence between indicators, and especially for independent confirmatory evidence to support client self-reports.

Evaluation is important in increasing the effectiveness of RET because it allows the practitioner to gauge how well the particular combination of RET strategies chosen for this client is working. If the therapy is leading to improvement, the "package" is effective (though the therapist has no way of knowing which components are the effective ones.) If no improvement is apparent, evaluation will lead the practitioner to initiate a change in the intervention.

When clients are brought into the evaluation process as joint evaluators with the practitioner, there can be two additional advantages: (1) rational scientific thinking is taught in a concrete way, and (2) the clients' attention is drawn to what has brought about the changes, namely, their efforts to implement the intervention strategies. It is hypothesized that feedback of this kind facilitates an internal locus of control in the clients as well as reminds them of effective strategies, so that if the problem recurs in the future, they may be able to reuse the strategies.

KEYS TO SUCCESSFUL RET CHILD TREATMENT

The following points are based on the collective experience of over two decades of working in schools with a wide variety of school-aged children and problems (Bernard & Joyce, 1984):

1. *Have onhand as many concrete-educational teaching aids as possible.* RET when applied to younger populations frequently incorporates a variety of structured-learning, didactic-teaching activities. It is important that the student be provided with visual aids to represent the different ideas being described, including "thought clouds," "self-concept drawings," and "happening–thought–feeling–reaction diagrams."

2. *Target one emotion and behavior for change in a specific situation.* A common problem is to work on a variety of emotional problems such as anger and anxiety along with the associated cognitions at the same time. It is best if you work on one problem at a time.

3. *For children older than 7, it is generally a good idea to illustrate with diagrams the relationship among activating events, thoughts, feelings, and behavior.* A common method is to use a "happening–thought–feeling–reaction chart": each category of event is written on a piece of paper or on the board, and specific examples are listed below it.

4. *Assess the young person for multiple cognitive errors.* It is important to get out and write down several errors of inference and evaluations before beginning to dispute.

5. *Allow the client the first opportunity to dispute cognitive errors.* This provides the child with the important insight that what he or she is thinking may be false and, importantly, that one can change one's thinking.

6. *Always tie the disputes with the client to the specific situation or event of*

concern. That is, make sure that the young person is considering whether his or her thoughts are sensible and true in terms of a specific situation: not "Where is the evidence you can't stand teasing?" but "Where is the evidence that you can't stand being teased by George when you arrive at school at 8:44 A.M.?"

7. *For children who are older than 7, make sure that they explain to the practitioner the relationship between changes in thinking and changes in feelings.* It is important that young clients learn that the way in which they can reduce their emotional upsets and feel good is by changing their thinking. This step can be bypassed with less intelligent, less articulate older students.

8. *Be animated when disputing.* It is important that the young client be stimulated to recognize and change irrational thinking. One way to do this is to modify your verbal behavior (e.g., change your voice tone, volume, speed, and accent) and your nonverbal behavior (e.g., getting out of your seat and walking around the room).

9. *Repeat the same disputational argument if the client does not seem to understand the dispute and still believes the erroneous or irrational idea.* Many young people require a repetition of arguments and evidence to dispute inferences and beliefs that they have held for an extended period of time and that they strongly believe.

10. *Project the same difficult situation into the future.* With the young client, generate coping and rational self-statements that he or she can use to modify his or her emotions and behavior in the future.

11. *Focusing on the same difficult situation, use role playing and modeling of rational self-statements. Then, have the young client overtly and then covertly rehearse rational self-statements and practice appropriate behavior, with the practitioner role playing aspects of the difficult situation.* That is, have the young person observe you while you think aloud in a difficult situation. He or she can play the role of an antagonist or help create the atmosphere of the difficult situation. Then, exchange roles.

12. *Assign homework.* During the time between sessions, the young client should be involved in some RET or other skill presented in the counseling session (e.g., self-observation of emotional upset, the use of rational self-statements that have been written down, and putting up with things the child thinks that he or she can't stand).

Working with Parents

As indicated earlier, parents can play an important role in the development of various problems of childhood. As well, they are vital adjuncts in bringing about an amelioration of the problem. RET has for many years recognized the importance of parental behavioral–child-management skills in the socializing and disciplining of children. There is plenty of research attesting to the lack of parenting skills in the parents of conduct-disordered children (e.g., Forehand, King, Peed, & Yoder, 1975; Patterson, 1981, 1982). RET practitioners routinely assess parenting skill assets and deficits and teach parenting skills.

The area in which RET has made the greatest contribution to an improvement in parent–child interaction, however, is *parental emotions*. One of RET's basic assumptions when working with parents is that, when parents become overly upset about their child's behavior, their behavior ceases to be effective at best and often brings about a negative result in the child.

When interviewing parents, the RET practitioner is on the lookout for extreme emotional reactions when parents observe their child misbehaving or experiencing a social, emotional, or learning problem. Typical parental emotions that impede effective child raising and problem solving are the following:

Guilt

When parents feel guilty, they are likely to (1) attribute their child's problem to themselves and (2) condemn themselves for being responsible.

Anger

Extreme anger (not just annoyance) is frequently encountered in the parents of children with conduct disorders. Parental anger is motivated by the idea that anger is an effective punishment tool and the irrational belief that "Children should always behave well and do as I say."

Anxiety

Parental anxiety is frequently encountered in the parents of children who experience "internalizing disorders" and learning difficulties. These parents believe that "It is awful that my child has a problem" and "My child cannot stand having the problem" (projected discomfort anxiety).

Low Frustration Tolerance

Many parents of children who experience adjustment difficulties in growing up have a low tolerance of the frustrations of bringing up children. They irrationally believe that "Parenting shouldn't be so hard" and that "It is too hard to solve my child's problems."

In working with parents, the RET practitioner spends a great deal of time helping parents modify their emotions by using standard RET disputational techniques. Clinical experience has shown that behavioral interventions with parents are not used effectively by parents because of their own intervening emotional reactions to their child's problems. RET teaches parents the importance of accepting themselves in the face of the problems that their children experience and of disciplining without anger; it also teaches that awfulizing about children's problems only aggravates the problems and distorts the severity of the problems, and that developing high frustration tolerance will help them to manage the hassles of child raising better.

Expectations of Parents

Parents vary in the expectations they bring to a consultation. Four groups of parents are now discussed, and the implications of their attitudes for the implementation of RET procedures are indicated.

1. *Parents who want their child "fixed."* The least "involved" parents are those who come seeking to have their child "fixed up." Such parents are not expecting to find their internal psychological processes being examined and may feel hostile to such an approach if it is embarked on without preliminary discussion. "Please fix up my child's problem" is often an unspoken attitude that may be associated with a number of thoughts: "I am helpless to solve this problem," "I don't want to have to face this problem," "I want this problem to go away," and "It's my child's problem— nothing to do with me." Attempting to engage these parents immediately in RET would most likely be ineffective unless these expectations are dealt with directly first.

2. *Parents who seek advice.* This second group of parents are more ready participants in a process of change because they see themselves as needing to change, but in a limited way ("Just tell us what to do"). Common thoughts of this group of parents may include "We just need to find out what to do—the right method," "Feelings? What could they have to do with it?" and "Don't go stirring up trouble in our family. We haven't come to you for that." These parents can be helped to expand their understanding of the child and the problem by being invited to reflect first on how the child may be *feeling,* and then to explore their own feelings in relation to the child. Awareness of how these feelings may be involved in the problem can then be discussed as a prelude to introducing RET.

Where advice-seeking parents resist such an exploration, they can be offered some behavioral strategies to implement. If, for example, parental anger is part of the problem, they may return at their next appointment without having had much success, and the way is opened to examine what could be getting in the way of their success, namely, their angry feelings.

3. *Parents who recognize that their feelings are part of the problem.* Some parents who come for help with their child's problem already recognize

that feelings are playing a part, if not in causing the problem, at least in maintaining it. This recognition does not mean that they know how to bring about desired changes. This group of parents is ready for the implementation of RET procedures from the beginning.

4. *Parents with an emotional problem between them.* Parents sometimes present with an emotional conflict between them that is directly related to their child's problem. For example, parents may disagree concerning the best way to discipline their child. With the child's growing noncompliance, they may experience anger, guilt, self-blame, or anxiety. One parent may be angry about the other's perceived weakness, and the other parent may feel worried and down about the ongoing problem. Disputation of the parents' underlying irrational beliefs will help them to deal with the feelings that have arisen around the child's problem.

Other parents present with both a child problem and a relationship problem that exists independent of the child. Remediation of the parents' problem is sometimes necessary if one is to make progress with the child. This is particularly the case where the parents are displaying poor emotional coping patterns to the child and such patterns have become part of the child's own problem. The most common example is low frustration tolerance (LFT) between the parents existing alongside child problems that include LFT in the child.

Nonverbal Obstacles to Changes in Parenting

Caring and well-meaning parents come to counseling to learn how to change their relationship with their child who is having a problem. They are aware or become aware that their "attitude" is part of the problem. Through RET techniques, they learn to dispute, for example, their anger-inducing beliefs and their LFT. They also plan and practice new strategies in their practical problem solving, but for some parents, one important factor that remains unchanged may be the *nonverbal habits of communication of emotion.*

For example, a parent who has been habitually angry may dispute the cognitive demands underlying the anger and settle down his or her emotional level but *still look angry to the child*, because the facial expressions associated with the angry feelings persist. In such cases, parents who are trying hard to change are puzzled by their children's negative reactions. "The look on your face" can be most effectively discussed when trust in the psychologist is established; it is not then perceived as criticism. It is our experience that such a discussion is effective when held in the presence of both parents because the parent concerned is unaware of how he or she looks, and the spouse usually confirms the observations with great enthusiasm. It has been noticed but the parents have not known how to communicate about it. Examples of these nonverbal signs include the previously angry parent who still frowns a lot and shows displeasure, when smiling would be more appropriate. Another example is the previously weak and ineffective disciplinarian who still gives instructions with a facial expression and a voice showing anxiety and lack of confidence in the child's compliance.

RECOMMENDATIONS FOR TREATING SPECIFIC CHILDHOOD DISORDERS

The Child Who Is Depressed

A child who is feeling depressed probably won't volunteer much information and may be quite withdrawn. Such a child requires gentleness. In assessment, check out the child's eating and sleeping patterns, although if the child is young (in elementary school), depression may not always show up in such patterns. Change in activity level in the direction of passivity may be apparent. Always check for suicidal thoughts if the young client is depressed, and especially if she or he is an adolescent. (The youngest client in our experience to talk of suicide was a grade 4 child, but it is uncommon at that young age.) Often, such thoughts will not be volunteered, but it is a relief to the young person when they are elicited—it is usually the first time that they have spoken about these thoughts to anyone. After checking whether they have a detailed plan and the means to carry it out, we ask whether an attempt has been made. A very useful question at this point, if they have indeed gone that far, is to ask, "What stopped you?" In response, clients present their strengths or the positive thoughts that they had, even in the depths of unhappiness. These can be a good starting point for treatment. A further point worth noting is that clients who are depressed and *not* suicidal do not seem disturbed by being questioned about it.

Practitioners can also check other self-destructive or self-mutilating tendencies in depressed adolescents. Visible marks (cuts or scars) on their bodies may be observed. If so, ask about them. In our experience, referring agents (parents or teachers) rarely know about this behavior.

In approaching a depressed child or adolescent, it is worth remembering that the working assumptions of the client in relation to an adult will probably be something like "No one is really interested in me. Why would you be any different? I'm not worth it anyway. Even if you accept me at first, when you find out what I'm really like, you won't!"

Practitioners would do well to deliberately "fire up" their energy and activity levels when working with depressed clients. We have observed in supervision in clinical settings and in teaching therapy through role playing that the body language of depressed clients is "catching" and practitioners can easily begin to imitate their clients. Needless to say, this imitation does not add to their effectiveness!

When low frustration tolerance and anxiety are associated with the depression, we can expect young clients to set very low expectations regarding what benefit they can get from therapy and to give up easily. One 15-year-old boy who was depressed needed six sessions working on the belief that he would probably always feel as dispirited and hopeless. He said he thought that nothing would help. Motivating him to try was the hardest part. The combination of erroneous inferences and irrational beliefs elicited after much difficulty was as follows: "What if I try this (therapy) and it doesn't work? That would be awful—the end. I'd be stuck forever. That would prove nothing could ever help me." Among other responses by the practitioner, an explanation was provided of the variety of therapeutic approaches available, and he learned that if one approach did not help him, he could try others. Giving RET a try was not the "awful risk" he had thought it to be.

The Child Who Is Anxious

In initiating contact with highly anxious children or adolescents, be aware that they are likely to be anxious about coming to see you. Try to learn their reasons before expecting involved participation. It is not uncommon for an anxious adolescent to go through convoluted, ambivalent behavior about not coming (e.g., he or she may keep the appointment but stand at the door, decline to sit down, and spend the first 10 minutes explaining why he or she can't come in and will have to leave). If this happens, the adolescent's anxiety can be relieved by a number of factors. The first and most important of these is an obvious *absence of anxiety in the therapist* about this reaction. Second, the adolescent requires room to move, that is, to exercise choice, and the aim is to provide choices and to try to make withdrawal the most unlikely choice.

Specific suggestions for a practitioner in this situation are as follows: Stay sitting, with relaxed body language. Say something like "A person can easily feel uncertain about coming here. He (she) may be wondering what's going to be involved or feel rather uncomfortable at first with someone new. That's natural. Would you like to ask me anything at all?" (Pause and answer if there are questions.) "Why not take some time to think about what you will do; say, during this coming week, you could consider what sessions here might offer you, and whether you think any difficulties or risks would be worth it. I would like a few minutes of your time now to tell you what I can offer. You can listen, and it will give you something to go on when you are making up your mind. I suggest we meet again, at least next week, so that you can let me know what you are thinking. There may be some things you will want to clarify with me then."

In our experience, clients who present in this way take four sessions or so to overcome their initial ambivalence and anxiety. Working slowly and patiently with them in overcoming this anxiety is the groundwork for effective RET interventions later. The practitioner shows his or her credibility in dealing with this anxiety well and is then trusted by the young person to give help with other (frequently many and varied) anxieties.

The Child with Conduct Problems

Accounts have been given elsewhere (e.g., DiGiuseppe, 1983, 1988) on the RET and behavioral interventions appropriate to use with conduct-disordered children and adolescents. However, whether the young person is under direction by a court order or is attending because of the parents' choice or the school's insistence on counseling if they are to stay in the school, these young people usually do not come very willingly. As Di-Giuseppe (1983) pointed out, they in fact stand to lose a lot: they have been getting their way more often than most. The question frequently asked of us in the supervision and in-service training of practitioners and youth workers is how to get these clients motivated. They don't want to be there. Others have the problem, not them! The answer, put in its most general way, is that we "use" their egocentrism and bargain our way into allowing them to give us a chance to show what we have to offer. As will be apparent in the detailed account below, this process of getting them involved incorporates teaching many of the skills of interpersonal cognitive problem solving (Spivack & Shure, 1974) as an initial basis for later therapeutic work. The suitability of such allied cognitive interventions in combination with RET has been discussed in detail previously (Bernard & Joyce, 1984).

With very reluctant clients, it may be fruitful to begin by helping with some practical problem solving. They can be helped to negotiate a difficulty (e.g., with a teacher). A second such exercise that is very useful with young people from tenth grade and upward is to do an assessment of their career interests (e.g., Career Assessment Inventory, Strong-Campbell Interest Inventory, or the Self-Directed Search). Young people with conduct problems have not generally worked out their career aspirations, goals, and plans, so this assessment is not off the mark. In addition, because it pays attention to their uniqueness, it demonstrates the credibility of your interest in them, that you are not just "wanting to fix them up." It also has the potential to give them positive feedback about themselves that contrasts well with the large amounts of negative feedback they have generally received from many adults. Finally, it provides the practitioner with an empirical basis for assisting the young person with the next step in the plan: goal assessment.

Helping young persons explore their goals can be done very simply: by making a list. Guide them with questions such as "What do I really want to do, to become, to achieve, to have?" and teach the skill of brainstorming while doing this (e.g., Waters, 1982). (Point out that they can use the brainstorming technique for such diverse activities as school work, staying out of trouble, and working on a social problem, and return to this skill in later sessions.) Usually, they have not formulated their goals before and are prepared to give it a try.

The list of goals produced can be used as a basis for the discussion of long-term and short-term goals and the difficulties that arise from the pursuit of short-term at the expense of long-term goals. Questions can be asked to elicit the clients' thinking about this issue, which focuses on a key problem of conduct disorder children, namely, low frustration tolerance. The next step in exploring ways of resolving the conflict between the pursuit of long-term and short-term goals involves teaching alternative solution thinking and consequential thinking. Many alternatives are generated by brainstorming for a specific goal conflict (e.g., "staying out of trouble" and "doing my own fun thing"), and then the consequences of pursuing each are thought through and recorded alongside the alternative.

After the teaching of the two interpersonal cognitive problem-solving skills in the context of goal attainment, the clients can be introduced to the idea that these thinking skills can help them with particular problems that they are having, for example, "getting people off my back." If the young client agrees to pursue this tack, the additional skill of perspective taking can be developed, enabling the adolescent to go beyond an egocentric view of the problem. In general, it is only after these skills have been taught that the ABCs of rational thinking and disputational techniques are introduced. The motivation to assume emotional responsibility is not easily found in the beginning; others are blamed for the clients' problems.

As noted by DiGiuseppe (1988), there is a group of conduct-disordered children who have been severely mistreated—rejected by their parents and often physically abused. The methods described above are intended not for this group, but for those from less traumatizing backgrounds.

CONCLUSION

The use of RET treatment methods with young clients and their significant others in schools and in mental health settings has a history of over 20 years. And as RET itself continues to evolve, its important and basic insights, skills, and attitudes can be used by people to produce beneficial changes in their lives; so, too, the use of RET by practitioners continues to be refined. Although the basic model of change in RET is a relatively simple one, the reality of trying to help improve the thinking and attitudes of school-aged children is not straightforward. RET offers the practitioner an impressive array of methods and techniques to be used to solve childhood problems. The challenge for RET practitioners is to maximize their effectiveness. This we have found over the years to be a stimulating and rewarding experience.

References

Bard, J. A., & Fisher, H. R. (1983). A rational-emotive approach to underachievement. In A. Ellis & M. E. Bernard (Eds.), *Rational-emotive approaches to the problems of childhood*. New York: Plenum Press.

Beck, A., & Emery, G. (1985). *Anxiety disorders and phobias: A cognitive perspective*. New York: Basic Books.

Bernard, M. E. (1981). Private thought in rational-emotive psychotherapy. *Cognitive Therapy and Research, 5*, 129–142.

Bernard, M. E. (1984). Childhood emotion and cognitive-behavior therapy: A rational-emotive perspective. In P. C. Kendall (Ed.), *Advances in cognitive-behavioral research and therapy*, Vol. 3. New York: Academic Press.

Bernard, M. E., & Joyce, M. R. (1984). *Rational-emotive therapy with children and adolescents: Theory, treatment strategies, preventative methods*. New York: Wiley.

Bernard, M. E., Rosewarne, P., & Joyce, M. R. (1983). Helping teachers cope with stress: A rational-emotive approach. In A. Ellis & M. E. Bernard (Eds.), *Rational-emotive approaches to the problems of childhood*. New York: Plenum Press.

Bordin, E. S. (1979). The generalizability of the psychoanalytic concept of the working alliance. *Psychotherapy: Theory, Research and Practice, 16*, 252–260.

Chess, S., & Thomas, A. (1984). *Origins and evolution of behavior disorders: From infancy to early adult life*. New York: Brunner/Mazel.

DiGiuseppe, R. D. (1981). Cognitive therapy with children. In G. Emery, S. Hollon, & R. C. Bedrosian (Eds.), *New directions in cognitive therapy*. New York: Guilford Press.

DiGiuseppe, R. D. (1983). Rational-emotive therapy and conduct disorders. In A. Ellis & M. E. Bernard (Eds.), *Rational-emotive approaches to the problems of childhood*. New York: Plenum Press.

DiGiuseppe, R. D. (1986). Cognitive therapy for childhood depression. In A. Freeman, N. Epstein, & K. M. Simon (Eds.), *Depression in the family*. New York: Haworth Press.

DiGiuseppe, R. D. (1988). Cognitive-behavior therapy with families of conduct-disordered children. In N. Epstein, S. Schebinger, & W. Dryden (Eds.), *Cognitive behavior therapy with families*. New York: Brunner/Mazel.

DiGiuseppe, R. D. (1989). Cognitive therapy with children. In A. Freeman, K. Simon, L. Beutler, & H. Arkowitz (Eds.), *Comprehensive handbook of cognitive therapy*. New York: Plenum Press.

DiGiuseppe, R. D. (1990). Rational-emotive assessment of school-age children. In M. E. Bernard & R. D. DiGiuseppe (Eds.), *Rational-emotive therapy and school psychology. School Psychology Review* Mini Series, *19*, 287–293.

DiGiuseppe, R. D., & Bernard, M. E. (1983). Principles of assessment and methods of treatment with children. In A. Ellis & M. E. Bernard (Eds.), *Rational-emotive approaches to the problems of childhood*. New York: Plenum Press.

DiGiuseppe, R. D., & Zeeve, C. (1985). Marriage: Rational-emotive couples counseling. In A. Ellis & M. E. Bernard (Eds.), *Clinical applications of rational-emotive therapy*. New York: Plenum Press.

Dryden, W. (1987). *Current issues in rational-emotive therapy*. London: Croon-Helm.

Elkin, A. (1983). Working with children in groups. In A. Ellis & M. E. Bernard (Eds.), *Rational-emotive approaches to the problems of childhood*. New York: Plenum Press.

Ellis, A. (1962). *Reason and emotion in psychotherapy*. New York: Stuart.

Ellis, A. (1980). Rational-emotive therapy and cognitive-behavior therapy: Similarities and differences. *Cognitive Therapy and Research, 4*, 325–340.

Ellis, A., Moseley, S., & Wolfe, J. (1966). *How to raise an emotionally healthy, happy child*. New York: Crown; Hollywood: Wilshire Books.

Eyberg, S., & Ross, A. W. (1978). Assessment of child behavior problems: The validation of a new inventory. *Journal of Clinical Child Psychology, 7*, 113–116.

Forehand, R., King, A., Peed, S., & Yoder, P. (1975). Mother-child interaction: Comparison of a non-compliant clinical group and a non-clinic group. *Behavior Research and Therapy, 12*, 79–84.

Foreyt, J. P., & Kondo, A. T. (1983). Cognitive-behavioral treatment of childhood and adolescent obesity. In A. Ellis & M. E. Bernard (Eds.), *Rational-emotive approaches to the problems of childhood*. New York: Plenum Press.

Forman, S. G. (in press). The rational-emotive approach to teacher stress management. In M. E. Bernard & R. D. DiGiuseppe (Eds.), *Rational-emotive consultation in applied settings*. Hillsdale, NJ: Erlbaum.

Grieger, R. M., & Boyd, J. D. (1983). Childhood anxieties, fears and phobias. In A. Ellis & M. E. Bernard (Eds.), *Rational-emotive approaches to the problems of childhood*. New York: Plenum Press.

Halford, K. (1983). Teaching rational self-talk to help socially isolated children and youth. In A. Ellis & M. E. Bernard (Eds.), *Rational-emotive approaches to the problems of childhood*. New York: Plenum Press.

Hauck, P. (1967). *The rational management of children*. New York: Libra.

Hauck, P. (1983). Working with parents. In A. Ellis & M. E. Bernard (Eds.), *Rational-emotive approaches to the problems of childhood*. New York: Plenum Press.

Huber, C. H., & Baruth, L. G. (1989). *Rational-emotive family therapy: A systems perspective*. New York: Springer.

Joyce, M. R. (in press). Rational-emotive parent mental health consultation. In M. E. Bernard & R. D. DiGiuseppe (Eds.), *Rational-emotive consultation in applied settings*. Hillsdale, NJ: Erlbaum.

Kendall, P. C., & Finch, A. J., Jr. (1979). Developing non-impulsive behavior in children: Cognitive behavioral strategies for self-control. In P. C. Kendall & S. Hollon (Eds.), *Cognitive-behavioral interventions: Theory, research and procedures*. New York: Academic Press.

Kendall, P. C., & Fischler, G. L. (1983). Teaching rational self-talk to impulsive children. In A. Ellis & M. E. Bernard (Eds.), *Rational-emotive approaches to the problems of childhood*. New York: Plenum Press.

Knaus, W. J. (1974). *Rational-emotive education: A manual for elementary school teachers*. New York: Institute for Rational Living.

Knaus, W. J. (1983). Children and low frustration tolerance. In A. Ellis & M. E. Bernard (Eds.), *Rational-emotive approaches to the problems of childhood*. New York: Plenum Press.

Knaus, W. J. (1985). Student burnout: A rational-emotive education treatment approach. In A. Ellis & M. E. Bernard (Eds.), *Clinical applications of rational-emotive therapy*. New York: Plenum Press.

McInerney, J. (in press). RET indirect service to children and adolescents. In M. E. Bernard & R. D. DiGiuseppe (Eds.), *Rational-emotive consultation in applied settings*. Hillsdale, NJ: Erlbaum.

Meichenbaum, D. (1977). *Cognitive behavior modification*. New York: Plenum Press.

Spivack, G., & Shure, M. B. (1974). *Social adjustment of young children: A cognitive approach to solving real life problems*. San Francisco: Jossey-Bass.

Walen, S., & Vanderhorst, G. K. (1983). A rational-emotive approach to childhood sexuality. In A. Ellis & M. E. Bernard (Eds.), *Rational-emotive approaches to the problems of childhood*. New York: Plenum Press.

Walen, S., DiGiuseppe, R. D., & Wessler, R. (1980). *A practitioner's guide to rational-emotive therapy*. New York: Oxford University Press.

Waters, V. (1982). Therapies for children: Rational-emotive therapy. In C. R. Reynolds & T. B. Gutkin (Eds.), *Handbook of school psychology*. New York: Wiley.

Waters, V. (in press). Teaching parents and teachers RET through direct service to client. In M. E. Bernard & R. D. DiGiuseppe (Eds.), *Rational-emotive consultation in applied settings*. Hillsdale, NJ: Erlbaum.

Woulff, N. (1983). Involving the family in the treatment of the child: A model for rational-emotive therapists. In A. Ellis & M. E. Bernard (Eds.), *Rational-emotive approaches to the problems of childhood*. New York: Plenum Press.

Young, H. (1983). Principles of assessment and methods of treatment with adolescents: Special considerations. In A. Ellis & M. E. Bernard (Eds.), *Rational-emotive approaches to the problems of childhood*. New York: Plenum Press.

Index

ABCs of RET, 2, 26–27, 35, 45, 57–58, 70–74, 308–309, 312–316
Adolescents. *See* Children and adolescents
Alcohol rehabilitation, 306–307
Anger, 99–100, 204–205, 207, 338
Anxiety, 96, 101–103, 255, 338, 342–343
Assertion, 201–206, 295
Assessment, 20–22, 56–57, 138–139, 152–157
  child and adolescent, 324–328
  depression, 240–247
  direct, 160–164
  dynamics, 155
  epistemology, 160–162
  hypothesis-driven, 162–164
  irrational beliefs, 165–169

Behavioral methods, 46–48, 141, 143
Brainstorming, 312

Children and adolescents
  anxiety, 342–343
  assessment, 324–328
  conduct problems, 343–344
  depression, 341–342
  evaluation of treatment, 334–336
  relationship building, 322–324
  theory of maladjustment, 319–321
  treatment, 328–334
Client characteristics
  age, 13–14
  cultural background, 16–17
  expectations, 18–20
  intelligence, 15
  nonverbal, 340–341
  personality disorders, 20–22
  religious background, 17–18
  self-efficacy, 295–296
  SES, 15–16
  sex, 11–13

Depression, 97, 232–236
  assessment, 240–251
  childhood, 341–342
  definition, 232–237
  family, 237–239, 257–258
  medication, 227–231
  seasonal affective disorder syndrome, 236–237
  treatment, 104, 247–254
Diagnosis. *See* Assessment
Disputing, 2, 31, 45, 48, 95, 111, 119–125, 174–176, 177, 188–193
  abstraction, level of, 186–188
  children, 328–334, 341–342
  depression, 247–254, 341–342
  heuristic, 180–181
  inferential, 140–141, 176–177, 179, 332–333
  logical, 179
  mad-dog, 111
  metaphorical, 185–186
  philosophical, 8–10, 178–179
  powerful, 64–65
  scientific thinking, 4
  Socratic, 121–125, 182–183
  style, 120–121

Elegant RET, 5, 27, 103
Emotional episode, 85–95, 174–176
Emotional responsibility, 54–56, 116–118, 126–127, 129–131
Emotions, 3–4, 6, 7, 71–75, 85–95, 174–176
Evaluation, 104–108, 280, 334
Expectations of client, 18–20

Fear, 205–206

Gestalt therapy, 308

Goal setting, 56, 74, 118–119, 131, 279–282, 292
Group therapy, 5, 291–298
Guilt, 98, 205, 338

Happiness, 59
Homework, 3, 48, 83–102, 125–126, 143–145, 294
Humor, 180

Irrational and rational beliefs, 41, 43, 45, 65, 78–79, 96–103, 181–182
Irrational Beliefs Test, Jones, 83–85

Jealousy, 101

Love, 269–270, 283–285
Low frustration tolerance, 36, 81, 209, 211, 338–339
  professional, 313

Medication, 28–29, 227–231, 259
Multi-Modal Therapy, 116–119

Pain, 224
Parents, 337–341
Perfectionism, 314
Performance appraisal, 310
Personality disorders, 9, 20–26
Philosophical RET, 8, 27–28
Physiology, depression, 222
Practitioner. See Therapist characteristics

Rational beliefs. See Irrational and rational beliefs
Rational self-statements, 333–334
Reinforcement, 200
Relationship, therapist and client, 24–26, 111–116, 128–129, 164–165, 226–227, 256
  bond, 134–136
  children and adolescents, 322–324
  goals, 137–138
  self-disclosure, 157–158
  tasks, 137
  therapeutic alliance, 133–134
Relationship therapy, 61–62, 286, 321
Religion, 17–18, 216
Resistance, 49, 51, 292–293

Responsibility, 54–56, 116–118, 126–127, 129–131

Sales training, 311
Self-acceptance, 65, 82–83, 98–99, 103–104, 266, 294
Self-efficacy, client, 295–296
Self-esteem. See Self-acceptance
Sexuality, 289–290
Suicide, 222
Symptom stress, 254

Therapist characteristics, 62–66, 111–113
  commitment, 66
  empathy, 26, 256
  errors, 5–8, 29–31
  female, 296–297
  flexibility, 63–64
  knowledge of RET, 23, 35
  low frustration tolerance, 313
  microcounseling skills, 112
  rapport, 113–114
  response to depression, 226–227
  role, 35
  styles, 1, 2, 24–26, 182–185
  values, 23–24
  warmth, 6, 26
Therapy. See Disputing
Treatment. See Disputing

Women
  assertion, 294
  disputing, 285–293
  physical image, 272, 289–290
  sex–love relationships, 270
  sex-role stereotypes, 267–278
  victimization, 274, 290–292
  work, 273, 286–288
Work
  alcohol rehabilitation, 306–307
  communication training programs, 313
  employee assistance programs, 305–309
  human resource personnel, 312–314
  leadership training, 311–312
  perfectionism, 314
  performance appraisal, 308
  sales training, 311
  training and development, 309
  women, 286–288